Paediatrics and Child Health

Paediatrics and Child Health

To our children: Aaron and Rebecca Krom;
Alysa, Katie, Ilana, Hannah and David Levene.

To our spouses: Michael and Sue.

To those individuals who over the course of years
have influenced our approach to children in health
and disease; Ben Berliner, Victor Dubowitz, Ze'ev Hochberg,
Hugh Jolly, Esther Rudolf, Hedva Steiner,
Myron Winick.

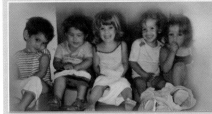

Paediatrics and Child Health

MARY RUDOLF

MB BS BSc DCH FAAP FRCPCH
Consultant Community Paediatrician
Leeds Community and Mental Health Trust
Belmont House, Leeds

MALCOLM LEVENE

MD MB BS FRCP
Professor of Paediatrics
Department of Paediatrics and Child Health
The General Infirmary, Leeds

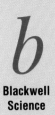

**Blackwell
Science**

© 1999 by
Blackwell Science Ltd
Editorial Offices:
Osney Mead, Oxford OX2 0EL
25 John Street, London WC1N 2BL
23 Ainslie Place, Edinburgh EH3 6AJ
350 Main Street, Malden
  MA 02148 5018, USA
54 University Street, Carlton
  Victoria 3053, Australia
10, rue Casimir Delavigne
  75006 Paris, France

Other Editorial Offices:
Blackwell Wissenschafts-Verlag GmbH
Kurfürstendamm 57
10707 Berlin, Germany

Blackwell Science KK
MG Kodenmacho Building
7–10 Kodenmacho Nihombashi
Chuo-ku, Tokyo 104, Japan

The right of the Authors to be
identified as the Authors of this Work
has been asserted in accordance
with the Copyright, Designs and
Patents Act 1988.

First published 1999

Set by Excel Typesetters Co., Hong Kong
Printed and bound in Italy by
Rotolito Lombarda, SpA, Milan

A catalogue record for this title
is available from the British Library

ISBN 0-86542-957-X

Library of Congress
Cataloging-in-publication Data

Rudolf, Mary J.
  Paediatrics and child health /
Mary Rudolf, Malcolm Levene.
     p.   cm.
  Includes index.
  ISBN 0-86542-957-X
  1. Pediatrics. 2. Children—Health
and hygiene. I. Levene, Malcolm
II. Title.
  [DNLM: 1. Pediatrics. 2. Child
Welfare.
    WS 200 L657p 1999]
RJ45.L38   1999
618.92—dc21
DNLM/DLC
for Library of Congress   98-24257
                    CIP

DISTRIBUTORS
Marston Book Services Ltd
PO Box 269
Abingdon, Oxon OX14 4YN
(*Orders*: Tel: 01235 465500
          Fax: 01235 465555)

USA
Blackwell Science, Inc.
Commerce Place
350 Main Street
Malden, MA 02148 5018
(*Orders*: Tel: 800 759 6102
            781 388 8250
         Fax: 781 388 8255)

Canada
  Login Brothers Book Company
  324 Saulteaux Crescent
  Winnipeg, Manitoba R3J 3T2
  (*Orders*: Tel: 204 837-2987)

Australia
  Blackwell Science Pty Ltd
  54 University Street
  Carlton, Victoria 3053
  (*Orders*: Tel: 3 9347 0300
            Fax: 3 9347 5001)

For further information on
Blackwell Science, visit our website:
www.blackwell-science.com

Contents

Preface, vii

Acknowledgements, ix

1 Nature and Nurture, 1

2 History Taking and Clinical Examination, 14

3 Health Promotion and Child Health Surveillance, 44

4 The Acutely Ill Child, 100

5 Common Symptoms and Complaints of Childhood, 142

6 The Newborn, 232

7 Developmental Problems, 261

8 Emotional and Behavioural Problems, 289

9 Emergency Paediatrics, 297

10 Chronic Medical Conditions of Childhood, 315

11 The Adolescent, 345

12 Clinical Investigations, 357

Index, 366

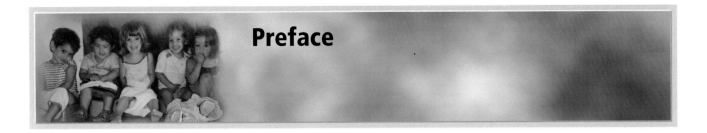

Preface

Experience is the child of Thought, and Thought is the child of Action. We cannot learn men from books.

Benjamin Disraeli

Medical education in Britain has radically changed in recent years. The General Medical Council has pointed a way forward into the 21st century with the document *Tomorrow's Doctors*. This acknowledges the 'information overload' within the medical curriculum and proposes radical changes involving the definition of a core body of knowledge, supplemented by self-directed learning according to students' own interests. It also recognizes that hospital-based medical education is becoming less appropriate as medical services are being directed into the community.

We have tried to adhere to the General Medical Council's guidelines when we planned this book. Recognizing that only a highly selected few of the children who present to their General Practitioner are referred to hospital, we have attempted to describe the problems of children presenting both in a primary health care setting as well as in hospital. Inevitably modern paediatrics requires some forms of sophisticated care to be undertaken in the hospital and these are described as appropriate.

The focus of this book is on helping the medical student develop a working approach to paediatric problems and child health. It has been written from the angle of symptoms and problems as they present to the primary care physician. This format is different to most undergraduate texts and it is apparent that some conditions such as convulsions may be discussed in different sections (e.g., the presentation of a child with fits, faints and funny turns is considered in a separate section to the management of epilepsy). In order to aid learning, the book has been extensively cross-referenced to avoid apparent disruption. We are confident that the student will soon appreciate the advantages of the symptom orientated approach. Working their way through the book, students can develop an approach to diagnosis in a logical and consistent manner, applying guidelines provided within the structure of each chapter.

The key to understanding paediatrics is a working knowledge of child development, growth and the acquisition of clinical skills. A number of chapters have been especially written with this in mind so that the student can appreciate how paediatrics differs from other medical specialties.

We have tried to slim down the factual information presented to the undergraduate. Many diseases of children are discussed only briefly and some not at all as we feel that if the medical student wants to delve more deeply into a subject there is a wide range of detailed textbooks available.

The basis for the acquisition of the art and skills of any branch of medicine must be clinical experience. We hope that, in the words of Benjamin Disraeli, this book can 'learn' students and in helping them to get the most out of their clinical experiences, lead them to appropriate Thought and Action.

MCJR
MIL

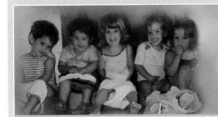

Acknowledgements

We are grateful to Dr Michael Stein for his help with the conception of this book and Mr John Oldham for his support.

We are also grateful to the following who have contributed illustrations: Dr Rosemary Arthur, Mr P.D. Bull, Dr Tony Burns, Professor Martin Curzon, Dr Mark Goodfield, Dr Phillip Holland, Mr Tim Milward, Dr P.R. Patel, Dr John Puntis, Dr Mark Stringer, Ms Clare Widdows, Dr Susan Wyatt and Dr Jane Wynne and to the Child Growth Foundation for permission to reproduce their growth charts.

1 Nature and Nurture

Introduction, 1
Physical growth, 1
Psychomotor development and

social interaction, 2
Nutrition, 5
Child care and education, 10

Social disadvantage, 10
Ethical issues in paediatrics, 11

And one man in his time plays many parts,
His acts being seven ages. At first the infant,
Mewling and puking in the nurse's arms.
And then the whining schoolboy, with his satchel,
And shining morning face, creeping like a snail
Unwillingly to school.

William Shakespeare

Introduction

Paediatrics is the branch of medicine that covers the childhood years. In general, the younger the child the more their physiology and metabolism differ from that of adults, but for older children these differences become less pronounced. There are, however, two areas that are unique to paediatrics: physical growth and development. A good understanding of how children change in terms of growth and development in the early years is very important and without this understanding it is not possible to practice paediatrics well. This chapter discusses how the child develops physically, neurologically, psychologically and emotionally from birth through to full maturity. The chapter also discusses how nutritional needs change through childhood as well as the way the child's environment influences well-being. Finally, ethical issues as they relate to paediatrics are discussed.

Physical growth

Growth vs. development

Growth and development are intimately related, but are not necessarily dependent on one another. Growth is a combination of increase both in the number of cells (hyperplasia) and in the size of cells (hypertrophy). Development is an increase in complexity of the organism due to the maturation of the nervous system. A child may develop normally, but be retarded in growth and vice versa. Brain injury does not necessarily cause impaired somatic growth although many children who are severely intellectually retarded are small.

Growth can be measured accurately but the measurement of development is much more difficult to quantify.

Factors that affect growth

Growth is influenced by a number of semi-independent factors, but growth itself is a continuum from early fetal life through to the end of adolescence. The following are the major factors affecting growth:
- *Genetics*. Growth patterns and final height are largely determined by genetic factors. A normal child's final height can be predicted as falling close to the centile midway between the parents' centiles.
- *Hormones*. The principal hormones influencing early growth are growth hormone and thyroid hormone. Growth hormone in childhood and the sex hormones play an important part in the pubertal growth spurt. Disturbance of any of these affects a child's growth (see Hypothyroidism, p. 58).
- *Nutrition*. World-wide, malnutrition is an important factor that influences children's growth, and is the major factor accounting for the differences in height observed between populations in developing countries and in the developed. In many developed countries (including Britain and the USA), malnutrition is still a cause of poor growth, and is sometimes associated with neglect. Overnutrition, a leading cause of obesity, is on the increase.
- *Illness*. Illness causes a child's growth to slow down. If the illness is short-lived, rapid catch-up occurs. Chronic illness can irreversibly and profoundly affect growth.
- *Psychosocial factors*. Sociodemographically, children and adults from higher socioeconomic classes are taller than their peers from the lower classes. An adverse psychosocial environment, particularly if there is emotional neglect, can have a profound negative effect on a child's growth.

Growth in infancy

The rate of growth in the first year of life is more rapid than at any other age. Between birth and 1 year of age, children on average increase their length by 50%, and triple their

Focal points
Factors necessary for normal growth

- Genetic potential (mid-parental height)

- Optimal intrauterine nutrition

- Appropriate postnatal nutrition

- Good health

- Normal psychosocial factors (nurture)

- Normal hormonal milieu

birthweight. Head circumference increases by one third. During the second year of life the rate of growth slows down and the baby changes shape to take on the appearance of the lean and more muscular child.

Growth in the preschool and school years

In the preschool years the child continues to gain weight and height steadily. Beyond the age of 2 or 3 years until puberty, the growth rate is steady at about 3–3.5 kg and 6 cm per year.

Growth in adolescence

Adolescence is characterized by a growth spurt which occurs under the influence of rising sex hormone levels. During the 3 or 4 years of puberty boys grow about 25 cm and girls 20 cm. Growth in the pubertal years is discussed in Chapter 11.

Catch-up growth

During a period of illness or starvation the rate of growth is slowed. After the incident the child usually grows more rapidly so that catch-up towards, or actually to, the original growth curve occurs ('catch-up growth'). The degree to which catch-up is successful depends on the timing of the onset and the duration of slow growth. This is particularly important in infants who have suffered intrauterine growth retardation (see p. 60), and who may have reduced growth potential.

In nutritionally compromised children, weight falls before height is impaired and head growth is the last to be affected. If growth has been slowed for too long or into puberty, complete catch-up is not achieved. There are important therapeutic implications in the early detection of children with abnormal growth velocity patterns. Early treatment is more likely to ensure that acceptable adult height is achieved.

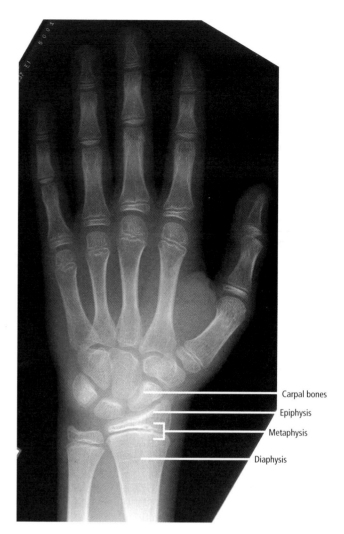

Carpal bones

Epiphysis

Metaphysis

Diaphysis

Fig. 1.1 X-ray of the left wrist taken for bone age. The development of the various bones are assessed, to give an estimate of the child's skeletal maturity.

Organ growth

Not all body systems grow at the same rate and in some respects the growth rates of some organs are independent of others. Full maturation is not complete until the end of the second decade.

Psychomotor development and social interaction

The newborn child is born into a social world and learns to interact initially with the mother, then other close relatives and eventually with other children and adults. Social

DIFFERENTIAL ORGAN GROWTH AT A GLANCE

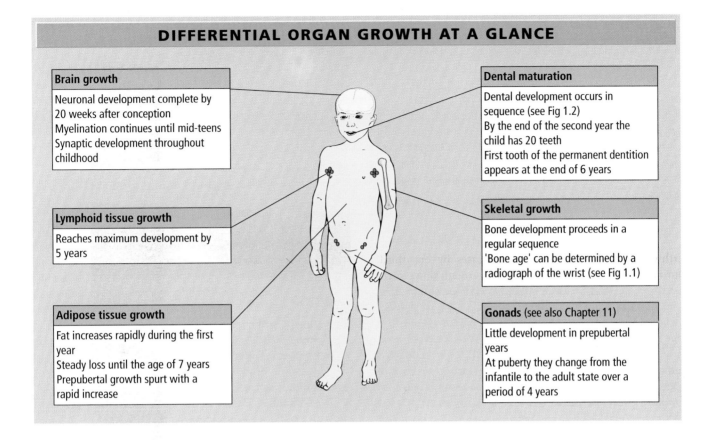

Brain growth

Neuronal development complete by 20 weeks after conception
Myelination continues until mid-teens
Synaptic development throughout childhood

Lymphoid tissue growth

Reaches maximum development by 5 years

Adipose tissue growth

Fat increases rapidly during the first year
Steady loss until the age of 7 years
Prepubertal growth spurt with a rapid increase

Dental maturation

Dental development occurs in sequence (see Fig 1.2)
By the end of the second year the child has 20 teeth
First tooth of the permanent dentition appears at the end of 6 years

Skeletal growth

Bone development proceeds in a regular sequence
'Bone age' can be determined by a radiograph of the wrist (see Fig 1.1)

Gonads (see also Chapter 11)

Little development in prepubertal years
At puberty they change from the infantile to the adult state over a period of 4 years

development is dependent on achieving important neuro-developmental landmarks which gives the child contact with the outside world.

Early social development is divided into discrete periods of time corresponding to developmental landmarks; each period can be considered to be an important milestone in the development of the child into a social being. These milestones and their assessment are discussed in Chapter 2.

The baby and preschool child

0–2 months

The mother of a new baby learns to 'bond' with the baby during the first hours and days after birth. It is not an automatic process and is facilitated by close physical contact. Mothers who are separated from their babies after birth (because they are premature and require admission to a neonatal unit) find bonding more difficult. Such mothers should be encouraged to handle their babies even if the baby is receiving intensive care. Mothers who find they do not immediately love their babies often suffer feelings of guilt because they have never been told that this is a common experience.

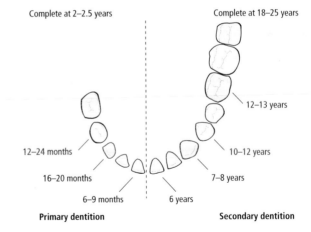

Complete at 2–2.5 years   Complete at 18–25 years

12–13 years
12–24 months   10–12 years
16–20 months   7–8 years
6–9 months   6 years

Primary dentition   **Secondary dentition**

Fig. 1.2 Dental development.

The infant is born with a variety of needs which must be met by the parents, usually the mother. In the first 2 months the baby starts to adapt his or her behaviour into states of arousal. Sleep and wake cycles begin to emerge at this time and are influenced by the routine in the house. The longest period of sleep usually occurs in the night.

The infant shows a great degree of alertness and is particularly attracted by the human face and the spoken word. Contact is achieved with the mother particularly during feeding when patterns of interaction occur. The mother and baby coordinate their behaviour and take turns to initiate contact by means of alternating sucking with pauses for eye contact. It appears that the infant is programmed to respond to his or her carer in particular ways, and in turn the carer is profoundly influenced by her own programming to stimulate her infant in certain ways and to respond to the baby's contact. A major milestone in the development of the baby as a social being in these early weeks is the beginning of the baby's first smile (at around 6 weeks).

2–5 months

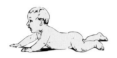

The major developmental change that occurs at the beginning of this period is the infant's visual development. At 2 months the baby can sustain eye contact and this is the first evidence of individuality that the infant shows to his or her mother. This is clearly a vital stimulus for the parents to interact with *their* child. With increasing development the infant shows progressively more gaze interaction. The baby develops patterns of gaze and looking away and the mother responds to her infant's gaze with stereotyped facial movements, speech and intonation patterns.

Another important aspect of this stage of development is the beginning of vocalization. When the child starts to babble the parents respond in an interactive verbal manner almost as if engaging the child in a conversation. The baby may initiate vocalization and the mother responds by questioning or talking to the infant with pauses for the baby's responsive babble. Although the infant clearly does not understand the meaning of his or her parent's speech, its pattern and interaction is essential for the child's own speech and social development. It has been shown that if the mother does not respond appropriately to her infant by smiling and talking when in an *en face* position, the baby becomes distressed and may withdraw from further interaction. The mother's sensitive responses to her baby at this age are essential for normal social development.

5–8 months

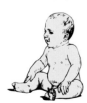

At this age the child begins to pay more detailed attention to objects. The child begins to reach for toys and so begins to explore the inanimate world. The mother now interacts with her child through objects as well as directly. At this stage simple play patterns start to emerge. At 6 weeks of age the baby spends approximately 70% of contact time

regarding his or her mother, but by 6 months two-thirds of the time is taken up with looking at the rest of the world.

The baby begins to initiate contact with an object by gaze and later by pointing. At this stage the infant is transforming from a completely egocentric creature to one who realizes that he or she lives in a world which is shared with many objects and people.

8–18 months

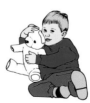

At this age mobility is rapidly developing and the child starts to leave the safety of his or her mother to interact further with his or her environment. The child begins to initiate contact rather than simply reacting to it. It is an age in which the concept of reciprocating begins to emerge. The child can initiate an enjoyable game such as 'peek-a-boo' and can control the game by reciprocating his or her response to that of the adults. He or she is 'learning the rules' both of the game and of social interaction in general. The child begins to be able to use the adult to obtain desired objects, and can also manipulate objects to attract the adult's attention.

The child has learnt to associate his or her cry with response and, for example, knows that if he or she is uncomfortable with a wet nappy, relief will be provided. Babies who are institutionalized become apathetic if their cries are unanswered because the communicative role has been extinguished.

In the first half of the second year the baby begins to take more interest in other children. Initially children play side-by-side, occasionally sharing a toy, and by 18 months may play together, but there is much less vocal contact than the child has with an adult at that age. The adult, particularly the parent, is the main influence in social training at this stage.

18 months and beyond

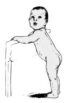

By 18 months the child begins to communicate verbally using speech to describe an event or effect a wish.

Make-believe play develops by 2 years and the child uses familiar objects to reconstruct observed or experienced events. The child develops the ability to recognize shapes, including letters (which is the first stage of reading), and then to copy shapes with a pencil.

The school-age child

Motor, language and social skills continue to develop rapidly during the school years. Horizons are broadened by starting school and often for the first time the child has to learn to function outside the security and safety of his or her own home.

Socialization is particularly important at this age and the child has to learn to relate to a variety of children and adults. Playing games is part of this process and observing and developing rules and taking turns encourages the child to learn about positive adaptation to society at large. Along with this, expectations for appropriate behaviour in a variety of situations increase. During school years the child also begins to develop a conscience and an understanding of right and wrong.

The adolescent

Adolescence, the period which bridges childhood and maturity, is a period of biological, psychological and sociological maturation. This is discussed in detail in Chapter 11.

Nutrition

Milk is the food of babies and it is capable of meeting the infant's nutritional needs for the first 4–6 months of life. Breast milk is the ideal food for human babies, but may be unavailable for some infants, in which case alternative formulae are available.

Nutritional requirements in infancy

Water
Over 70% of the newborn infant's weight is water, compared with 60% for an adult. Infants are less able to conserve water and consequently their fluid requirements are considerably higher than that of older children.

Energy
The newborn infant requires approximately 110 kcal/kg/day (462 kJ/kg/day) for normal growth and these energy requirements are provided by a balance of carbohydrate, fat and protein.
• *Carbohydrate.* Almost all the carbohydrate in both human and formula milk is lactose and about 40% of the total energy requirement comes from carbohydrate sources.
• *Fat.* Fat is the most important source of energy in milk and provides approximately one half of the infant's energy requirement.

• *Protein.* Milk protein can be divided into curd and whey. Curd consists predominantly of casein and precipitates in the stomach. Whey contains mainly lactalbumin and lactoferrin. Colostrum is the very thin watery milk produced by the breast in the first few days after giving birth. It has a very high proportion of immunoglobulins.

Minerals
The mineral requirements change as babies mature. At birth the renal conservation of sodium is poor and newborn babies lose more in their urine than older infants. Premature babies, in turn, require a higher sodium intake than full-term babies because of the functional immaturity of the kidneys.

Calcium and phosphate absorption in infancy is high as a result of the rapid growth rate. The relative ratio of these two minerals is important in determining adequate absorption.

Vitamins
All babies require essential vitamins. Surprisingly, breast milk is deficient in vitamin K. All newborn infants should be given vitamin K at birth to prevent haemorrhagic disease of the newborn.

Trace elements
There are a large number of essential trace elements present in milk which are essential for normal growth and development. Iron is one of the most important and breast milk contains sufficient iron for dietary needs over the first 6 months of life.

Breast-feeding

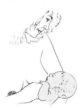

The proportion of women breast-feeding varies widely throughout the world. The World Health Organization reports that in some countries it is usual for all mothers to breast-feed for up to 1 year. In Britain only two thirds of women offer their babies any breast milk at all, and less than half continue to breast-feed by 4 months of age. These figures are influenced by socioeconomic class; 97% of women in the highest socioeconomic class feed their first baby compared with less than 50% in a group of less advantaged women.

The factors that predict successful breast-feeding are shown in Table 1.1.

In developed countries the positive reasons to breast-feed babies are psychological as much as the promotion of physical health. Breast-feeding is also free of cost which may be important in some parts of modern Britain. In developing countries the argument for breast-feeding is very

Table 1.1 Factors associated with successful breast-feeding

High socioeconomic class
Intention to breast-feed whilst pregnant
Paternal support
Whether the mother herself has been breast-fed

strong: formula feeds may easily be contaminated by polluted water used in making up the feed, with the risk of fatal gastroenteritis.

Physiology of lactation

During pregnancy there is a marked increase in the number of ducts and alveoli within the breast, in response to changes in maternal and placental hormones. The size of the nipple also increases. In the third trimester prolactin sensitizes the glandular tissue causing small amounts of colostrum to be secreted.

At birth, oestrogen levels fall rapidly while prolactin rises. This is stimulated further by the infant sucking at the breast. The prolactin secretion from the anterior pituitary maintains milk production from the breast alveoli. The volume of milk produced relates to the frequency, duration and intensity of sucking.

The flow of milk from the breast is under the control of the let-down reflex. The baby rooting at the nipple causes afferent impulses to pass to the posterior pituitary which secretes oxytocin. This acts on the smooth muscle fibres surrounding the alveoli so that milk is forced into the large ducts. As the baby takes less milk, the stimulus for prolactin production reduces and lactation is inhibited. The hormonal maintenance of lactation is summarized in Fig. 1.3.

The let-down reflex is stimulated by contact with the baby, including hearing the baby cry and handling the child. Dripping of milk from the breast not being suckled is caused by the reflex action; this diminishes after the first few weeks. Anxiety and embarrassment suppress the reflex by action of the sympathetic nervous system. Every step possible should therefore be taken to put the mother at her ease and avoid unnecessary anxiety.

Colostrum The milk produced in the first few days after birth is called colostrum and is a thin, yellowish fluid. It is particularly valuable for the establishment of lactobacilli in the bowel and contains less fat and energy but more immunoglobulins than later milk.

The constituents of milk do not reach their mature proportions until 10–14 days after birth. The secretion from the breast between colostrum and mature milk is referred to as transitional milk.

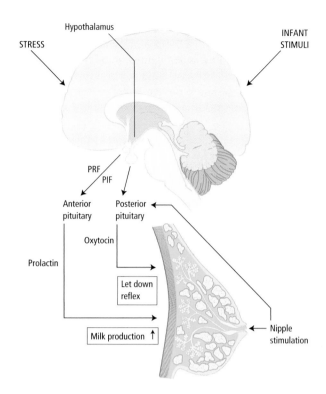

Fig. 1.3 Physiology of lactation. PIF, prolactin inhibiting factor; PRF, prolactin releasing factor.

Technique of breast-feeding

The majority of the milk taken by a baby from the breast is consumed in the first 5 minutes of the feed. Much of the rest of the time at the breast is spent in non-nutritive sucking. The mother should be aware of the feeling of her breast being 'emptied' by her baby shortly after commencement of suckling, but the time spent at the breast following this is also very important.

The mother should be encouraged to put her baby to the breast immediately after birth and the normal baby attempts to suck. Little milk is produced, but the stimulation is important in the establishment of lactation. The mother should be encouraged to put her baby to the breast on demand and she should also feed her baby during the first night if she is not too tired. The time the baby spends on the breast should be gradually increased so that the nipples become accustomed to the baby sucking.

Trauma to the nipple in the first few days after birth should be minimized. The baby exerts strong suction on the nipple and a baby should never be pulled off the breast. The mother should be shown how to release the baby by using her finger to depress the breast away from the corner of the baby's mouth. Each feed should be commenced on alternate breasts.

Babies are often given complement formula feeds in the early days of life by well-meaning staff in order to let the mother rest, but this is counterproductive and should be avoided. If the baby appears to be hungry and it is considered not appropriate to put him or her to the breast, then he or she may be given a solution of dextrose and water.

Advantages of breast-feeding

The advantages of breast-feeding are summarized in Table 1.2.

Breast-fed infants have a significantly lower risk of respiratory and gastrointestinal infections in the early months of life compared with formula-fed infants. Breast milk contains a number of important anti-infective properties which are summarized in Table 1.3.

Contraindications to breast-feeding

For the average healthy infant there are no disadvantages to breast-feeding. Infants born with anomalies such as severe cleft lip and palate and obstructive bowel problems may not be able to feed, although every effort should be made to provide them with expressed breast milk rather than formula feeds.

Similarly, there are very few contraindications to breast-feeding for the mother. The most important reason to prevent a mother from breast-feeding is if she is

HIV-positive: the risk of transmitting the HIV virus to her baby is doubled by breast-feeding. A mother who is excreting *Mycobacterium tuberculosis* should also not breast-feed.

Mastitis (inflammation of the breast) is a common problem, but far from being a contraindication it is alleviated by continued and frequent breast-feeding.

Drugs in breast milk

Most drugs given to the mother are excreted to some degree in her milk, but the exposure to the infant is usually so little that the risk is minimal. Examples of drugs that are definitely contraindicated include tetracyclines (staining developing teeth), antimetabolites (impair cell growth) and opiates (drug addiction).

Formula feeds

Formula milks are based on cow's milk, but are highly adapted to meet the basic nutritional requirements of growing immature infants. A variety of components of cow's milk are utilized. Skimmed milk is produced by removing the fat content, and the curd can be separated leaving whey and lactose together with minerals. These are the building blocks of infant milk formula.

Virtually all formula feeds have added carbohydrate, usually lactose or maltodextrins. Most milk manufacturers replace the fat with polyunsaturated vegetable oil or butterfat blend. This alters the fatty acid profile to resemble breast milk more closely. The protein base of formula milk is usually demineralized whey to which is added the appropriate mixture of minerals, vitamins and trace elements. Casein-predominant milks are usually given as a

Table 1.2 Advantages of breast-feeding

| Perfect balance of milk constituents |
| Little risk of bacterial contamination |
| Anti-infective properties |
| Ideal food for brain growth and optimal development |
| Convenience |
| No expense to purchase milk |
| Psychological satisfaction |
| Possibly reduces risk of atopic disorders |

Ways to encourage successful breast-feeding

- Introduce the concept to both parents antenatally
- Place the baby on the breast immediately after delivery
- Allow the baby to feed on demand in the early days especially
- Avoid offering any formula feeds
- Ensure the mother receives good nutrition and plenty of rest

Table 1.3 The role of anti-infective agents in breast milk

Cells	Milk is teeming with white cells, mainly macrophages, polymorphs and both T- and B-lymphocytes
Immunoglobulins	Secretory IgA is the predominant immunoglobulin Particularly high concentration in colostrum
Lysozyme	Lyses bacterial cell walls
Lactoferrin	Binds iron necessary for the replication of some bacteria and reduces bacterial growth
Interferon	In low concentrations in breast milk and has antiviral properties
Bifidus factor	The carbohydrate bifidus factor encourages lactobacilli to flourish in the bowel which inhibits overgrowth of *Escherichia coli*

supplement to babies of 4–6 months who are perceived to be still hungry. This process produces a formula milk product that is similar in its basic proportions to that of mature breast milk.

It is clear that although there are similarities between breast and formula milks, the constituents are chemically quite different. The protein in formula milk is based on cow's milk protein and the fat content is quite different to breast milk fat content. The major differences between breast and formula milk are shown in Table 1.4.

Additives

Formula or bottlefed babies require no vitamin supplementation.

Table 1.4 Comparisons between breast and formula milk

Breast milk	Formula milk
Sterile	May be contaminated by 'bad' water
Contains anti-infective properties (see p. 7)	
Reduces risk of infection	
No cost	Expensive
Perfectly adapted for human babies	Foreign protein
	Non-human fat content
Allergic disorders reduced	May increase risk of allergy
Possible IQ enhancement	

Fluoride drops should be given to the baby from 2 weeks to 2 years if the drinking water is not fluoridated.

Preparation of feeds

The preparation of a formula feed is summarized in Fig. 1.4. Some mothers find it more convenient to make up the day's supply of feeds at one time. This is a satisfactory method provided the milk can be stored in a refrigerator. Mothers must be instructed to use a level measure of powder and not a heaped one, which produces too concentrated a feed, especially in its electrolyte content, which may cause hypernatraemic dehydration (see p. 117). To obtain a level measure the excess powder is removed with the blade of a knife.

Scrupulous attention should be paid to sterility: bottles and teats should be sterilized by either boiling or by an anti-septic solution such as mild sodium hypochlorite (Milton). It is essential that the bottles are filled with the solution and the teats are totally immersed. The Milton solution should be made up each day.

Most mothers like to give the milk warm, although babies will take a cold feed just as well. To ensure that the feed is not too hot it should be tested by shaking out a little onto the back of the hand. The teat should not be touched or it will become contaminated. The hole in the teat should be of such a size that when the bottle is inverted, milk comes out rapidly in drops, but not a stream. Too large a hole causes the baby to choke on the feed and too small a hole leads to

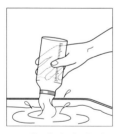

1. Sterilize the feeding bottle

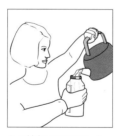

2. Add the appropriate volume of cooled boiled water to the bottle

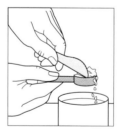

3. Add 1 level scoop of milk powder to each 30 ml of water

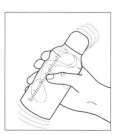

4. Shake bottle well

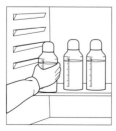

5. Keep in fridge until ready to feed

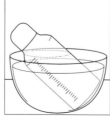

6. Rewarm the feed to room temperature or body temperature prior to feeding

Fig. 1.4 Preparation of formula feed.

excessive air swallowing as a result of the baby vigorously sucking to obtain the milk.

Weaning

Healthy infants do not require weaning until 4–6 months of age. Breast or formula milk provide all their nutritional requirements in the early months. Some prematurely born infants do appear to require weaning relatively earlier than babies born at term, and relatively early introduction of mixed feeds may be necessary to satisfy them. Too early an introduction of mixed feeding may be associated with obesity.

In developed countries there is a wide choice of weaning feeds. In Britain cereals and rusks are the favoured first solid food, but package foods to which water is added may also be used. All modern cereals for babies are gluten free and this may be associated with a fall in the incidence of coeliac disease (p. 166). The semisolid food is given by spoon before offering the bottle or breast. Its timing should be whatever suits the mother. Alternative weaning foods are purées of cooked vegetables, fish or meat. These can be purchased in preprepared containers or be liquidized at home in a food blender.

Babies are conservative individuals and dislike change. The earlier a new tasting food is introduced, the more likely it is to be accepted. Only one new food should be introduced at a time, and if disliked it should be withdrawn for a few weeks and then tried again. When weaning the child, cup and spoon feeding should be introduced early in order to make the change easier and reduce the possibility of the baby refusing to give up the bottle.

As the child gets older the diet will become more like that of the parents. The child will now begin to try to hold the spoon him- or herself although he or she is likely to go through a stage of wanting to use fingers only. Once the baby starts to chew his or her fingers, and even before any teeth have erupted, the baby can be given toast or a hard rusk to chew on. At no time should the child be left alone while feeding for fear of choking.

By the age of 9 months, most babies are ready to eat at least one meal a day with the family. The food should be similar to the rest of the family group, but presented in an attractive and appropriate way: cut up into small pieces or mashed. It will, of course, be necessary for the food to be given to the baby on a spoon or a fork.

Babies can be given undiluted and unboiled bottled cow's milk from 12 months of age. This can be served cold, but as many infants are used to warm milk the child may initially reject it.

At 6 months a multivitamin preparation should be started with weaning to ensure adequate intake and should be continued until the child is 2 years old.

Focal points
Weaning

0–4 months	Breast or formula milk only
4–6 months	Introduce puréed or liquidized foods
6–9 months	Give more soft feeds before milk feeds. Encourage finger feeding. Give fruit juices in a cup
9–12 months	Three meals a day, at least one with the family
1 year and beyond	Undiluted cow's milk in a cup

Focal points
Infant nutrition

- Breast milk is the ideal sole feed for the first 4–6 months
- Continue breast or formula milk for the first year
- Puréed (weaning) food should be offered by spoon from 4 to 6 months
- Only one new food should be introduced at a time
- Once a baby begins to chew, mashed and then cut up food can be given
- Babies can usually feed themselves biscuits or rusks at 7 months
- Cup feeds should replace breast-feeds and bottles discouraged beyond the age of 1 year
- Vitamin supplements should be given from 6 to 24 months

Nutrition in the preschool years

As a toddler the child becomes increasingly dextrous and coordinated and no longer needs to be fed, but eats independently using a spoon and drinking from a cup. Along with this independence comes a change in eating habits and it is normal for a toddler to eat unpredictably, consuming large meals on some occasions and almost negligible amounts at others.

Milk is now no longer the main source of nutrition, although the child should still drink 1 pint of milk per day. In these early years, it is important to ensure that the child becomes used to eating a well-balanced diet. This should include foods from the four basic food groups:
1 meat, fish, poultry and eggs;
2 dairy products (milk and cheese products);
3 fruits and vegetables;
4 cereals, grains, potatoes and rice.

In encouraging a good diet, it must be stressed that children of this age have different requirements from adults. A diet low in fat and high in fibre is unlikely to provide the calorie content that is essential for the active, rapidly growing child. For this reason whole fat milk, rather than skimmed milk should be given until the age of 5 years. It is also important to discourage children from developing a taste for sweet and salty foods.

The development of independence and inconsistent eating habits often causes problems within the family (see p. 292). Parents may become very anxious about the child's diet and resort to a variety of tactics to make their child eat. This can be extremely stressful for all concerned and may be associated with failure to thrive (see p. 67).

The other common problem of this period is iron deficiency anaemia (see p. 90) resulting from low iron stores. These may be inadequately maintained by the toddler's low intake of iron-rich foods and so fail to keep up with the growth of the child. Excessive milk intake may contribute by leading to a reduction in appetite for other nutrients, and may also be responsible for poor weight gain.

Nutrition in the school years

In the school years children have to learn to eat food other than that provided at home, and usually have a midday meal at school. The principles of healthy eating should be maintained, although this may become more difficult as children are introduced to snacking on sugary and salty foods by their peers. Schools are well placed to educate about nutrition and provide well-balanced meals. Unfortunately this is often offset by tuckshops and drink and snack machines on the premises.

The rapid growth rate in the adolescent years leads to increased requirements for energy, calcium, nitrogen and iron. Unfortunately, in this critical period, when good nutrition is so important, the modern teenager often develops a lifestyle which leads to a very poor nutritional intake. Particular problems include an increase in snacking and skipping meals, an inappropriate consumption of fast foods, dieting and restrictive cult diets. The problems of obesity (see p. 68) and eating disorders (see p. 351) often have their onset at this time, while teenage pregnancy has nutritional consequences for both the baby and the mother.

Principles of good nutrition in young children

- Allow only 1 pint of milk each day
- Encourage a diet with food from each of the basic four food groups
- Give three meals and two nutritious snacks each day
- Avoid added salt
- Minimize sugar in the form of sweet drinks and sweets
- Avoid foods which are likely to be aspirated, e.g. nuts, boiled sweets
- Avoid food battles

Child care and education

Increasingly mothers are working outside of the home, and have to find alternative care for their young children. Options include a nanny or minder in the home, or child care outside of the home. Child-minders who take other children into their own home have to be legally approved and registered with the Department of Social Services.

Alternative care is available in **day nurseries** staffed by nursery nurses. These may be run by Social Service departments, privately or by voluntary organizations. Unfortunately they are in limited supply and are often expensive. In disadvantaged areas family centres may be provided, which not only provide child care but are also attended by parents with the aim of improving parenting skills.

The majority of children grow up away from an extended family network, and many parents appreciate the opportunities for their children to mix with other children from a young age. **Mother and toddler groups** and **playgroups** are available in most areas. The former are attended by children accompanied by a carer. Playgroups are run by trained and registered leaders, where children attend for a few sessions per week and have the opportunity to meet, play and socialize with others.

In Britain compulsory education begins at the age of 5 years, although there is limited availability of **nursery school** places from the age of 3 years. From 5 to 11 years children attend **primary school** and then move to **secondary school** until the school leaving age of 16 years. At 16 years teenagers have the option to continue their education in a **secondary school sixth form, sixth form college** or **college of further education**.

Educational provision for children with special needs is discussed on p. 275.

Social disadvantage

A large and increasing number of children, in both developed and developing countries, grow up socially disadvantaged. Disadvantage may arise as a consequence of poverty, poor housing, homelessness, inadequate parenting and problems resulting from immigration. It is important to appreciate that these all have a significant impact on children's health. Alleviation of these problems are mainly political issues for society, but physicians need to understand the impact of these problems, and where necessary and possible, to act as the child's advocate in improving their circumstances.

Poverty

It is hard to bring up a family on a low income. Not only is it hard to feed and clothe children, and provide them with the care and conditions required for them to develop and thrive, but poverty also often diminishes the capacity of parents to be supportive, consistent and involved with their children.

Poverty has a strong effect on the physical health of children, and children from poor families have higher than average rates of death and illness from almost all causes (Table 1.5). Many factors are responsible for the increased morbidity, including overcrowding, poor hygiene and health care, poor diet, environmental pollution, poor education and stress.

Housing

Housing conditions have a profound effect on children's health and development. Dampness and mould are associated with an increase in a wide variety of symptoms and illnesses. Overcrowding and poor sanitary conditions are related to the spread of gastroenteritis and respiratory infections. Inadequate housing may lead to parental depression affecting a child's psychosocial development and behaviour. Poor housing is also linked to a higher rate of accidents, including road traffic accidents as a result of a lack of safe supervised areas for play outside.

Homelessness

Homelessness exacerbates the problems of poverty. Homeless families have very restricted facilities, often living in bed and breakfast or hostel accommodation, with little space or privacy and little possibility of cooking. Moves are frequent with disruption in the provision of health and social services and schooling for the children. Homeless children suffer from increased frequency of illness (infections, anaemia), neurological conditions and learning disorders, fits, mental illness, dental problems, trauma and substance abuse, and are more likely to be victims of abuse and neglect.

Family structure

There have been major changes in the structure of society in recent years. Only 80% of children in developed countries now live with both natural parents, and there are increasing numbers of parents bringing up children single-handedly. Although this does not necessarily imply that the children are disadvantaged, single parenting is difficult, particularly if it is associated, as it often is, with a reduced income, lack of support with resultant stress and depression, and family tensions and arguments. These all may have an effect on the child.

Ethnic minorities and immigrants

The other major change that has occurred in developed countries is absorption of a variety of different ethnic and cultural groups. While immigrant families are often well supported within their cultural framework, children may be disadvantaged in a variety of ways of which health professionals need to be aware.

Language and cultural barriers often lead to high degrees of social stress and isolation, and families may find it difficult to access services including health care. Specific health problems affecting some groups include nutritional deficiencies, higher perinatal and infant mortality rates, and inherited diseases if consanguinity is common practice.

Ethical issues in paediatrics

Ethics is the science of morals, and morals are the personal framework that dictate right and wrong. The law defines what an individual in a society may and may not do, and a moral approach to a situation depends on an individual's conscience, religious views and previous experience.

Paediatrics is a speciality where there are many ethical issues to be considered, such as withdrawal of intensive care, consent and parental rights. The medical student should be aware of some of these issues and it is the responsibility of every practising doctor to have established his or her own *modus vivendi* for working in these difficult areas.

Three important concepts underlie an understanding of ethical issues. These are the sanctity of life, omission vs. commission, and the quality of life. Each is briefly discussed here.

Table 1.5 Morbidity associated with poverty

Low birthweight
Poor growth
Respiratory infections
Iron deficiency anaemia
Lead poisoning
Poor vision
Hearing disorders
Psychological problems
More and longer hospitalizations
Lower survival in some malignancies (e.g. leukaemia)
Lower educational attainment
More likely to attend special school

Sanctity of life

Life is sacred and any act intended to end a life is illegal. It is thought by those with a particular religious point of view that every effort must be made to preserve life, under all circumstances, but this is not accepted by others. Most people would agree that to offer an anencephalic baby intensive care would be wrong because the prognosis for life is so poor; intensive care simply delays the time for the heart to stop beating. Others believe that not feeding a patient in a persistent vegetative state is acceptable so that the patient dies of dehydration, albeit appropriately sedated. Therefore the concept of the sanctity of life is too broad to be the ultimate moral benchmark as there is much scope within the law for making decisions that affect life and death.

Omission vs. commission

This concept considers the method of a patient's death. It is illegal to undertake an act that kills a patient: this is an act of commission. An example would be giving a patient a lethal injection: this is both illegal and immoral. Many would argue that giving a powerful narcotic injection to a patient who is dying in extreme pain is acceptable, knowing that an outcome of this injection is death by respiratory depression. This is not illegal as the primary aim of treatment is to alleviate pain and not to kill.

There is a moral difference between causing someone to die by a positive action and allowing death to occur by failing to act. An example of the latter is leaving septicaemia untreated in a patient on a ventilator who has a very poor prognosis, knowing that death will occur as a result of non-treatment with antibiotics. This is legal and most would argue is ethical. An act of omission may be illegal if failing to treat causes a patient to die who might otherwise have fully recovered.

Both acts of commission and omission may therefore be acceptable in one framework and unacceptable (and illegal) in another.

Quality of life

Most people would agree that ventilating a baby who has no chance of independent survival without a ventilator is wrong. The quality of life the child would have if he or she were to survive is a factor to be considered. This usually causes the most controversy within an ethical context.

'Quality of life' is a nebulous concept. It has been suggested that the quality of life is encapsulated within the idea of individual 'humanhood'. The qualities of humanhood are those that make us individual. These include:
- awareness of oneself;
- concept of time, both future and past;
- ability to communicate;
- care and concern for others;
- curiosity.

Withdrawal of intensive care

Uncritical application of intensive care is one of the most frequent areas of ethical uncertainty in medicine and is particularly relevant to paediatrics. The physician must consider the following issues within the ethical context of offering or continuing intensive care:
- *What is the prognosis?* Intensive care that only acts to put off the time of death is unlikely to be in the best interest of the patient, but this may help relatives come to terms with the impending death. Long-term intensive care of a patient with a hopeless prognosis is often thought to be wrong. Withdrawal of intensive care should be considered and refocuses the emphasis of care from the child to the family to help the parents with the process of mourning.
- *Quality of life.* If the patient survives, will the quality of life be acceptable? The answer to this question often depends on whom it is being addressed to. Some parents may say that life of any quality is acceptable even if their child is very severely damaged with blindness, severe spasticity and very low intelligence. Other parents may find a child with only moderate disability unacceptable.
- *Pain and suffering.* One may question whether treatment which is very painful or where the child has to suffer severely to overcome a life-threatening disorder is justified. The management of cancer is an example of a protracted course of unpleasant and distressing treatment. If the ultimate prognosis is good then this may be easy to justify, but if the prognosis is uncertain or poor then it may be unfair to put the child through the distress of treatment.
- *Use of scarce resources.* In most developed health care services there is an unequal balance between demand on facilities and their availability. There may only be one intensive care ventilator with two patients requiring it. This often causes major dilemmas in neonatal intensive care where a less acceptable form of therapy must be given because the resources are limited. A judgement may have to be made as to which patient is most likely to benefit from the treatment.

Guidelines from the Royal College of Paediatrics and Child Health

Recommendations have recently been produced by the Royal College of Paediatrics and Child Health to help doctors decide when medical treatment should be withdrawn from children. The situations when this should be considered include:
- when the child is brain dead;

- when the child is in a permanent vegetative state;
- when care delays death without easing suffering;
- when the child survives so physically or mentally impaired that it is unreasonable to expect him or her to suffer further;
- when the illness is so progressive and irreversible that further treatment is intolerable.

Consent and parental rights

Another area of ethical concern is the issue of consent. For adults, it is accepted that a competent patient has the right to accept or refuse health care. Many paediatric patients are not competent to make their own decisions and therefore parents traditionally have made such decisions on their behalf. This is acceptable in most situations and the majority of parents act in the best interests of their child, but the issue arises regarding the age at which an individual becomes competent to make his or her own decisions.

Whereas many people feel that a child's views should be taken into account, it becomes impossible to define an age at which a child will have the maturity to decide whether he or she wishes to be investigated or treated for an illness, particularly if this is at variance with the parent's views.

A particularly controversial issue regarding consent concerns the prescription of contraceptives to adolescents. Strict requirements for parental consent may deter adolescents from seeking health care, with consequences in terms of teenage pregnancies and sexually transmitted disease. In Britain a legal precedent has been set, such that the physician may prescribe contraceptives without parental consent, provided the adolescent is deemed mature enough to understand the risks and benefits of the treatment.

Another difficult issue concerns situations where parents fail to act in the best interests of their child. Not many years ago it was accepted that parents had absolute rights over their child and that these rights should not and could not be interfered with by external agencies. In fact, the first court case prosecuting a parent for abusing a child had to be brought on the grounds of cruelty to an animal as there was no procedure to prosecute a parent abusing a child. Society has changed its views and laws now exist whereby children can be protected and parental rights and authority curtailed (p. 97). However, debate continues as to the extent to which society and the law can intervene in parental practices, particularly where cultural issues are involved. An example of this is female circumcision.

Ethical conflicts

The nature of ethical dilemmas means that there can be no right or wrong answers. Each case is different and its circum-stances must be carefully reviewed. The parents' wishes must be very carefully considered and it is, in general, unwise to act against their wishes. Sometimes, however, it is necessary to do so if the parents' wishes are clearly unreasonable or unrealistic. In these circumstances it is usually appropriate to take the legal precaution of making the child a ward of court so that the decision is taken out of the clinician's direct control.

A second major source of ethical conflict arises when one clinical view conflicts with another. An example may be in withdrawing care, when the doctor thinks it a reasonable option but a senior nurse disagrees. These differences must be reconciled and it is a failure of medical management if major disagreement continues to exist. It is important that the opinion of every member of the clinical team is heard and that no-one feels left out of the process. Ultimately a decision must be made by the senior clinician but it is his or her role to ensure, as far as possible, that no-one feels that the decision is wrong.

The essence of decision making in medical ethics is effective communication. Communication should involve the child, when appropriate, parents, other relatives and staff, and, if necessary, lawyers and possibly clergy. Decisions cannot be made by committee but neither can they be made by dictat. Sometimes prolonging intensive care with no prospect of the patient surviving is the appropriate course of management in order to buy time for relatives to accept the appropriateness of the decision.

Focal points
Medical ethics

- The clinician can only act within the legal code

- Ethical decisions need not be made rapidly and only after full discussion and consideration

- It is usually inappropriate to make decisions which conflict with the views of the patient's relatives

- All members of staff must be involved in discussions before a decision is made

- Discuss all options with the parents so that they know that all the possible courses of treatment have been considered

- Where the child is mature enough, he or she should be involved in ethical decisions

- Adolescents may receive treatment without parental knowledge, provided they are deemed mature enough to appreciate its consequences

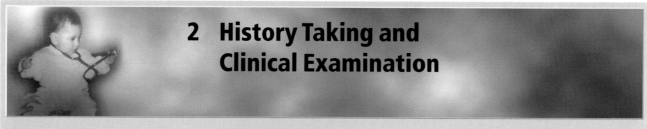

2 History Taking and Clinical Examination

Introduction, 14
An approach to examination, 17
Assessment of growth, 17
General observation, 21
Neurological assessment, 21

The visual system, 27
The ear, nose and throat, 28
The reticuloendothelial system, 29
The respiratory system, 31

The cardiovascular system, 33
The abdominal system, 36
The musculoskeletal system, 38
Developmental assessment, 39

Studies of medical outpatient consultations show that 86% of diagnosis depends entirely on what the patient says; their own story. What doctors find on examination adds a further 6%; and technical investigations (X-rays, blood tests, etc.) add another 8%.

British Medical Journal 1975

Introduction

In clinical medicine, history taking and physical examination are the keystones of diagnosis and subsequent therapy. The first contact between the child, the family and the doctor sets the scene for the future professional relationship. Very little may be remembered by the child and his or her family about the first visit except whether the doctor gave the impression of being an approachable and sympathetic person. When the patient is a child, the doctor's approach is of special importance and techniques must be altered in light of the patient's age.

Every child should have a personal child health record (see p. 45) held by a parent. This should be maintained as an individual record on a child's growth, health and development as well as contacts with doctors and health care workers. The record is particularly useful when the child is the subject of a new referral to a doctor and should be brought to the appointment so that details of immunization, growth and development are readily available.

History taking

Most patients make first contact with a doctor in a GP surgery or in an outpatient clinic. The child needs to be put at ease and made to feel welcome. The child should usually be greeted first, provided that this is not likely to embarrass him or her. Call the child by his or her name and introduce yourself. If the family have been waiting for some time apologize for the delay. The aim is to become friends and help the child to make contact with the doctor.

The consulting room should have age-appropriate toys and the child be encouraged to play with them. The doctor should not be seated across a desk from the family, but they should sit side by side. During the interview it is helpful to maintain as much eye contact with the child and his or her family as possible. If the child is old enough, questions should be directed at him or her; and the younger child should be involved in the discussion.

A major feature of the interview is observation of the child and his or her family. The following points should be specifically ascertained:
• How do the parents relate to the child and vice versa?
• Does the mother or father appear depressed, anxious or tearful?
• Does the child separate from the mother?
• Does the child play constructively?
• Is the child unusually distractable?

The interview

The medical history often provides more information on which to make a diagnosis than the clinical examination. The aim of the history is to build up a picture of the child, his or her problem(s), family and environment.

When taking the history, the doctor must decide whether it would be better for the child to leave the room to play rather than to hear him- or herself being discussed, but he or she should always come into the consulting room initially to prevent fear of the unknown while waiting to be called. A sensitive doctor will often anticipate the parents' wish for them not to talk in front of the child. Some parents feel too embarrassed to make the request with the result that they may withhold important information.

Many parents and children cannot express their particular fears. For example, the presenting complaint of headache may represent fears about brain tumour, and enlarged glands may arouse anxiety about cancer. It is very important for the doctor to anticipate these problems and ask specifically about them. These fears can be elicited by asking questions such as: 'Is there anything in particular you are worried about?' or 'In my experience some parents worry about cancer in a child with tummy pain. Is this a fear of yours?'

It is often very helpful at the end of the interview to ask the parent(s) what they think the cause of the problem is. Their answer may reflect their anxieties or guilt that they may be in some way responsible for the child's condition.

The history

A structured approach to taking the history is important. Asking questions in a fixed sequence is necessary in order to avoid forgetting important points, but this must not become too rigid as sometimes it is necessary to pursue a different line in questioning to elicit important information.

Presenting complaint(s)

Record the chronology of the presenting complaint in a systematic manner with a heading for each date line starting from when the child was last '100%' or 'their normal self':

- 4 weeks ago: onset of cough;
- 3 days ago: sore throat;
- today: convulsion.

Never write the days of the week in the history as they give no indication of the duration of the disease. It is important for the person taking the history to have a clear idea in his or her own mind of the chronology of the presenting complaint. If you are confused, ask direct questions to clarify the point.

Previous medical history

The GP's referral letter is often helpful in determining previous visits to the doctor's surgery and details of any medication the child has been given. All previous admissions to hospital must be enquired about and noted. It may be necessary to write to other hospitals to determine the exact nature of investigations and treatment that had been carried out previously. Enquire about allergies and determine how severe any previous allergic reactions had been. Ask specifically about asthma, eczema and hay fever.

Perinatal history

Record the duration of pregnancy. Enquire into specific problems during the pregnancy such as hypertension, smoking, drug ingestion, influenza-like illnesses. Details of the birth must be recorded such as birthweight, type of delivery, presentation of the child and condition at birth. Specific questions may be required as the mother may not be able to describe the infant's condition at delivery. The following questions are helpful:

Schema for history taking

Presenting complaint

Previous medical history
Details of hospital admissions
Problems addressed by the GP
Drug history
Allergies
Perinatal history
Details of pregnancy (smoking and alcohol intake) and labour
Condition at birth. Did the child need to be taken away for resuscitation/special treatment?
Birthweight and gestation
Breast or bottle feeds in the neonatal period
Neonatal problems

Developmental history (see also p. 39)
Establish the ages at which developmental milestones were reached

Immunization history
All immunizations with dates

Family history
Father and mother: record first names, ages and occupations. Ask about any medical problems
Siblings: record names, ages and any medical problems. Any sibling deaths? Miscarriages or terminations?
Other people living in the house. Ask about their illnesses
Family illness and allergies
Pets in the home

Social history
Type of housing
Do other families live with them?
How long has the family lived at that address?
Does anyone in the house smoke?
Family arrangement
Is there a man in the household. Is he the father of the children?
Who is the main carer?
Are there financial problems or unemployment?
Is the family receiving social support or other benefits?
School or nursery the child attends. Are there any problems?

System review
ENT: ear ache, hearing impairment, recurrent sore throats, enlarged glands
Respiratory: cough, wheeze
Cardiovascular: faints, murmurs, cyanosis
Neurological: headaches, fits, faints or funny turns
Gastrointestinal: vomiting, diarrhoea, constipation, abdominal pain
Genitourinary: enuresis, dysuria, frequency, age of menarche, dysmenorrhoea
Skin rashes

• Did the baby need any special treatment at birth, for example, help with breathing?
• Was the baby taken away from you after birth? If so, for how long?
• How long was it before you could feed your baby?
• How old was the baby when he or she went home?
• Did the baby suffer from any fits in the newborn period?
• Did the baby have breathing problems requiring oxygen?

Family history

When recording the members of the family it is best to draw a family tree as shown in Fig. 2.1.

Ask specifically about the following:
• Whether there is a member of the family with a similar condition to that being complained of by the child.
• Consanguinity. This is particularly common in some ethnic groups.
• Establish how the family works. Who is the breadwinner? If there is a man in the house, is he the father of the patient or the other children?

Social history

Social problems may strongly influence the health of children in a family. An absent father may be a source of unhappiness for the child and enquiries should be made into the relationship the child has with his or her natural father. School is another potential source of conflict and anxiety for the child. Bullying may be a particular problem which is unknown to the parents. Determine whether the symptoms that the child complains of are related to school days and whether he or she misses time from school.

Clinical examination

The approach to the clinical examination depends on the age and cooperation of the child. The examination of the newborn is discussed in Chapter 6. Older children are examined in a manner very similar to the adult; by organ system in a systematic manner. The young child, particularly if fretful or anxious, must be approached quite differently. Any

uncomfortable procedure such as examination of ears and throat should be left to last in order to avoid upsetting the child as much as possible. Time spent initially gaining the child's confidence is never wasted.

A young child may be put at ease if the doctor keeps up a 'running commentary' during the examination. The doctor asks questions as the examination proceeds, but if the child fails to answer he or she should immediately pass on to another question. A child can become acutely embarrassed by the silence after a doctor's question, whereas he or she may be reassured by the doctor's continuing chatter.

The mother should be left to undress the child because he or she is liable to get upset if a stranger does this. The doctor must be prepared to vary his or her routine to suit the child, and it may be necessary to examine the back of the chest before the front or the abdomen before the chest. This variable routine has the disadvantage that parts of the examination may be forgotten, but this can be avoided by a strictly systematic method of recording so that it is immediately obvious if any part of the examination has been overlooked.

Before applying a stethoscope to a young child's chest it is often helpful to put it first on the chest of the mother or a teddy bear to show the child that it is not frightening.

Formulation of the problems and plan of action

Problem list

After taking the history, a list of relevant problems should be compiled as part of formulating the history. Following the examination and investigations, further problems may be identified and are added to the list. All the factors including family and school difficulties that may affect the presenting complaint should be considered. It is important to compile a list of all the problems that impinge on the presenting complaint. An example of a problem list is:
• abdominal pain;
• constipation;
• single unsupported mother of the child;
• bullying at school;
• sibling has cerebral palsy.

At the end of the first consultation it is important to identify to the parents and the child what the problems are and then to discuss further steps to be taken. These should be considered under the following headings:
• Investigations to be carried out.
• Therapy.
• Contract with the parents:
   • Ensure that the parents understand what the doctor's view of the problem is.
   • Agree on what needs to be done.

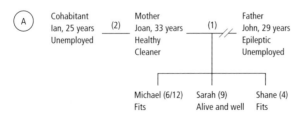

Fig. 2.1 Example of family tree to illustrate family history.

- Agree on when the child should be seen again.
- Provide information leaflets.
- Contact with support organizations of families with similar problems where appropriate.

AN APPROACH TO EXAMINATION

Assessment of growth

Accurate measurement of height, weight and head circumference is a vital part of the assessment of all children referred for a medical opinion. Growth can only accurately be assessed by taking at least two measurements of various growth parameters (e.g. length, weight and head circumference) and observing the relative points at which these measurements fall on a growth chart appropriate for the child's age and sex.

Measurement of height

The measurement of height should be precise and is only accurate if made with care using the appropriate equipment.

In the first 2 years of life, length is measured on a measuring frame or mat (Fig. 2.2). From the age of 2, providing the child can stand, vertical height is measured against a specially calibrated standing frame. Consistent technique is necessary to estimate standing height accurately (Fig. 2.3).

Weight

Weight is measured by weighing scales. Infants should be laid in a pannier scale and older children can stand or sit on the weighing machine. These scales must be calibrated accurately on a regular basis. Babies should be weighed naked with their nappy off and older children weighed wearing only their underclothes.

Head (occipitofrontal) circumference (OFC)

This can be measured accurately to the nearest millimetre. A flexible, non-stretchable tape measure is used and is put around the occipitofrontal region of the head. Three successive measurements are made at slightly different points and the widest is taken to be the OFC.

Growth standards

In order to interpret a child's growth, comparison must be made with population standards. These standards are presented in the form of growth charts, which demonstrate the population's growth in the form of centiles. The growth charts currently in use are the 1993 Child Growth Standards, which were constructed from detailed data collected on children across the country.

Separate charts are available for girls and boys and are divided into three age groups: 0–1 year, 1–5 years, and 5–18 years. Age is given along the x axis which, depending on the chart, may be shown in months or decimally. Height, length, weight and head circumference measurements lie along the y axis. Nine centiles ranging from the 99.6th to the 0.4th centile are shown as continuous or dotted lines (Fig. 2.4).

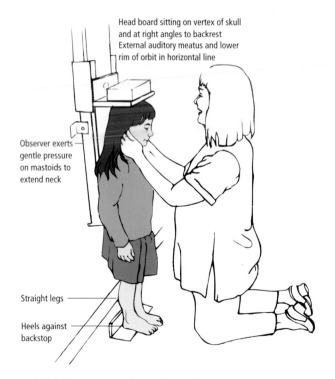

Head board sitting on vertex of skull and at right angles to backrest
External auditory meatus and lower rim of orbit in horizontal line

Observer exerts gentle pressure on mastoids to extend neck

Straight legs

Heels against backstop

Fig. 2.3 Measurement of standing height.

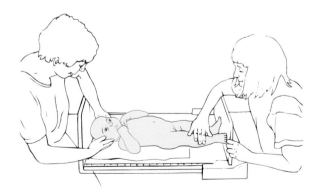

Fig. 2.2 Measurement of length using a frame.

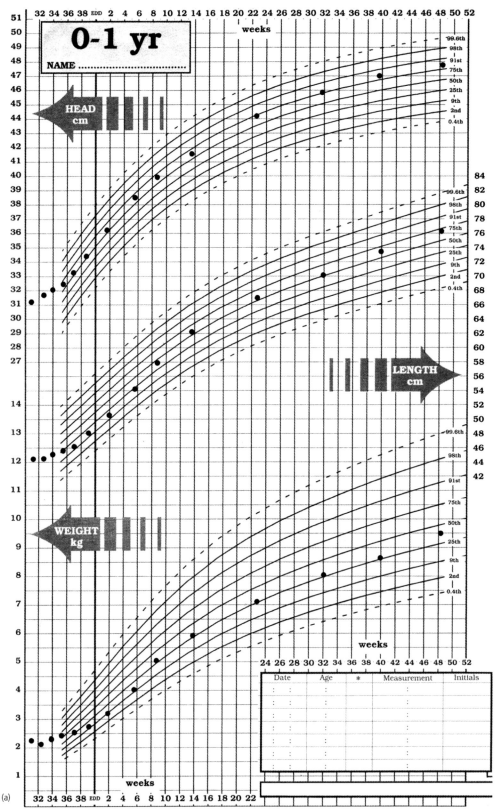

Fig. 2.4 (a–c) Child Growth Standard charts showing a baby's growth at 28 weeks' gestation until 2 years corrected for prematurity. © Child Growth Foundation.

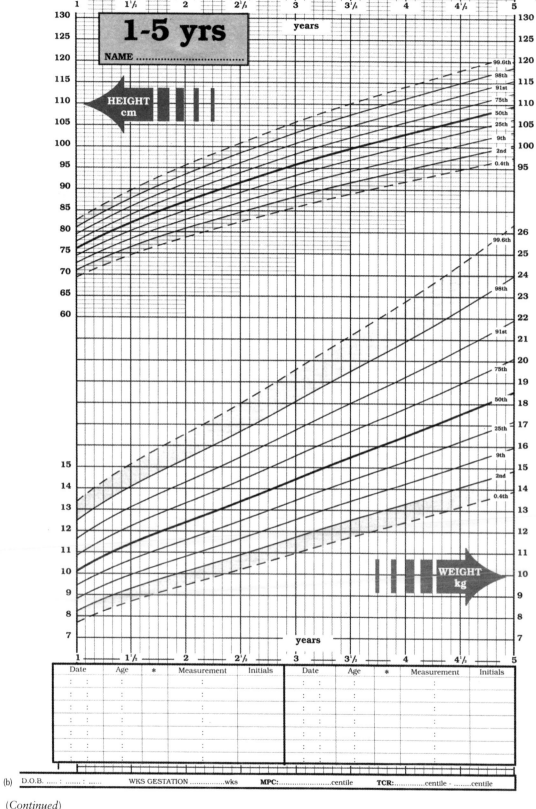

(b) D.O.B. ..... : ...... : ......   WKS GESTATION ....wks   **MPC**:......................centile   **TCR**:.............centile - ....centile

Fig. 2.4 (*Continued*)

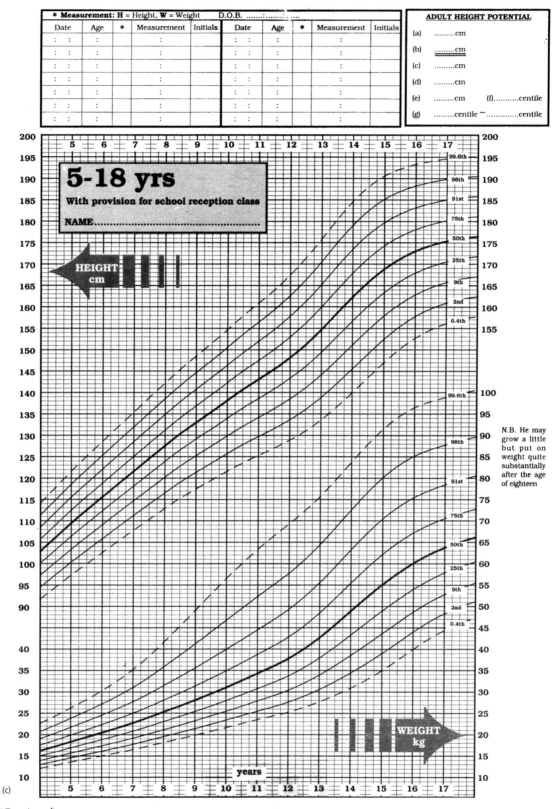

Fig. 2.4 (Continued)

Plotting a child's growth

In order to interpret a child's growth measurements, they must be plotted on the appropriate growth chart. If the child was born prematurely, the child's age should be corrected up to the age of 24 months, so that the post-term age is plotted rather than the chronological age (see Fig. 2.4a). The centile along which the point falls relates the child's growth to the rest of the population. Thus, if a boy's weight falls on the 50th centile, he is average, and 50% of the population will be heavier and 50% lighter than him. If his height falls on the 9th centile, he will be relatively short with 91% of the population taller and only 9% smaller.

The further a child's growth falls away from the normal population the more likely it is that he or she has a problem. Thus, measures falling between the 0.4 and 2 centiles may be normal, whereas those below the 0.4th centile are more likely to be abnormal. Furthermore, when a child's growth is followed over time, crossing centiles (other than in the first 2 years or at puberty) is concerning and needs evaluation. Interpretation of growth in babyhood and at puberty is important and requires skill.

Interpretation of growth charts

After the first 2 years of life a child should continue to grow along the same centile, although infants in the first few months of life may follow a centile quite different to their subsequent growth centiles. It is important to relate the height with weight and head circumference on centile charts, so obtaining an idea of the build of the child. Interpretation of children's patterns of growth is discussed in Chapter 3.

General observation

Much can be learnt by watching the child while he or she is being undressed and by how the child plays. Observation starts from when the child and his or her family enters the room and should not be confined to the course of the physical examination.

Formal observation should include:
• Examination of the child's hands. Observe the palmar creases, and the nail beds for colour (cyanosis, anaemia). The most sensitive way to detect early clubbing is to look at the profile of the nail bed as the normal angle is lost very early in the clubbing process (Fig. 2.5). The commoner causes of clubbing are listed in Table 2.1.
• Examine the lips and tongue for central cyanosis. Evert the lower eyelid to assess the colour of the mucosal membrane for anaemia.

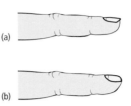

Fig. 2.5 Nail bed angle: (a) normal and (b) clubbing.

Table 2.1 Commoner causes of finger clubbing

Familial	Benign condition
Cardiovascular disease	Cyanotic heart disease e.g. Fallot's tetralogy
Respiratory disease	Chronic suppurative lung disease e.g. cystic fibrosis
Bowel disease	Chronic inflammatory bowel disease e.g. ulcerative colitis

Focal points
The examination of organ systems

• Observation

• Palpation

• Percussion

• Auscultation

• Observe the child's facies for evidence of dysmorphic features or asymmetry.

Neurological assessment

Neurological assessment in infants is discussed on p. 24.

Observation

Abnormal movements
These may occur in children with neurological disorders. The commonest is choreoathetosis (writhing movements of the limbs) usually associated with facial grimacing. Sudden jerking movements may be due to myoclonic epilepsy or, in infants, infantile spasms (pp. 181, 333).

Gait
In ambulant children, observation of the way they walk (gait) is very important. This may give clues to the neurological disorder. Abnormal gait patterns include:

Stiffness This is the commonest major gait abnormality and suggests an upper motor neurone lesion, usually cerebral palsy (Fig. 2.6). In mild cases it may be exaggerated by asking the child to run. The patterns of abnormal movement in different types of cerebral palsy are discussed in Chapter 10.

Waddling The child with spastic diplegia has a more waddling gait (Fig. 2.7). The predominant feature is adduction of both thighs, so that the knees are flexed and knock together with the ankles apart. The child tends to take weight on the toes or anterior part of the foot.

Weakness because of a neuromuscular problem This may be suspected if the child finds it difficult to get up from a sitting position. The characteristic feature of this is the Gower's sign where a weak child will 'climb up his legs' to a standing position (p. 269).

Ataxia The child walks in an unsteady manner with a broad-based gait.

Muscle bulk

Muscle bulk is assessed by observation, comparison of one side with the other and palpation. Wasting of muscle groups occurs in both upper motor neurone disorders (cerebral palsy) and in lower motor neurone lesions (spina bifida, nerve palsies).

Tone

Muscle tone is defined as the resistance to passive stretch. Determination of whether tone is normal or not depends on the examiner's experience and the age of the child. Tone in various muscle groups can be assessed by the examiner moving the limb with the child relaxed.

With the child lying on his or her back, the major limb joints should be put through their passive range of movements and resistance to movement is assessed. Tone in the lower limb can be elicited by lifting the leg a few centimetres from the couch and letting it fall back.

Increased tone suggests an upper motor neurone lesion and reduced tone (hypotonia or floppiness) a lower motor neurone lesion. Spasticity is the term used to describe spasm in a muscle group with increased tone. In spasticity of the lower limbs the thigh adductors are more usually affected. The tone of these muscles can be elicited by lying the child on his or her back with the examiner grasping the ankles. The legs are then rapidly abducted by the examiner and the tone assessed by the resistance to this movement (Fig. 2.8a). The tone in the gastrocnemius muscle, which is also particularly affected in spastic cerebral palsy, is assessed by passively dorsiflexing and plantarflexing the foot (Fig. 2.8b). Hypertonia in this muscle group causes resistance particularly in plantarflexion.

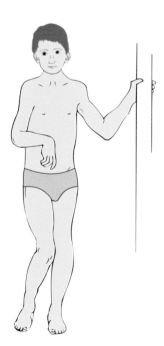

Fig. 2.6 Hemiplegic gait exaggerated by asking the child to run.

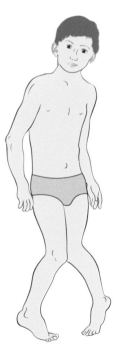

Fig. 2.7 Waddling gait in a child with spastic diplegia.

Muscle power

In cooperative children muscle power should be formally assessed by testing opposing muscle groups in both upper and lower limbs. The muscle power around each joint should be assessed.

Sensation

In older cooperative children sensation is tested in the same way as it is for adults. The following modalities should be assessed:
- light touch using cotton wool;
- pain with a blunt needle;
- temperature;
- proprioception (position sense).

One side should be compared with the other. The child should either close his or her eyes or the examiner should shield the area under examination so the child cannot pick up visual clues.

Sensory loss is not a common finding in children with upper motor neurone lesions.

Coordination

This is best tested in the upper limb by the nose–finger test and in the lower limb by the heel–shin test.

Nose–finger test The child is asked to touch lightly the tip of the nose and then the tip of the examiner's finger. Once the child has established the idea he or she is asked to do this as rapidly as possible while the examiner moves his or her finger. The accuracy of the pointing is assessed. In ataxia the child finds it difficult to touch accurately either finger or nose. Both hands should be tested separately.

Heel–shin test (Fig. 2.9) With the child lying on his or her back he or she is asked to straight leg raise and then bend the leg so that the heel accurately touches the patella. The child should then be instructed to run the heel down the front of the shin. Both sides should be tested separately.

Reflexes

A tendon jerk is detected by slightly stretching the muscle and tapping the tendon in a direction perpendicular to the tendon. The degree of muscle contraction that occurs as a result of the stimulus is described in terms of normal, exaggerated (UMN), weak (LMN) or absent. Before concluding that a reflex is absent, distraction (reinforcement) should be attempted to elicit the reflex. This is done by asking the child either to clench their teeth very hard together or to interlock the fingers of both hands and try and pull them apart. The manoeuvre to elicit the reflex is then repeated.

Tendon jerks should be formally assessed for the following tendons:
- biceps;
- triceps;
- supinator;

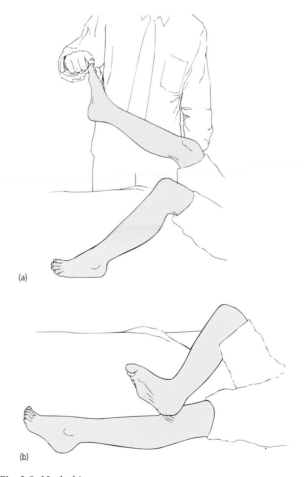

(a)

(b)

Fig. 2.9 Heel–shin test.

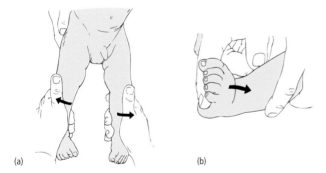

(a)   (b)

Fig. 2.8 Assessment of tone in the lower limbs: (a) assessment of adductor tone and (b) tone assessed at ankle by dorsiflexion/plantarflexion.

- knee;
- ankle.

In young children the ankle jerk is most easily elicited by gently holding the foot in a slightly dorsiflexed position with the examiner's thumb over the ball of the foot. The examiner's thumb is tapped by the hammer and the elicited plantarflexion of the foot observed (Fig. 2.10).

Normal tendon activity is learnt by experience. Increased reflexes suggest an upper motor neurone lesion.

Plantar reflex It is best to leave this until last as children do not enjoy it. This is elicited by using the examiner's thumb nail to stroke the lateral border of the sole of the foot firmly from heel to little toe. The response is normally up-going in infants until the age of 8 months, but thereafter a down-going response is normal. An up-going response (a positive Babinski reflex) or an asymmetrical response in a child over 8 months is abnormal.

Cranial nerves

In older children the cranial nerves are elicited in exactly the same way as they are in adults. Some information about cranial nerve function in young children can be obtained by observation (see below).

It is important for the undergraduate to assess the following cranial nerves routinely. This may not be possible in uncooperative children.

Cranial nerves II, III, IV, VI Examination of these is described in the section on The visual system (p. 27).

Cranial nerve V (trigeminal) The motor component of this nerve is the masseter muscle. This can be assessed by the bulk of the masseter muscle while asking the child to bite hard.

Cranial nerve V provides sensation to much of the face and it is divided into three divisions: ophthalmic, maxillary

and mandibular. Sensation to light touch should be tested in each of these areas.

Cranial nerve VII (facial nerve) Ask the child to screw up his or her eyes as tightly as possible. Weakness (inability to bury the eyelashes on one side) or inability to close the eye fully may indicate cranial nerve VII weakness. The child is also asked to show his or her teeth. Drooping of the corner of the mouth suggests facial nerve palsy.

Neurological examination in babies

The main difference between neurological examination as described above and examination in younger children is the inability or unwillingness of young children to co-operate with the examiner. Consequently the assessment is based much more on observation while playing with the child.

Schema for neurological examination in the older child

Observation
Abnormal movements
Gait (ask child to attempt to run). Assess evidence of:
  stiffness
  weakness
  ataxia
Muscle bulk:
  wasting
  pseudohypertrophy (see Duchenne
  muscular dystrophy, p. 267)
Cranial nerves
Tone (assess multiple muscle groups)
  Normal
  Hypotonia
  Hypertonia
Power (assess multiple muscles)
Sensation
  Light touch
  Pain
  Temperature
  Proprioception
Coordination
  Nose–finger test
  Heel–shin test
Reflexes
  Tendon jerks
  Plantar reflex
  Parachute reflex (see Fig. 2.15)

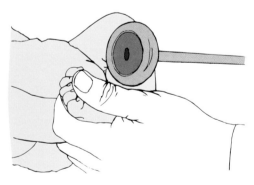

Fig. 2.10 Eliciting the ankle jerk in young children. The hammer percusses the examiner's thumb.

Observation

This is very important in learning about neurological function. Particular points to observe (or enquire about) include:

• *Irritability.* Can the baby be consoled by cuddling?

• *Spontaneous movement.* Reduced movement suggests muscle weakness.

• *Position at rest.* A severely hypotonic baby lies in a frog position (Fig. 2.11). A stiff baby may have a retracted neck (opisthotonos) with scissoring of the legs when held upright (Fig. 2.12).

Palpation

Palpation of the fontanelle in children of 6 months and below may give some useful information. A bulging fontanelle suggests raised intracranial pressure and is a late sign in meningitis (p. 109).

Handling

The child should be picked up to assess tone. The floppy baby tends to slip through the examiner's hands like a rag doll and the stiff baby does not yield to gravity when being moved through the air.

Tone is assessed by the baby's responses to gravity. Tone should be assessed while holding the baby in a number of positions.

• Ventral suspension. The examiner puts his or her hand under the abdomen and lifts the child off the couch. A hypotonic baby will droop over the examiner's hand.

• Pull to sit. The examiner holds the infant's hands and pulls him or her into a sitting position. Head lag on pulling to sitting (see below) indicates a hypotonic infant.

• Limb tone is assessed by passive movement such as measuring the popliteal angle. If tone is low there is little resistance whereas if high the leg resists extension (Fig. 2.13). If tone is low there is little resistance whereas if high the leg resists extension.

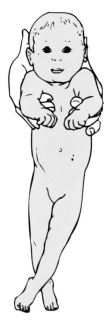

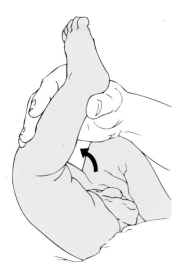

Fig. 2.12 Scissoring of the lower limbs.

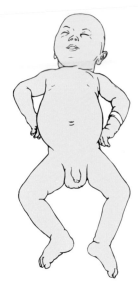

Fig. 2.11 A hypotonic child lying in the frog position.

Fig. 2.13 The popliteal angle.

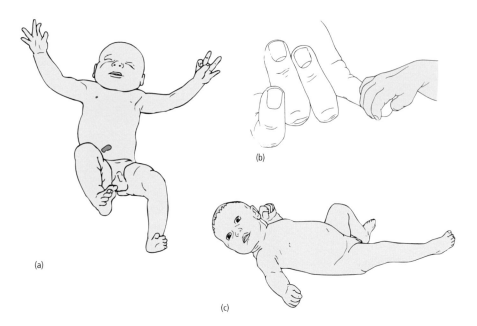

Fig. 2.14 Elicitation of primitive reflexes: (a) Moro reflex; (b) palmar grasp reflex; and (c) asymmetrical tonic neck reflex

Reflexes

Tendon jerks are elicited as described for older children.

Primitive reflexes (Fig. 2.14) appear and disappear at different times as shown in Table 2.2. Their absence or their persistence beyond a given period signifies neurological dysfunction.

The parachute reflex appears at 9 months of age and is elicited by pitching the baby forward. It comprises extension of both arms with extension of the hands (Fig. 2.15). Asymmetry of this reflex may be an early sign of a unilateral upper motor neurone lesion (spastic hemiplegia).

Table 2.2 Age at which primitive reflexes appear and the latest age by which they should have disappeared. Persistence after this time is definitely abnormal

	Appearance	Disappearance
Stepping	Birth	1 month
Moro	Birth	4 months
Palmar grasp	Birth	2 months
Asymmetrical tonic neck reflex	Birth	6 months
Parachute reflex (Fig. 2.15)	9 months	Persists

Schema for neurological examination in babies

Observation
Irritability
Reduction in spontaneous movement
Hypotonia (frog position)
Hypertonia (opisothotonus)
Symmetry of facial appearance

Palpation
Fontanelle

Tone
Assess tone by:
   ventral suspension
   pulling to sitting
   assessing popliteal angle

Reflexes
Tendon jerks
Primitive reflexes

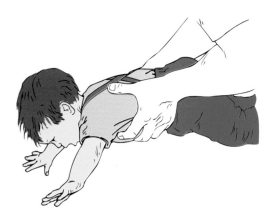

Fig. 2.15 The parachute reflex.

The visual system

Elicitation of the red reflex (p. 47) is essential in the newborn ocular examination. Each eye must be assessed separately. It is possible for a child who has no vision in one eye to appear to have normal visual function if both eyes are assessed together.

Observation

• The iris, sclera and pupil should all be inspected. A red eye will be recognized by scleral or conjunctival injection. A cataract may be detected by observing some opacity of the lens.
• The pupillary reflex is assessed by shining a bright light momentarily into the eye from about 10cm distance. Note the pupillary reaction in the stimulated eye and the consensual constriction in the other eye.
• The corneal light reflex must be tested in the assessment of a squinting eye. If a bright pen torch is directed towards the child's eye at a distance of about 45cm then a reflection of the light is seen in both corneas (the corneal light reflex). Normally the reflection is seen in the centre of the child's pupils when the child is looking straight at the light source. If the reflection is asymmetrically placed in the two eyes then the visual axes are not parallel suggesting that a squint is present (Fig. 2.16).

Assessment of visual acuity

Visual attention may be tested in newborn infants by gaining their attention with a visually interesting object (usually the examiner's face) and moving the object to see if the child follows.

There are a variety of formal vision testing kits available for young children. The Stycar rolling ball test is most widely used where small white balls of different diameters are rolled across the floor to detect the limit of the child's visual resolution.

Simple screening tests of vision should be routinely employed in assessing a newly referred child. Can the child see small blocks and does he or she reach for them? Can he or she see tiny beads such as 'hundreds and thousands'? The vision in each eye should be tested separately. Older children can be asked to count fingers as a simple screening test of vision. Each eye should be tested separately.

Ocular movements-

Once the visual attention of the child has been obtained, testing the range of movements is simple. The visually interesting object should be moved through the eight positions of

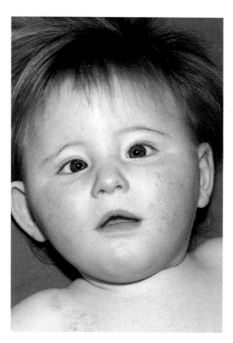

Fig. 2.16 A 6-month-old baby with a convergent squint. Note the asymmetrical corneal light reflex which confirms that the visual axes are not parallel and that this child has a squint rather than simply a wide bridge to the nose.

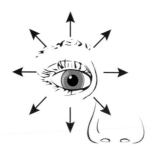

Fig. 2.17 The eight positions of gaze.

gaze (Fig. 2.17). The examiner should watch the visual axes during these movements to detect limitation in the movement of one or both eyes.

Visual field

The visual field can be simply assessed in most children of 5 years and older by the 'wiggly finger test'. The child sits opposite the examiner, approximately 1m apart. The child is asked to look at the examiner's nose and to hold his or her hand over his or her right eye. The examiner covers his or her own left eye with his or her left hand. The examiner then gradually brings his or her other hand into the range of vision of the child with a finger wiggling and the child is asked to say when he or she first sees the wiggly finger (Fig. 2.18). The examiner will be able to compare the child's

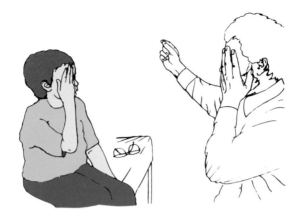

Fig. 2.18 'Wiggly finger' test.

visual field with his or her own as a normal control. This is repeated with the examiner's hand being moved from different angles. The test is then conducted in the same way but with the other eye covered.

Fundoscopy

The use of the ophthalmoscope is an essential skill in clinical medicine. It is more difficult in children, particularly babies who do not like having a bright light shone into their eyes and will try to look away. Particular attention should be paid to the lens (presence of cataracts) and the retina.

Assessment of a squint

It is essential to be able clinically to assess a young child for a squint. Squints are discussed on p. 77.

Examination for a squint comprises the following stages:
- Corneal light reflex at different angles of gaze (p. 27).
- Ocular movements. Is there an increasing angle of squint in particular angles of gaze suggestive of a paralytic squint?
- Visual acuity.
- The cover test.
- Fundoscopy.

The cover test

This is a useful test to confirm whether there is a subtle squint. It is necessary first to decide which eye is thought to be squinting. The examiner asks the child to look at a visually interesting object (Fig. 2.19a). The examiner then covers the normal eye without touching the child's face (Fig. 2.19b). The squinting eye will rapidly flick to fix on the object. This is a positive cover test. When the cover is removed the squinting eye will again flick in the other direction as the covered eye becomes the dominant eye again (Fig. 2.19c).

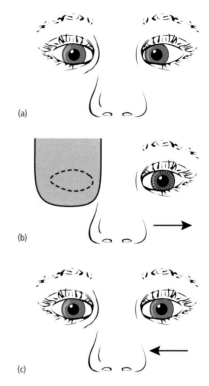

Fig. 2.19 Cover test to assess a squint.

Examination of the visual system

- Observation of the eyes
- Assessment of visual acuity
- Assessment of ocular movements
- Testing of visual fields
- Fundoscopy

A latent squint is also detected by the cover test. In this case the eyes appear to have parallel axes on direct observation. When the eye with the latent squint is covered it will move to the nasal direction if the squint is convergent, and when the cover is removed, the eye will flick back to its normal position.

The ear, nose and throat

Examination of the ear

Every doctor involved in the care of children should be able to examine the ear competently. Examination of the ears is

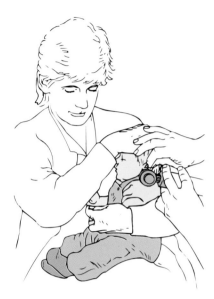

Fig. 2.20 Position to hold a baby for otoscopic examination.

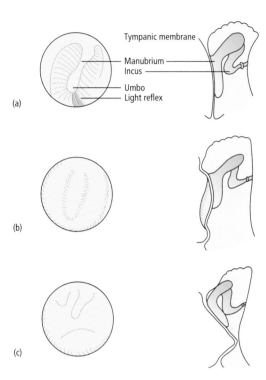

Fig. 2.21 Tympanic membrane appearances: (a) normal; (b) otitis media with a bulging drum; and (c) glue ear with a retracted drum.

traditionally left to the end of the examination as it is most likely to upset the young child. The child should be held by the mother on her lap with the child's head against her chest. If the child is likely to struggle the mother's other hand should restrain his or her arms, and his or her legs can be gripped gently between the mother's legs (Fig. 2.20).

The examiner should hold the auroscope with the hand resting against the child's temple so that the instrument will move with the child. The top of the pinna is grasped by the examiner's other hand and pulled up to straighten out the external auditory meatus. The largest possible speculum is chosen which will comfortably enter the meatus and is not advanced more than 0.5 cm in infants and 1 cm in older children. If wax is present, an attempt should be made to remove it gently.

The tympanic membrane should be carefully inspected. The normal appearances are shown in Fig. 2.21a. The membrane is normally white in colour and translucent, with a light reflex at its anterior lower pole. Some middle ear structures can be observed through the membrane including the handle of the malleus and the umbo. The normal drum lies in a neutral position. If there is increased pressure in the middle ear as results from otitis media the drum bulges forward and is inflamed (Fig. 2.21b). If the drum is retracted, as occurs in some cases of glue ear, the light reflex is lost, the drum is dull and both the malleus and the umbo are very obvious (Fig. 2.21c). In some cases, a fluid level can be seen through the membrane and air bubbles may also be present. Assessment of drum mobility is a specialized examination technique not carried out routinely.

Examination of the throat

In older cooperative children this is done in the same way as for adults. Young children do not like to have their throats examined and this is best done with the child sitting on the mother's lap as shown in Fig. 2.22. If the child is uncooperative and will not open his or her mouth the wooden spatula is gently used to part the lips and teeth and the tongue is depressed. If the child cries this facilitates the examination.

The tonsils should be examined for size, redness and exudate. Normal tonsillar size varies enormously. The tonsils are lymphoid tissue and are very small at birth and grow to maximal size by 4–5 years, getting smaller in the early teens. Normal tonsils can appear very large in preschool children. If they meet in the midline they are probably abnormally large. The signs of tonsillitis are discussed on p. 104.

In addition the oropharynx should be observed for redness (pharyngitis).

The reticuloendothelial system

Lymph node enlargement is very common in childhood and glandular tissue should be routinely assessed as part of the

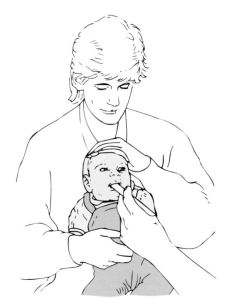

Fig. 2.22 Position for holding a child to examine the throat.

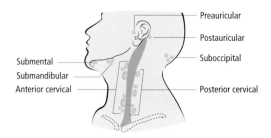

Fig. 2.23 The cervical lymph nodes.

physical examination. In many cases an enlarged lymph node is a response to a localized infection and its origin should be sought. The spleen is the largest lymphoid organ in the body and is examined as part of the abdominal assessment (p. 36). The sites of superficial lymph node position should be systematically examined as described below.

Neck

The sternomastoid muscle divides the neck into the anterior and posterior triangles and the site of lymph node enlargement is shown in Fig. 2.23. The neck is examined from the front and behind and the two triangles carefully assessed. The region under the jaw is best examined from the front by placing both hands in the angle of the jaw and working them initially forwards and then down the posterior triangle to the clavicle. Enlargement of nodes behind and under the ear and in the occipital region are best examined by standing behind the child. In preschool children, small (usually no larger than the size of a pea), firm, mobile and discrete swellings are very common. These are often described as 'shotty'. They reflect relatively recent infection and the parents should be strongly reassured that they are, first, benign and, second, that they will eventually resolve spontaneously even though they may persist for many months in some cases.

If a single node is enlarged the following qualities should be recorded:
• position;
• diameter;

> ### Focal points
> ### The lymph node enlargement
>
> *Shotty mobile nodes:*
> are common and of no concern
>
> *If one gland is found to be enlarged:*
> carefully examine for lymphadenopathy elsewhere
>
> *If lymphadenopathy is generalized:*
> examine for hepatosplenomegaly
> blood tests are essential

• whether it is mobile or fixed;
• consistency: hard or rubbery.

Enlarged cervical glands are most commonly caused by tonsil or, less commonly, middle ear infection and both should be carefully inspected. Occipital nodes enlarge as a result of scalp infection (eczema is a common cause) and rubella causes occipital node enlargement.

Axillae

Each axilla is examined separately with the child sitting and facing the examiner. Explain to the child what you are going to do. The examiner supports the flexed arm at the elbow with his or her left hand holding the right arm and places his or her right hand in the right axilla. Palpate for the presence of enlarged nodes against the chest wall. The process is reversed to examine the other side. Localized axillary lymphadenopathy indicates infection in the hands (paronychia is common) or arms.

Groin

With the child lying supine, the examiner gently palpates the groin for enlarged nodes. The nodes are usually small, discrete and mobile. Localized enlargement of groin nodes suggests infection in feet or legs.

The respiratory system

In children interpretation of physical signs relating to the respiratory system requires care. The child with obvious sounds on auscultation may have no significant disease, whereas the child with more subtle signs, such as tachypnoea and intercostal recession, is likely to have a significant respiratory condition even if auscultation is unremarkable.

Observation

Is there an audible wheeze or stridor? Look for signs of respiratory distress; namely tachypnoea (count respiratory rate), use of accessory muscles, nasal flaring or recession. Restlessness and drowsiness suggest hypoxia/hypercapnoea (increase in CO_2). Normal respiratory rate varies with age and is shown in Table 2.3. The sites of chest recession are summarized in Fig. 2.24.

Examine the hands for evidence of clubbing, cyanosis or anaemia. The causes of clubbing are listed in Table 2.1.

Describe the chest shape. The commoner abnormalities in chest shape are illustrated in Fig. 2.25:
• Barrel chest (because of air trapping) has an increased anteroposterior diameter and is best observed by looking at the chest from the side (Fig. 2.25a).

Table 2.3 Normal respiratory rate at different ages

Age	Awake respiratory rate (breaths per minute)
0–12 months	25–40
1–5 years	20–30
6 years and above	15–25

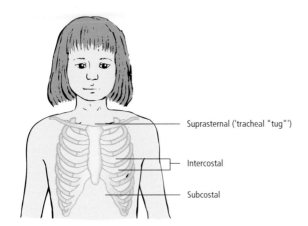

Fig. 2.24 Sites of chest recession in a young child with respiratory distress.

Suprasternal ('tracheal "tug"')

Intercostal

Subcostal

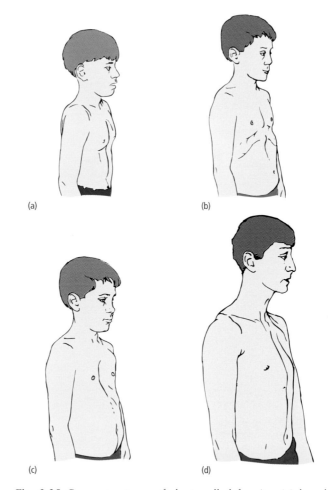

(a) (b) (c) (d)

Fig. 2.25 Commoner types of chest wall deformity: (a) barrel chest; (b) Harrison's sulcus; (c) pectus excavatum; and (d) pectus carinatum.

• Harrison's sulcus is caused by diaphragmatic overactivity and is shown by grooves parallel to and 2–3 cm above the costal margin. It is seen in chronic asthma (Fig. 2.25b).
• Pectus excavatum (also known as funnel chest) is a common deformation and may be without significance (Fig. 2.25c).
• Pectus carinatum (also known as pigeon chest) may be associated with various forms of congenital heart disease (Fig. 2.25d).
• Chest asymmetry with one half of the chest more prominent than the other may be a result of scoliosis and is assessed by examining the spine (pp. 38, 89).

Palpation

Mediastinal deviation is assessed by looking for deviation of the trachea and/or the apex impulse. The tracheal position is palpated by identifying the trachea in the suprasternal notch between two fingers (Fig. 2.26). The apex impulse is detected by the method described on p. 33.

Chest expansion is also assessed by palpation. The examiner's hands are placed on the child's chest with the thumbs just touching each other at the sternum and the fingers lightly resting on the skin over the ribs (Fig. 2.27). The child is asked to take a deep breath and the distance the thumbs move apart determines the degree of chest expansion. In a 5-year-old child 1 cm expansion or more is normal.

Percussion

The chest is percussed to assess its degree of resonance. The middle finger of the left hand (if the examiner is right handed) is placed along the line of the rib and is then struck with the first finger of the right hand as if it were a hammer hitting a small nail. The quality of the resonant note is compared with other parts of the chest. The entire chest, back and front, should be percussed in a systematic way. Normal liver dullness is detected anteriorly, commencing just below the nipple. Apart from the area of liver dullness the percussion note should be symmetrical across the chest. Percussion is not very useful in children below 1 year of age.

The resonant note is increased with hyperinflation because of air trapping. This is particularly seen in chronic asthma. A dull percussion note may be because of underlying consolidation or lung collapse. Pleural effusion causes a stony dull percussion note.

Auscultation

Auscultation of the breath sounds should be carried out with the diaphragm of the stethoscope. Start at the top of the chest anteriorly, comparing one side with the other and then listen over the back in a similar manner.

There are two main types of breath sound; vesicular and bronchial. Vesicular sounds are heard when air enters and leaves normal lung tissue. There is a distinct interval between inspiration and expiration. Bronchial breathing is normally heard over the trachea and is continuous throughout the breath cycle. The sound is harsher than that heard in vesicular breathing.

Adventitious sounds include either crackles (crepitations) or wheezes (rhonchi). Crepitations are discontinuous noises that sound like the soft rustling of leaves. They are more likely to be normal if cleared by coughing. Wheezes are usually expiratory but may be heard on inspiration as well. They indicate bronchial narrowing or intraluminal oedema.

In young children, sounds transmitted from the upper airway may be confused with lower respiratory sounds, particularly wheezes. Listen first to the noise of breathing without the stethoscope. Sometimes, when the upper airway sounds are soft, applying the stethoscope close to the child's mouth, nose or larynx may help to clarify the nature of the upper airway noise to avoid confusing it with the noises coming from the chest itself.

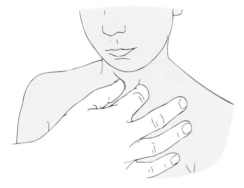

Fig. 2.26 Examining the position of the trachea.

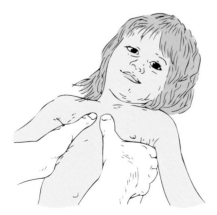

Fig. 2.27 Assessing chest expansion.

Focal points
The respiratory system

- In children, the observation of respiratory distress is more important than auscultatory findings

- The respiratory rate in infants is normally faster than in older children

- Percussion and auscultation may be unreliable in delineating consolidation in the young child

- In children, transmitted sounds from the upper airways may easily be confused with adventitious sounds

Schema for examining the respiratory system

Observation

Look for signs of respiratory distress:
    alar flaring
    tachypnoea
    inter/subcostal recession
Look for clubbing
Is the shape of the chest abnormal?

Palpation

Check for mediastinal deviation:
    tracheal position
    apex beat
Assess chest expansion

Percussion

Assess whether the note is equal and resonant
Define the upper edge of liver dullness

Auscultation

Listen for breath sounds
Define any adventitious noises:
    crepitations?

The cardiovascular system

Observation

Cyanosis is a major sign of cardiovascular disease. Cyanosis also occurs as the result of respiratory disease and both systems should be examined sequentially. Central cyanosis is always abnormal. This is determined by examination of the tongue. Lips and fingers may be blue because of non-cardiac causes such as cold, and are not uncommon in babies. Anaemia and clubbing can both be determined by examination of the child's hands as described above.

General inspection should also comment on general growth, the presence of breathlessness (this may be a result of cardiac as well as respiratory disease) and chest shape. Pectus carinatum is the only abnormal shape associated with heart disease.

Palpation of the pulse

The peripheral pulse should be examined for rate, rhythm and character. It is easier to assess the right brachial pulse in young children rather than the radial.

Rate The rate should be timed over 15 seconds and converted to a rate per minute. Normal heart rate depends on the child's age (Table 2.4).

Rhythm Sinus arrhythmia is normal and is a variation in rate with the respiratory cycle. Occasional ectopic beats are also normal in children.

Pulse character This is detected by the pulse volume. There are a number of abnormalities seen in non-acutely ill children.

• *Collapsing pulse (waterhammer pulse)*. This is because of a wide pulse pressure most usually in children with patent ductus arteriosus. The increased pulse volume is best felt by elevating the limb.

• *Slow rising pulse*. This is self-descriptive with a slow upstroke and rapid fall off in the impulse. It is caused by left ventricular outflow obstruction.

Radiofemoral delay It is always important to compare the radial or brachial pulse in the right limb with the femoral pulse. In coarctation of the aorta the pulse in the right limb is either felt before the femoral (or left radial pulse) or the femoral pulse is absent.

Palpation of the praecordium

The apex beat should be palpated by one fingertip. The examiner's hand is placed over the chest with the fingertips in the anterior axillary line (Fig. 2.28). The maximal lateral impulse is determined with one fingertip. This is the apex beat and is normally in the mid-clavicular line in the fifth intercostal space (fourth interspace in children less than 5 years old). A forceful apex or displacement of the apex to the left suggests left ventricular hypertrophy or lung disease distorting the mediastinal position.

Right ventricular hypertrophy can be detected on palpation by placing the palm of the hand over the lower half of the sternum (Fig. 2.29). An abnormal impulse is felt by a heaving sensation under the heel of the hand.

A thrill is a palpable murmur felt as a vibration and is

Table 2.4 Range of heart rates in normal children

Age	Normal heart rate (beats per minute)
<3 months	100–180
3–24 months	80–150
2–10 years	70–110
>10 years	55–90

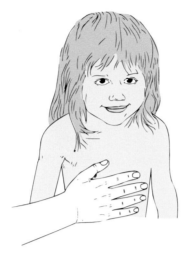

Fig. 2.28 Palpation of the apex beat by the index finger.

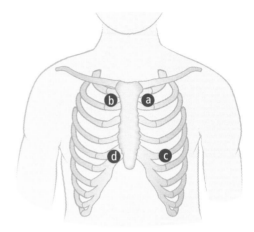

Fig. 2.30 Valve areas: (a) pulmonary, (b) aortic, (c) mitral, (d) tricuspid.

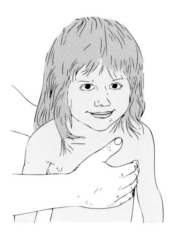

Fig. 2.29 Position to place hand to assess for a parasternal heave.

always abnormal. The fingertips should be placed over the four valve areas on the praecordium and in the suprasternal notch (Fig. 2.30).

Auscultation

The chest should be auscultated carefully with both the bell and diaphragm of the stethoscope. The bell is particularly important in picking up low-pitched murmurs. The examiner must discipline him- or herself to listen first for heart sounds and then for murmurs. The chest should be auscultated in five areas; the four valve areas (see Fig. 2.30) and over the back. If a murmur is heard its intensity should be assessed with the child lying and turned onto his or her left side.

Heart sounds

The first heart sound comprises closure of the mitral and tri-cuspid valves. The second sound occurs with closure of the aortic and pulmonary valves. These two valves do not close simultaneously. On inspiration blood is sucked into the right side of the heart and right pulmonary ejection is prolonged causing the pulmonary valve to close slightly after the aortic valve. During expiration the two valves close together. Normally, splitting of the second heart sound is heard in the pulmonary area on inspiration. Fixed splitting of the second heart sound (this does not vary with respiration) is caused by overfilling of the right ventricle usually because of an atrial septal defect. A loud and single second heart sound is heard when pulmonary vascular resistance is raised, usually because of a large left to right shunt (e.g. a large ventricular septal defect). A third heart sound is heard in up to a quarter of normal children and is caused by rapid filling of the ventricles. An ejection click is caused by aortic or pulmonary valve stenosis.

Murmurs (see also p. 80)

Murmurs are caused by turbulence of blood flow and may be innocent or associated with cardiac pathology. In infants there may be no murmur despite major cardiac anomalies.

Murmurs can be graded according to their loudness and presence of a thrill into six grades (Table 2.5). The loudness of the murmur does not correlate with the severity of the lesion.

The murmur may occur during systole or diastole. Diastolic murmurs denote cardiac pathology. Systolic murmurs may be either ejection (diamond-shaped in intensity) or pansystolic (Fig. 2.31). In the latter case the term may be misleading as the murmur does not always occur throughout systole.

Distinguishing vibratory murmurs and venous hums from pathological murmurs are discussed on p. 80.

Table 2.5 Grading of cardiac murmurs. Grades 1 and 2 are usually innocent, Grades 5 and 6 are always significant and Grades 3 and 4 are suspicious

	Murmur	Thrill
Grade 1	Barely audible	None
Grade 2	Soft and variable in nature	None
Grade 3	Easily heard	None
Grade 4	Loud	Present
Grade 5	Very loud	Present
Grade 6	Heard without a stethoscope	Present

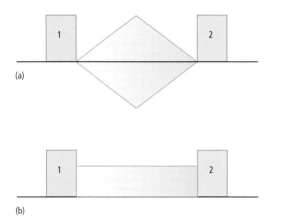

Fig. 2.31 Shape of cardiac murmurs: (a) ejection systolic murmur; and (b) pansystolic murmur. 1, 2 denote the first and second heart sounds.

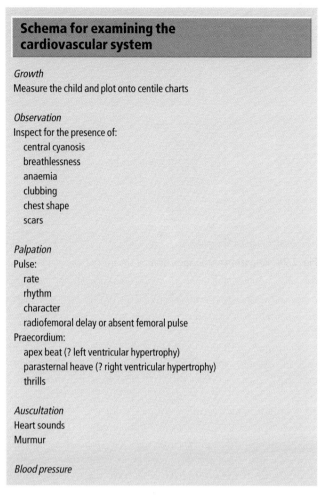

Schema for examining the cardiovascular system

Growth
Measure the child and plot onto centile charts

Observation
Inspect for the presence of:
   central cyanosis
   breathlessness
   anaemia
   clubbing
   chest shape
   scars

Palpation
Pulse:
   rate
   rhythm
   character
   radiofemoral delay or absent femoral pulse
Praecordium:
   apex beat (? left ventricular hypertrophy)
   parasternal heave (? right ventricular hypertrophy)
   thrills

Auscultation
Heart sounds
Murmur

Blood pressure

Focal points
The cardiovascular system

- Sinus arrythmia is normal in children

- Radiofemoral delay or absent femoral pulses are always abnormal

- A systolic ejection murmur denotes no cardiac pathology in at least 50% of cases

- A thrill is always abnormal

Diastolic murmurs may be caused by:
- increased blood flow through a normal atrioventricular valve;
- narrowing (stenosis) of an atrioventricular valve;
- incompetence (leak) of the pulmonary or aortic valves.

Blood pressure

Measuring the child's blood pressure is an essential part of the physical examination, but is left to last to avoid upsetting the younger child. An appropriately sized cuff must be used. It should be wide enough to cover two-thirds of the upper arm and the bladder of the cuff should completely encircle the arm. It is important to have a range of cuff sizes available in every paediatric clinic. Systolic pressure is measured at Korotkoff phase 1 and diasystolic at Korotkoff phase 4.

In very young children where measurement of blood pressure by traditional methods is difficult a Doppler probe may be used to detect systolic pressure. Another method is the flush technique. The cuff is applied and the child's hand and lower arm wrapped in a bandage or squeezed by the examiner's hand. The cuff is then inflated to above expected systolic pressure. The bandage is removed and the child's hand looks white as the blood has been squeezed out. As the cuff is slowly deflated the colour will suddenly flush back when systolic pressure has been reached.

The upper limit of normal for blood pressure in childhood is shown in Table 2.6.

Table 2.6 Upper limit of normal (>2 standard deviations from the mean) for systolic blood pressure through childhood

Age of child	Abnormal systolic pressure (mmHg)
Neonate	90
1–12 months	100
1–5 years	110
6–9 years	120
10–12 years	130
13–14 years	140

The abdominal system

This section discusses examination of the abdomen in children with non-acute problems. The child with an acute abdominal problem requires a different approach and this is described on p. 132.

Examination of the abdomen does require the child to be relaxed, otherwise the abdominal muscles are contracted and palpation becomes difficult. The best way to ensure relaxation is to examine the child while he or she is lying on a couch. The examiner should be at eye level with the abdomen, which usually means kneeling beside the couch. Alternatively, the young child may be laid on his or her mother's lap. It may be necessary to examine some children standing up if the alternative is to have them crying when lying down.

Observation

General observation should include evidence of the following:
• *Jaundice.* If subtle it is best seen in the sclerae. The colour of the urine should also be observed (Table 4.19, p. 131).
• *Oedema.* This may be a feature of renal or liver disease. In children oedema is first noticed in the face and the mother may remark on puffy features. Unlike oedema in adults it is not usually seen early in the feet or over the sacrum.
• *Skin lesions.* Pruritus is a common feature of cholestatic jaundice and scratch marks may be very obvious. Spider naevi are seen in children with chronic liver disease. These are small surface blood vessels that radiate out from a central point and sometimes resemble a small red spider. They blanche on pressure (unlike petechial haemorrhages) and then rapidly refill once the pressure is removed.
• *Wasted buttocks.* Look for loose skin folds over the buttock, which suggest recent significant weight loss.

In toddler-age children the abdomen is normally protuberant because of an exaggerated lordosis and relaxed abdominal musculature. Umbilical herniae are common particularly in black infants. These usually require no treatment as they rarely obstruct or incarcerate.

Any distension (either generalized or localized) and visible peristalsis should be noted in particular. The groin should be observed for the bulge of an inguinal hernia or maldescended testes.

Palpation

The aim of palpation is to;
• determine whether the abdomen is tender;
• determine whether there are any masses in the abdomen;
• to evaluate whether there is enlargement of the four major organs available for palpation (liver, spleen and kidneys).

Before touching the child's abdomen, the examiner should warm his or her hands and enquire of the child whether the abdomen is tender. Initially palpate the abdomen lightly with two to four fingers depending on the size of the child. All four quadrants should be palpated for tenderness or obvious masses. If the abdomen is not tender then deeper palpation of the four quadrants should be carried out.

Liver examination
The liver enlarges downwards to the right iliac fossa. Examination should therefore start in the right lower quadrant. The patient should be examined from the right with the right hand if the examiner is right handed. The liver is palpated with the lateral aspect of the whole right index finger (Fig. 2.32) and the examining hand is gradually moved up to the right costal margin until the liver edge is felt. When a child is fretful and does not permit thorough palpation of the abdomen, he or she can often be persuaded to cooperate if the doctor places the child's hand on his or her abdomen and then, covering it with his or her own hand, palpates through it.

In children up to 2 years the liver is normally palpable 1–2 cm below the right costal margin and feels smooth and soft. The upper limit of the liver can be detected by percussion. The liver may appear to be enlarged if there is lung overinflation.

Spleen
The spleen enlarges towards the right iliac fossa and is examined with the hand initially in the right iliac fossa. It is progressively moved up towards the left costal margin (Fig. 2.33) while the child is taking deep breaths. On inspiration the enlarged spleen will be pushed down by the diaphragm towards the examiner's hand.

Usually the spleen is only modestly enlarged and palpable just under the left costal margin. There are two useful tech-

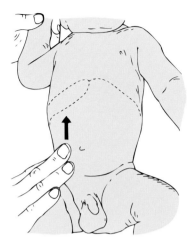

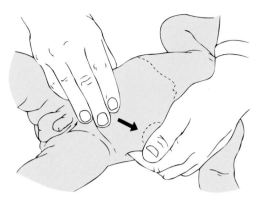

Fig. 2.34 Bimanual examination for a moderately enlarged spleen.

Fig. 2.32 Palpation for an enlarged liver.

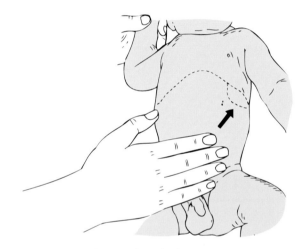

Fig. 2.33 Palpation for an enlarged spleen.

niques to increase the chance of detecting a modestly enlarged spleen.

1 Bimanual palpation with the left hand in the left loin and pushing the spleen up towards the palpating right hand (Fig. 2.34).

2 Turn the child onto his or her right side while palpating with the right hand. This causes the spleen to drop towards the examining right hand. Ask the child to take deep breaths and the spleen is palpable on inspiration.

Kidneys

These are examined by bimanual palpation. One hand is placed on the loin pushing up and the other on the anterior aspect of the flank on the same side pushing down. The lower end of the normal kidney may be felt between the two hands and an enlarged kidney should be palpable by this technique.

Percussion

The abdomen should be percussed. A distended bladder will be dull to percussion. Bowel distended with gas will be hyper-resonant.

Ascites can be diagnosed by detecting shifting dullness. Ascitic fluid can be suspected by dullness on percussion in the flanks with a resonant note over the midline. The child should then be rolled over to lie on his or her side and the same midline point percussed after a few moments. If the note has become dull then this indicates that ascitic fluid has shifted with the change in the child's position to give a dull note.

Auscultation

Auscultation of the bowel is useful in children who present with an acute abdomen (p. 132). Listen in the same spot for 1 minute to assess whether bowel sounds are absent because of an ileus. Partial or full bowel obstruction is associated with increased or tinkling bowel sounds.

Rectal examination

This is not routinely performed. If required it should be carried out last. The anus should be inspected for fissures or signs of trauma. The lubricated tip of the index finger should then be pressed flat against the edge of the anus before insertion. This method causes much less discomfort than insertion direct into the centre of the orifice. The examiner's little finger should be used in infants.

Genitalia

In girls the vulval lips should be gently parted to exclude any abnormality of the lower vagina.

In boys the scrotum should be inspected and the testes palpated. An underdeveloped scrotum suggests undescended testicles. The testes may be visible in the scrotum but may

Schema for examination of the abdominal system

Observation
Inspect for:
　jaundice
　oedema
　scratch marks
　spider naevi
　abdominal distension

Palpation
Establish whether the abdomen is tender prior to palpation
Light palpation for obvious masses
Deep palpation for other masses
Specifically palpate for:
　liver
　spleen
　kidneys
Groin for hernia or maldescended testicles

Percussion
Resonant note
Shifting dullness (ascites)

Auscultate
Note whether bowel sounds are:
　absent
　tinkling

Rectal examination
Not a routine part of the physical examination

Focal points
The abdominal system

- A protuberant abdomen is normal in toddlers

- Light palpation precedes deep palpation to assess areas that are acutely painful

- The liver edge is normally palpable in children below 2 years

- An underdeveloped scrotum suggests undescended testes

retract rapidly and disappear if the scrotum is roughly handled. First examine the testicles with the child lying down. If the testes are retracted they can often be gently milked down into the scrotum. If this is unsuccessful then the child should be examined while squatting and again gentle coaxing is necessary to encourage the testicle into the scrotum.

The groin should also be examined for swellings (p. 86) which are most likely to be caused by an enlarged lymph node, a gonad or a hernia. Undescended testicles are discussed on p. 87.

The musculoskeletal system

Examination of the musculoskeletal system is very specialized. The undergraduate is only expected to examine a major joint such as the knee and to assess clinically for the presence of scoliosis.

Scoliosis (see also p. 89)

This may be obvious by inspection of the back while the child is standing upright. The shoulders should be level and any asymmetrical prominence of a scapula should be noted. If a scoliosis (curve) is present and is significant it remains when the child is asked to bend to the side.

The most sensitive way to examine for a subtle scoliosis is to bend the child forward while observing the child's back. A fixed scoliosis causes prominence of the posterior ribs on the convex side of the bend (Fig. 2.35).

Examination of a large joint

Observation

- Observe the joint for swelling or redness. An effusion causes loss of definition of the joint. In the knee the outline of the patella is lost and if the effusion is mild then the normal concavity is lost first along its medial side.
- Observe the muscle bulk above and below the joint for wasting.

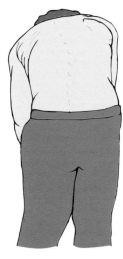

Fig. 2.35 Detection of scoliosis by asking the child to bend forward.

Palpation

• Palpate the joint for an effusion. This is most likely to be apparent in the knee. First look for the 'bulge sign' by milking fluid in the medial aspect of the knee into the lateral recess. The lateral side of the knee is then firmly stroked in a downward direction to push the fluid back into the medial compartment. The movement of the fluid causes a 'bulge' to be seen in the medial recess.

• If the effusion is large then use the 'patella tap' sign. This is done by pressing firmly on the suprapatellar pouch with one hand to empty any fluid from this compartment and with the other hand pushing firmly downward on the patella. If fluid is present in the knee then a bulge is seen in the suprapatellar pouch when the kneecap is pushed down.

Range of movements

Move the joint through its normal range of movements to assess any limitation or contractures.

Developmental assessment

Developmental assessment is an integral part of the paediatric examination and it is important for the undergraduate to know a number of age specific milestones so that he or she can clinically assess the developmental age of a child of 2 years or below.

Developmental assessment should be carried out after a careful neurological examination as a child with cerebral palsy may not be able to perform a variety of motor tasks such as reaching or walking. The child's developmental assessment will clearly be impaired by any motor disability, yet his or her intellectual capacity may be normal.

Development is a continuous process from conception to maturity, but its rate varies greatly in different, though still normal, children. There are also racial differences; the Afro-Caribbean baby at birth is developmentally more mature than the Caucasian in motor items, and remains ahead for the first year.

Development is not a smooth continuous process but made up of lulls and spurts. Moreover, having achieved a skill, this may go into abeyance while another is being learned. Some skills develop separately, becoming coordinated later. The achievement of a new stage is dependent on the growing maturity of the nervous system so that development cannot be accelerated from outside sources, but external factors, particularly environment and to a lesser extent illness, can retard it.

It is convenient to divide development into four major areas:

1 gross motor;
2 fine motor;
3 speech and language;
4 social.

Major milestones of development for the first 2 years in each of the four assessment areas are summarized in Figs 2.36–2.39.

Major delay in all four areas of development usually denotes intellectual retardation (p. 269), unless it is caused by severe emotional deprivation, but an isolated delay in any one area is often not abnormal. Delay in walking alone (p. 267) is common and may have been present in siblings or parents. Acquisition of speech is another common isolated delay, and in all children with speech delay, deafness must be excluded.

Gross motor development (Fig. 2.36)

At birth the infant assumes a naturally flexed posture and when prone the baby flexes the hips and tucks up the bottom. By 6 weeks the pelvis is flatter on the table, but by 4 months he or she can lift the head and shoulders off the couch. By 6 months the arms are held extended supporting the chest off the couch (Fig. 2.36a).

Sitting is achieved gradually with progressive improvement in neck and trunk tone. On pulling the child to a sitting position the degree of head lag is less with advancing age (Fig. 2.36b). The average age for sitting unsupported is 6–7 months and at this age the child needs the hands for support. By 9 months the baby can get into the sitting position alone. By 11 months the child can pivot while sitting to reach toys (Fig. 2.36c). The child moves from a sitting to crawling position at 7–9 months, but some babies never pass through the crawling phase. Pulling to standing occurs at 10 months and walking around while holding onto the furniture by 11 months.

Some children (especially boys) become adept at getting about by bottom shuffling and a history of bottom shuffling can usually be obtained from at least one family member.

Around 12 months the baby can walk with one hand held and can stand unsupported. Independent walking is achieved on average at 12–13 months but this is very variable.

At 15 months the baby can reach a standing position without support and can clamber up stairs.

By 18 months the child can walk upstairs holding the banister and is very steady on the feet. He or she should be able to throw a ball without falling over. Failure to walk independently at 18 months requires investigation (p. 267).

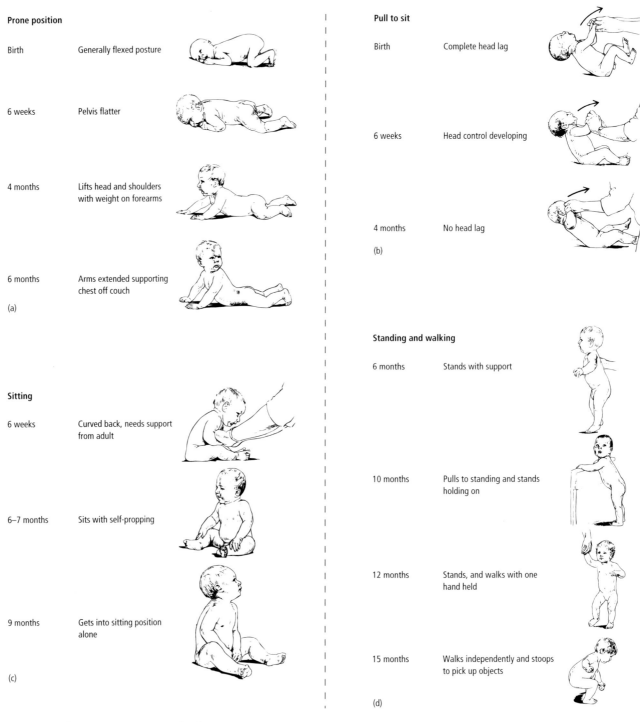

Prone position

Birth — Generally flexed posture

6 weeks — Pelvis flatter

4 months — Lifts head and shoulders with weight on forearms

6 months — Arms extended supporting chest off couch

(a)

Sitting

6 weeks — Curved back, needs support from adult

6–7 months — Sits with self-propping

9 months — Gets into sitting position alone

(c)

Pull to sit

Birth — Complete head lag

6 weeks — Head control developing

4 months — No head lag

(b)

Standing and walking

6 months — Stands with support

10 months — Pulls to standing and stands holding on

12 months — Stands, and walks with one hand held

15 months — Walks independently and stoops to pick up objects

(d)

Fig. 2.36 (a–d) Stages in gross motor development.

Fine motor development (Fig. 2.37)

At 1 month the infant's hands are closed most of the time but by 2 months the hands are largely open. By 3 months the grasp reflex has disappeared and the baby holds objects in the midline and will rattle a toy purposefully. At 5 months the child starts to reach for objects, initially with both hands embracing them towards the body and by 6 months starts to be able to use the hands independently and transfers from one hand to the other.

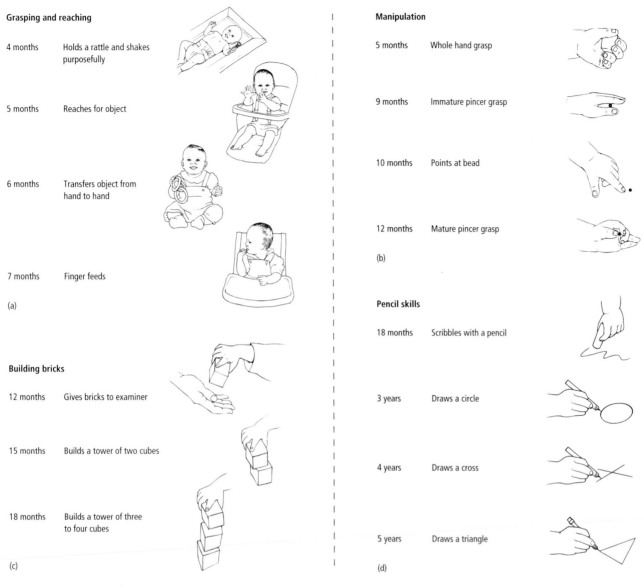

Grasping and reaching

4 months	Holds a rattle and shakes purposefully
5 months	Reaches for object
6 months	Transfers object from hand to hand
7 months	Finger feeds

(a)

Building bricks

12 months	Gives bricks to examiner
15 months	Builds a tower of two cubes
18 months	Builds a tower of three to four cubes

(c)

Manipulation

5 months	Whole hand grasp
9 months	Immature pincer grasp
10 months	Points at bead
12 months	Mature pincer grasp

(b)

Pencil skills

18 months	Scribbles with a pencil
3 years	Draws a circle
4 years	Draws a cross
5 years	Draws a triangle

(d)

Fig. 2.37 (a–d) Stages in fine motor development.

By 7 months the hands are able to undertake useful tasks and are used in play and exploration. The baby should be able to grasp an object and bring it to the mouth, e.g. feeding him- or herself with a biscuit. Passing an object from one hand to another also develops at this time (Fig. 2.37a).

By 9 months the finger movements become refined. At 8–9 months there is a raking grasp, which by 10 months has developed into a scissor grasp using thumb and first finger and by 12 months finger–thumb apposition, also known as a pincer grasp, has been fully achieved (Fig. 2.37b).

By 1 year, the baby will give a 2 cm square wooden block to the examiner and release it. He or she can build a tower of two wooden cubes at 15 months and three to four cubes at 18 months (Fig. 2.37c). At this age the child scribbles with a pencil and turns the pages of a book. Fine motor development advances rapidly after this time and by the age of 3 years the child can draw a circle, a cross at 4 years and a triangle at 5 years (Fig. 2.37d).

In the fourth year the child draws a circle for a face and then progressively add limbs directly from the face with one or two facial features such as eyes and mouth. It is not until 5 years that the child draws a body to which arms and hands are attached.

Speech and language development
(summarized in Fig. 2.38)

Vocalization starts at about 3 months and at this age a baby enjoys playing with his or her voice. By 7 months the baby should be making four different consonant sounds such as 'da', 'ba', 'ma' and 'ka' and by 8 months he or she should be combining these sounds together in repetitive sequences ('double babble').

The first recognizable word is spoken on average at 11 months and by 12 months the baby has two or three words which he or she uses with meaning. These words may be indistinct to any one other than the mother. Jargon (unintelligible but highly expressive 'language') develops at about 15 months of age. By 18 months the average child has 10 recognizable words and by 24 months they are linked into two-word sentences. From then speech develops rapidly so that by the age of 3 years the child can form full sentences and talks incessantly.

An isolated speech delay is relatively common but before assuming it is benign, two factors must be determined. First, does the child hear normally (p. 48)? Secondly, does the child understand commands. This should be testable from 1 year of age.

Social development (summarized in Fig. 2.39)

This is an assessment of how the child interacts with the people around him- or herself. Sights and sounds are the most important stimuli that elicit reactions in the child. By 4 weeks the baby quietens to speech, or eyes open widely in

Table 2.7 Milestones that it is essential to memorize

Age	Milestone
4–6 weeks	Smiles responsively
6–7 months	Sits unsupported
9 months	Gets to a sitting position
10 months	Pincer grasp
12 months	Walks unsupported
	Two or three words
	Tower of two cubes
18 months	Tower of three of four cubes
24 months	Two to three word sentences

Table 2.8 Developmental warning signs

At any age
Maternal concern
Discordance in different developmental areas
Regression in previously acquired skills

At 10 weeks
No smile

At 6 months
Persistent primitive reflexes
Persistent squint
Hand preference
Little interest in people, toys, noises

At 10–12 months
No sitting
No double syllable babble
No pincer grip

At 18 months
Not walking independently
Fewer than six words
Persistent mouthing and drooling

At 2½ years
No two to three word sentences

At 4 years
Unintelligible speech

Speech

3 months	Vocalizes	ooh, aah
8 months	Double babble	dada baba mama
12 months	Two or three words with meaning	Mummy
18 months	10 words	Teddy Ta Bottle Bed Dog No Daddy Bikky
24 months	Linking two words	Daddy gone
3 years	Full sentences, talks incessantly	Teddy goes to sleep Teddy's tired Good night Teddy

Fig. 2.38 Stages in speech and language development.

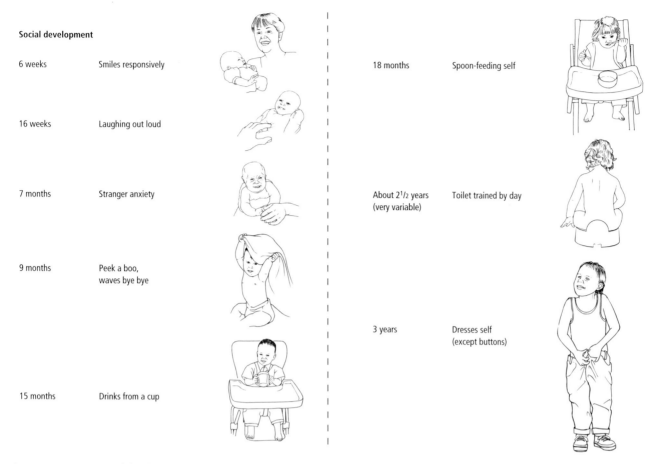

Social development

6 weeks	Smiles responsively	
16 weeks	Laughing out loud	
7 months	Stranger anxiety	
9 months	Peek a boo, waves bye bye	
15 months	Drinks from a cup	
18 months	Spoon-feeding self	
About 2½ years (very variable)	Toilet trained by day	
3 years	Dresses self (except buttons)	

Fig. 2.39 Stages in social development.

response to the spoken word. At 6 weeks the baby smiles responsively. For this to be considered a social reaction the child must smile in response to the examiner's (or parent's) smile. Failure to smile by 8 weeks is definitely abnormal. By 12 weeks the baby squeals with pleasure, and by 16 weeks laughs out loud. By 20 weeks the child will smile at him- or herself in a mirror.

At 7 months the infant begins to show 'stranger anxiety' and may be upset when picked up by the examiner. 'Permanence of objects' develops on average by 9 months. At this stage an infant will search for an object that drops from view. By 9 months the baby should play 'peek-a-boo' and by 10 months the baby should understand the meaning of the word 'no'. Other important social items include waving bye-bye (9 months), playing pat-a-cake (12 months) and drinking from a cup (15 months). At 18 months the child will attempt to bring a spoon to his or her mouth, but drops

much of what is on it and at 24 months will start to indicate toilet needs. Toilet training by day is usually achieved by 2½ years, although nocturnal enuresis is usual for some time beyond this. A baby starts to help with dressing by 1 year of age and by 3 years should be able to dress and undress fully.

Essential milestones

It is impossible to remember all the milestones that children acquire in the course of development, but the medical student should appreciate the sequence of developmental stages in each of the developmental areas. The milestones that are essential to know are shown in Table 2.7.

In addition, it is also important to know at what stage the lack of certain skills becomes abnormal and requires further investigation. These are summarized in Table 2.8.

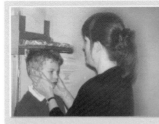

3 Health Promotion and Child Health Surveillance

Introduction, 44
Child health surveillance procedures, 45
Health education and promotion, 50
Immunization, 51
Diseases routinely immunized against, 51
Growth, 54
Child protection, 56

PROBLEMS COMMONLY DETECTED OR PRESENTING IN THE COURSE OF CHILD HEALTH SURVEILLANCE, 56
Growth problems: short stature, 56
Physiological causes of short stature, 58
Endocrine causes of short stature, 58
Chronic illness as a cause of short stature, 59
Genetic causes of short stature, 59
Intrauterine growth retardation as a cause of short stature, 60
Psychosocial causes of short stature, 61

Growth problems: plateauing in growth, 61
Growth problems: tall stature, 61
Growth problems: failure to thrive, 61
Organic causes of failure to thrive, 62
Genetic causes of failure to thrive, 67
Environmental/psychosocial causes (non-organic failure to thrive), 67
Obesity, 68
Causes of obesity, 69
The large head, 71
Pathological causes of a large head, 72
The small head (microcephaly), 75
Pathological causes of microcephaly, 76
Visual problems, 77
Refractive errors, 77
Squint (strabismus), 77
Disorders of vision, 78
The teeth, 78
Heart murmurs, 80
Innocent (functional) murmurs, 81

Pathological murmurs: defects causing a left to right shunt, 81
Pathological murmurs: obstructive lesions, 83
Genitalia: scrotal swellings, 85
Causes of scrotal swellings, 85
Genitalia: swellings in the groin, 86
Genitalia: absent testes, 87
Causes of impalpable testes, 87
Other genital findings, 88
Musculoskeletal problems: concerns about gait, 88
Causes of odd gaits, 89
Musculoskeletal problems: scoliosis (curvature of the spine), 89
Pallor and anaemia, 89
Causes of anaemia in childhood, 90
Abuse and neglect, 95
Types of abuse and neglect, 97

The fundamental objective of pediatrics is to guide children safely and happily through childhood so that they will become healthy, well adjusted, normal young adults — to enable them to achieve their maximum potential physically, intellectually, psychologically and socially.

James G. Hughes, MD

Introduction

Child health surveillance is a programme that overviews the physical, social and emotional well-being of all children, with the aim of promoting their optimum health and development and preventing illness.

The programme has many facets which include:
• guidance on important child health topics such as development, behavioural problems, nutrition and the use of services for children;
• measurement and recording of physical growth;
• monitoring of developmental progress;
• prevention of disease by immunization;
• detection of abnormalities through physical examination and screening tests, and by facilitating early recognition by parents;
• health promotion and education;

• identification of children in need, whether socially disadvantaged or with disabilities.

Professionals involved in child health surveillance

Health visitors
Health visitors are nurses who are specially trained in child care and development. They work either in the framework of a baby clinic or with GPs, and carry out the bulk of the child health surveillance and health promotion programme for preschool children. This includes running child health clinics, visiting at home and providing support, particularly for those children and families identified as being in need or at risk.

School nurses
School nurses are specially trained nurses who work in the framework of schools. They are responsible for identifying children with medical needs, facilitating their care at school, providing liaison between professionals and supplying medical information to school staff. As school doctors are no longer required to see every child at school entry, the school nurse is now responsible for reviewing all children and selecting those who need to be seen by the community paediatrician.

Community paediatricians

Community paediatricians are doctors who specialize in working in the community. Part of their work involves routine surveillance, although this side of the work is now increasingly being carried out by GPs, health visitors and school nurses. They are responsible for evaluating children identified as having problems through the child health surveillance programme or school. Some have specialized roles such as audiology, child protection or developmental paediatrics.

General practitioners

In recent years GPs have taken over responsibility for the routine aspects of most of the preschool child health surveillance programme, i.e. routine examinations and immunizations, although community paediatricians may still run baby clinics in disadvantaged areas.

Parents

Parents have a central role in enhancing the health of their children and they should be seen as partners in child health promotion.

Child health records

Parent-held child health records

A recent development has been the issuing of child health records to parents. The advantages of this are that the child's record is available wherever and whenever the child is seen, confidentiality rests with the parents and, most importantly, it involves the parents centrally in the surveillance programme. The parent-held record consists of a record of child health surveillance checks, the child's growth chart, parental observations, a record of primary care and dental and hospital visits, and health education and advice. Parents have welcomed this development and have been shown to be responsible in ensuring that it is kept up to date.

Other records

In addition to the parent-held record, each professional keeps their own record of contact with the child. Computer-based systems are increasingly being used and are particularly effective in child health surveillance.

Special registers

Many districts keep registers of children with special needs or chronic illness. They are useful in providing parents with information about services, keeping track of referral and review, anticipating needs and auditing the service. The parents' permission is required before placing a child on a register.

Detection of medical and developmental problems

An important part of the child health surveillance programme involves identification of subtle or latent defects and disorders that may seriously affect the child later in life. These defects and disorders are usually identified in one of the following ways:
- Child health surveillance procedures.
- Follow-up of infants and children who have suffered various forms of trauma or illness.
- Detection by parents or relatives, who are often the first to recognize that their child has a problem. When such suspicions are reported to a health professional, they should be taken seriously as the parents are often correct.
- Detection by other professionals such as nursery nurses, playgroup leaders and teachers. Playgroup leaders and nursery nurses play an important part in child care, particularly in deprived areas, and become expert at recognizing the child whose health or development requires further evaluation.

CHILD HEALTH SURVEILLANCE PROCEDURES

Child health surveillance procedures involve the following methods:
- Formal screening tests.
- Routine physical examination.
- Developmental evaluations.
  These are summarized in Table 3.1.

Screening

Screening is the identification of unrecognized disease or defects by the application of tests, examinations and other procedures which can be applied rapidly. Screening tests sort out apparently well children who may have a problem from those who do not. A screening test is not intended to be diagnostic.

Various criteria have been established to determine whether there is a value for screening for a particular condition. These criteria include a recognizable latent or early symptomatic stage of the condition, and the availability of some form of treatment or intervention that can influence the course and prognosis. Cost inevitably must be considered and needs to be balanced against the cost of medical care as a whole and the cost of treatment if the patient does not present until later.

The following screening tests have been incorporated into the child health surveillance programme.

Age	Screening procedure	General examination	Health education
Newborn	Hip examination Testicular descent Red reflex Phenylketonuria (after 72 hours) Thyroid Hearing test if high risk	Weight, length Head circumference Full physical examination (see p. 234)	Feeding and nutrition Baby care Crying and sleep problems Car seats
10 days	Hip examination	Weight Prolonged jaundice	Nutrition Immunization Accidents—bathing, fires Passive smoking
6–8 weeks	Hip examination	Weight Head circumference Eyes Development	Nutrition Immunization Recognition of illness in babies Accidents—fires, falls and scalds

6–9 months	Hip examination
	Testicular descent
	Distraction test for hearing
		Eyes for squint	Accident prevention—choking,
			  burns, falls, safety gates, car
			  seats
			Nutrition
			Teeth
			Passive smoking
			Developmental needs

18–24 months	Hip examination	Gait
		Language
		Consider testing
		  haemoglobin level
			Accident prevention—falls from
			  heights, drowning, poisoning,
			  road safety
			Nutrition
			Developmental needs, language
			  and play
			Behaviour problems

36–48 months	Cardiac examination	Height, weight	Check on medical or development
			  problems that may interfere
			  with education

School entry	Vision (Snellen chart)
	Hearing (Sweep test)
		Nurse selects children
		  who require a medical
		  evaluation
			Parental and teacher concerns

8 years	Visual acuity	School nurse appraisal	Diet Dental care
11 years	Visual acuity Colour vision	School nurse appraisal	Health education in school Teenage counselling
14 years	Visual acuity	School nurse appraisal	Careers advice Self-referrals to school doctor or nurse

Table 3.1 The child health surveillance programme

Congenital hypothyroidism

- *Age at which the test is performed*. Neonates.
- *The test*. A few drops of blood are obtained by heel prick, dripped onto a filter paper and sent to a central laboratory for analysis of thyroid hormone (T_4) or thyroid-stimulating hormone (TSH) (Fig. 3.1).

- *Significance of the test*. Approximately one in 4000 infants is born with congenital hypothyroidism. If untreated, cretinism with severe learning disability (mental retardation) results (see p. 271). If treated early with thyroid hormone, the child grows and develops normally.

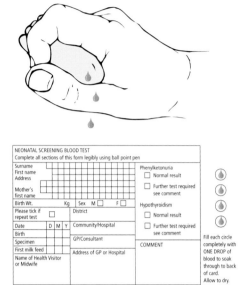

Fig. 3.1 Neonatal screening blood test for phenylketonuria (Guthrie test) and hypothyroidism.

- *Action if the test is abnormal.* The baby must be referred urgently to a paediatric endocrinologist.

Guthrie test for phenylketonuria

- *Age at which the test is performed.* Neonates (after 72 hours of age).
- *The test.* The test is carried out on the same sample as that taken for thyroid testing. The baby must be on full milk feeds for 3 days prior to testing.
- *Significance of the test.* One in 10 000 babies is born with phenylketonuria (PKU). This causes severe learning disability (mental retardation). Institution of a low phenylalanine diet prevents the build up of phenylalanine metabolites which cause brain damage.
- *Action if the test is abnormal.* Referral to a metabolic clinic for dietary advice and long-term follow-up.

Eliciting the red reflex using an ophthalmoscope
(see also p. 235)

- *Age at which the test is performed.* Neonates, 6 weeks.
- *The test.* The examiner looks through an ophthalmoscope, held approximately 50 cm from the baby, and directs the light into the baby's eyes. A red reflection is normally seen as the light is reflected back from the vascular retina (Fig. 3.2).
- *Significance of the test.* If white light is reflected instead of red, it is a serious sign and suggests the presence of a cataract or other intraocular pathology, preventing the reflex from being elicited.

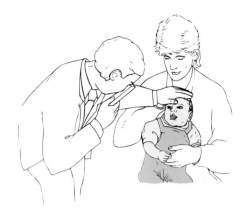

Fig. 3.2 Eliciting the red reflex using an ophthalmoscope.

- *Action if the test is abnormal.* Immediate referral to an ophthalmologist is required, as in those conditions that are treatable, amblyopia (p. 78) can only be avoided if treatment is given early.

Examination for congenital dislocation of the hips
(see also p. 239)

- *Age at which the test is performed.* Neonates, 10 days, 6 weeks, 6–9 months.
- *The test.* The Ortolani and Barlow procedures for babies up to the age of 3 months are described on p. 239. Limited hip abduction, shortening of the leg and limp (once walking) are sought beyond 3 months.
- *Significance of the test.* Approximately three per 1000 babies are born with dislocated, subluxed or dysplastic hips. Orthopaedic treatment given early is likely to be more effective in preventing limp in childhood and painful disability later in life.
- *Action if the test is abnormal.* Orthopaedic referral is required. Ultrasound is useful to confirm the diagnosis. Treatment involves the use of a harness or splint to maintain the hip in flexion and abduction. If this conservative treatment fails surgery is required.

Palpation for testicular descent

- *Age at which the test is performed.* Neonates, 6 weeks.
- *The test.* The testes are palpated when the baby is relaxed (Fig. 3.3).
- *Significance of the test.* Non-palpable testes suggest maldescent (see p. 87). If corrected early, the sequelae of infertility and malignancy are minimized.
- *Action if the test is abnormal.* If on repeat examination the testes are impalpable, referral to a paediatric surgeon is required. Surgery should be performed before the age of 2 years.

Distraction test for hearing

• *Age at which the test is performed.* Seven to nine months (valid to the age of 18 months).
• *The test.* The test requires two people working in collaboration, one to sit in front of the baby and hold the baby's attention and one behind the baby to present the sounds. The baby must be in a cooperative mood, and developmentally able to sit steadily on the mother's lap and turn the head from side to side. The test sounds used are usually minimal voice ('ooh, ooh') for low tones and a high-pitched rattle for high tones. The baby should identify the sounds by turning promptly to the source (Fig. 3.4).
• *Significance of the test.* Significant sensorineural hearing loss occurs in one to two births per 1000, and conductive hearing loss is more common (see p. 284). If hearing deficits are not identified early before language is acquired, permanent impairment of language development can result.
• *Action if the test is abnormal.* Referral to the audiology service is required so that more sophisticated testing can

be performed, and appropriate intervention provided (hearing aids, speech and language therapy for the sensorineurally deaf and grommets for conductive hearing loss) (see p. 285).

Sweep test for hearing

• *Age at which test is performed.* School entry.
• *The test.* Sweep audiometry tests the child's ability to hear sounds at a set level across the main speech frequencies.
• *Significance of the test.* As most cases of sensorineural deafness are detected earlier by distraction testing, this test principally identifies children with hearing impairment caused by secretory otitis media (see p. 105), which may have educational implications.
• *Action if the test is abnormal.* The ears should be examined for otitis media. Referral to an ENT surgeon and more sophisticated audiological evaluation is required.

Visual acuity using a Snellen chart

• *Age at which the test is performed.* School entry, 8, 11 and 14 years.
• *The test.* The child's visual acuity is tested 6 m from the Snellen chart, occluding each eye in turn (Fig. 3.5). In young children a letter matching card can be used instead of asking them to name the letters.
• *Significance of the test.* Myopia is very common in childhood. If the child can only read letter size 6/12 or less, he or she is likely to be myopic.
• *Action if the test is abnormal.* Referral to an optician for prescription of spectacles is required.

Ishihara colour vision test

• *Age at which the test is performed.* 11 years.

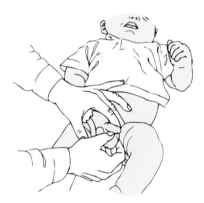

Fig. 3.3 Palpation for testicular descent.

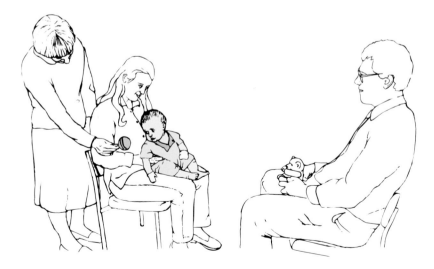

Fig. 3.4 The distraction test for hearing.

• *The test.* Screening cards with symbols which cannot be identified by the colour blind are presented to the child.
• *Significance of the test.* Colour vision defects can preclude people from entering certain careers and it is helpful to know of this defect early.

Other screening tests

Cystic fibrosis In some areas immunoreactive trypsin levels in blood, or protein testing of meconium at birth, are used as screening tests for cystic fibrosis.

Haemoglobinopathies (Sickle cell disease and thalassaemia). These are common among some ethnic communities. Screening is carried out in some parts of the country.

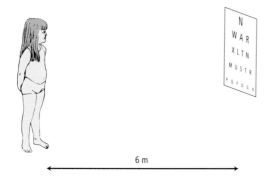

Fig. 3.5 Testing visual acuity using a Snellen chart.

Iron deficiency anaemia (see p. 90). Occurs in 5–10% of young children but in up to 50% in disadvantaged areas. Screening is not routinely performed at present, but health professionals need to be aware that it is common and should not hesitate to measure haemoglobin levels if anaemia is suspected.

Routine physical examination

In addition to formal screening tests, children undergo routine physical examinations. This allows identification of some important conditions as well as addressing parental concerns regarding their child's health and physical development. The key features to be examined in a routine examination are shown in Fig. 3.6.

Developmental examination

The developmental examination involves a developmental history, observation of the child's behaviour and the administration of tests (p. 39). The purpose is to ensure that the child's development is progressing at a normal rate and to recognize deviations from the normal pattern. It is usually performed by the health visitor, at the ages indicated in Table 3.1 (see column on General examination). If the child is delayed or is demonstrating abnormal development, referral to the appropriate therapist or, if difficulties seem to be complex, to a child development team is made (see p. 274).

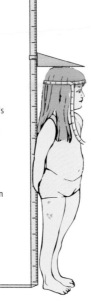

Height and weight
A child's growth reflects his or her general well-being. Deviations in the growth pattern can be an important indicator of a problem (see p. 17 for measurement, pp. 56–68 for interpretation)

Eyes
Visual defects must be identified early before permanent suppression of vision in the affected eye develops. The young baby's ability to fix and follow is tested and the cover test is performed if there is suspicion of a squint (see p. 28)

Heart examination
Identification of heart murmurs on routine examination is the commonest presentation of congenital heart disease (see p. 80)

Genitalia
Screening for undescended testicles is routinely performed. Other abnormalities may also be identified (see p. 85)

Head size
Measurement of the occipitofrontal circumference is of value in identifying macro- and microencephaly (see p. 17 for measurement, p. 71,75 for interpretation)

Teeth
Caries remains an important problem in childhood and its identification is important in terms of recommending dental treatment (see p.78)

Scoliosis
Scoliosis appears in the teenage years and may progress to serious deformity (see p. 38,89)

Signs of neglect and abuse
Routine physical examinations provide a good opportunity to identify children who are at risk (see p. 95)

Gait
A child's gait often arouses parental concern and usually has little significance. However, abnormal gait may indicate conditions such as congenital dislocation of the hip (see p. 239) or cerebral palsy that require attention (see p. 277)

Fig. 3.6 Key features to be examined on routine examination.

HEALTH EDUCATION AND PROMOTION

Increasingly, young families are growing up isolated and without the support of an extended family. Parenting skills and confidence are often lacking, and the child health programme is therefore particularly valuable in providing information and advice to inexperienced parents. The following issues are addressed by the programme.

Baby care

The young parent is likely to need advice about simple issues such as clothing, bathing, handling and positioning the baby. They need to know about common medical problems, and to learn the appropriate responses when the baby is unwell. As time goes by, they need to know about normal development, what to expect from their child, how to promote learning and how to recognize developmental difficulties.

Nutrition (see Chapter 1)

If a good nutritional environment is provided in the early years, the ground is laid for healthy eating later in childhood and beyond. Addressing nutritional issues forms a major part of a health visitor's work. It includes promotion of breast-feeding, advising about weaning, dealing with eating difficulties commonly encountered in toddlers and education about healthy diets for the entire family.

Behavioural problems

Behavioural concerns are universal. Advice and support in the early stages can avoid their developing into major problems. Crying, sleep problems and temper tantrums are particularly common issues of concern.

Dental care

Information should be provided about dental hygiene, the use of fluoride, and regular dental check-ups.

Passive smoking

Children exposed to passive smoking are at greatly increased risk of respiratory disorders. Avoidance of passive smoking is an important health promotion issue.

Accidents

Accidents are the commonest cause of mortality in the childhood years and an important cause of morbidity. The term accident is actually inappropriate as it implies the injury occurred by chance. In fact most accidents are predictable and could be avoided with appropriate strategies. As most accidents occur in the home, education of parents has an important impact on the prevention of accidents. Areas which should be addressed in the course of health education are shown in Tables 3.1 and 3.2.

Health promotion in school

School provides an invaluable opportunity to educate the young about healthy living. The school years are a time when adjustments in lifestyle can be made more easily than later on in life. Issues of particular importance which are addressed are:
- nutrition;
- physical activity;
- drugs and alcohol abuse;
- contraception and safe sex;
- sexually transmitted diseases;
- smoking;
- healthy relationships;
- parenting skills.

Table 3.2 Strategies for the reduction of injuries in childhood

Injury	Prevention strategy
Road traffic injuries	Use of car seats and belts
	Road safety instruction from age 2 years
	Cycle helmets
Falls	Gate on stairs
	Guards on windows
	Safe playground surfaces
Burns	Caution in the kitchen
	Reduce home hot water temperature
	Installation of smoke detectors
	Fire guards
	Flame-proof clothing
	Cover electric sockets
	Avoid trailing flexes on kettles and irons
Drowning	Never leave young children alone in bath
	Fence pools
	Swim only with lifeguard present
Poisoning	Keep medicines/poisons out of reach
	Locks on cupboards
	Safety caps on bottles
Choking	Keep small toys away from toddlers
	No nuts before age 5 years
	Teach Heimlich manoeuvre (p. 302)

IMMUNIZATION

Protection against some infectious diseases is provided by immunizations given at various stages during childhood. A high level of uptake of immunizations is important to ensure both protection for the individual but also, in some diseases, herd immunity. Table 3.3 shows the recommended schedule for immunizations at each age.

General immunization guidelines

- Immunizations should not be given at a younger age than that indicated in the schedule.
- Those vaccines which require repeat immunization should not be given at shorter intervals than indicated in the schedule.
- If for any reason a child misses an immunization or immunizations, it should be given at a later stage. There is no need to restart the course.
- Immunizations should not be given if a child is acutely unwell with fever.
- Immunizations should not be given if there has been a serious reaction following a previous dose of the same vaccine.
- Live attenuated vaccines (e.g. polio, measles, mumps, rubella, BCG) should not be given to immunodeficient children such as those on cytotoxic therapy or high-dose steroids because of the risk of severe generalized infection.

Table 3.3 National immunization schedule

Infant	
Birth	BCG for high-risk babies
2 months	DTP (diphtheria, tetanus, pertussis)
	Polio
	HIB (*Haemophilus influenzae* B)
3 months	DTP, polio, HIB
4 months	DTP, polio, HIB
12–15 months	MMR (measles, mumps, rubella)
Preschool	
3–5 years	DT, polio booster
	MMR
Secondary school	
11–14 years	BCG if Heaf test negative
13–18 years	Diphtheria, tetanus booster
	Polio booster

Diseases routinely immunized against

Diphtheria

The disease

Diphtheria is now very rare in developed countries. It is caused by the organism *Corynebacterium diphtheriae*. Infection occurs in the throat, forming a pharyngeal exudate, which leads to membrane formation and obstruction of the upper airways. An exotoxin released by the bacterium may cause myocarditis and neuritis with paralysis.

The vaccine

The vaccine is an inactivated toxin (toxoid), given as an intramuscular injection combined with tetanus and pertussis vaccines at 2, 3 and 4 months. A more dilute form is given to individuals over the age of 10 years.

Tetanus

The disease

Tetanus is caused by an anaerobic organism, *Clostridium tetani*, found universally in the soil, which enters the body through open wounds. Progressive painful muscle spasms are caused by a neurotoxin produced by the organism. Involvement of the respiratory muscles results in asphyxia and death.

The vaccine

The vaccine is an inactivated toxin (toxoid) given combined with diphtheria and pertussis, by intramuscular injection. After a primary course of three injections in infancy and a booster at school entry, a further two boosters 10 years apart are required. If a dirty wound is incurred more than 10 years after the last injection, a further booster is required. If a non-immunized individual sustains a dirty wound, tetanus immunoglobulin is given and a full course of the inactivated toxoid initiated.

Pertussis (whooping cough)

The disease

Whooping cough is caused by the bacterium *Bordetella pertussis*. It is an upper respiratory illness which lasts for 6–8 weeks, consisting of three stages: catarrhal, paroxysmal and convalescent. The child experiences paroxysms of coughing, followed by a whoop (a sudden massive inspiratory effort against a narrowed glottis), with vomiting, dyspnoea and sometimes seizures. Manifestations are most severe in the child under the age of 2 years, where there is a high morbidity and mortality. Complications include bronchopneumonia, convulsions, apnoea and bronchiectasis. The diagnosis must be suspected clinically, and confirmed by special culture of nasopharyngeal swabs. Erythromycin given early in the catarrhal stage shortens the illness, but is ineffective if given when the whoop is heard.

The vaccine
The vaccine is made from the killed organism, given in three doses with diphtheria and tetanus. Mild reactions consisting of local pain and swelling, irritability and pyrexia are common. The risks of naturally acquired pertussis far exceed any risks of the vaccination and it is recommended for all babies, other than when a severe reaction has followed a previous immunization or if a progressive neurological disease is present.

Polio

The disease
Polio is caused by the poliomyelitis virus, which produces a mild febrile illness, progressing to meningitis in some children. Paralysis in association with pain and tenderness develops as a result of anterior horn cell damage, and may lead to respiratory failure and bulbar paralysis. Residual paralysis is common in those who survive.

The vaccine
The vaccine used in Britain (Sabin) is a mixture of three live attenuated strains of poliovirus and is given orally. The vaccine establishes both gut and systemic immunity, and is excreted in the faeces, so contacts must be immunized

---

WHOOPING COUGH (PERTUSSIS) AT A GLANCE

Epidemiology
Endemic, with epidemics every 3–5 years

Aetiology/pathophysiology
Bordetella pertussis infection
Droplet spread

Prevention
Immunization with killed organism given at 2, 3 and 4 months and at school entry

History
Paroxysms of coughing
Characteristic inspiratory whoop at end of paroxysm (absent in infants)
Fever*
Vomiting at end of paroxysm*
Seizures*

NB *Signs and symptoms are variable

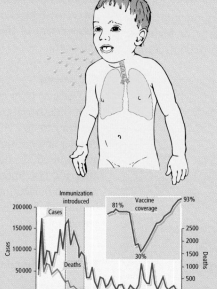

Physical examination
Very distressed during a paroxysm
Infant is very sick
Dyspnoea
Nasal discharge
Apathetic
Weight loss

Confirmatory investigations
Diagnosis is clinical
Confirmed by pernasal swab culture early in disease

Differential diagnosis
Pertussis is readily clinically recognized during the paroxysmal stage
Other causes of cough (see Table 5.21)

Management
Erythromycin given early shortens the illness, but is ineffective later

Complications
Bronchopneumonia
Convulsions
Apnoea
Bronchiectasis

Course/prognosis
Lasts 6–8 weeks
High morbidity and mortality for child <2 years

too. The vaccine is contraindicated in the immunodeficient child.

Haemophilus influenzae B

The disease
Haemophilus influenzae B is the main cause of meningitis (p. 107) in young children, leading to severe neurological sequelae such as profound deafness, cerebral palsy and epilepsy in 10–15% of cases and death in 3%.

The vaccine
The vaccine consists of the polysaccharide capsule of the killed organism conjugated with a protein, and is given three times in infancy. It is only effective against type B infection. The vaccine is highly effective with a low incidence of side-effects.

Measles

The disease
Measles is characterized by a maculopapular rash, fever, coryza, cough and conjunctivitis (see p. 193). Complications include encephalitis leading to neurological damage and a high mortality rate.

The vaccine
The vaccine is a live attenuated virus given at 12–15 months of age with mumps and rubella and again before school entry. It is common for children to develop a rash and fever 5–10 days after the immunization. Children who are immunodeficient and those severely allergic to eggs (the vaccine is grown on chick embryo tissue) should not receive the vaccine.

Mumps

The disease
Mumps causes a febrile illness with enlargement of the parotid glands (see p. 227). Complications include aseptic meningitis, sensorineural deafness and orchitis in adults.

The vaccine
The vaccine is a live attenuated virus grown on chick embryo tissue and is given with measles and rubella at 12–15 months of age. It should not be given to immunodeficient children or those severely allergic to eggs.

Rubella (German measles)

The disease
Rubella is a mild illness causing rash and fever (see p. 194). Its importance lies in the devastating effects it has on the fetus if infection occurs in the early stages of pregnancy. These include multiple congenital defects such as cataracts, deafness and congenital heart disease.

The vaccine
The vaccine is a live attenuated virus given with measles and mumps vaccines at 12–15 months of age. A mild form of rubella sometimes occurs following vaccination. In the past it was given to girls only at the age of 11 years, but this policy has changed in order to try to achieve herd immunity and stop epidemics. The vaccine, as for all live virus vaccines, is contraindicated in pregnancy.

Tuberculosis

The disease
Tuberculosis (TB) remains a major problem in many developing countries and still occurs in developed countries, particularly in immigrant communities from endemic areas such as Asia and Africa. Most children with TB are identified because they are contacts of infected adults. Tuberculosis affects many organs including the lungs, meninges, bones and joints. The diagnosis is not always easy, and often relies on demonstration of tuberculin sensitivity, which develops within 4–8 weeks after infection. This is demonstrated by Heaf or Mantoux testing. Active TB requires treatment which must be continued over many months.

The Heaf test
Purified protein derivative (PPD) is 'shot' into the skin using a Heaf gun with a disposable head. The result is read 3–10 days later. Tuberculin sensitivity causes severe induration at the site (Fig. 3.7) and if found the child requires a chest X-ray and follow-up. In most parts of the country Heaf testing is performed at 10–14 years and vaccination is offered to those who are tuberculin negative.

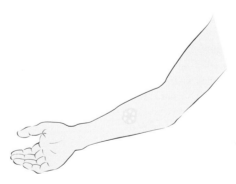

Fig. 3.7 The Heaf test. In tuberculin-positive individuals six raised papules surrounded by a wheal are seen at 3–10 days.

TUBERCULOSIS AT A GLANCE

Epidemiology

TB still occurs in the UK, especially in the Asian community

Aetiology/pathophysiology

Infection with *Mycobacterium tuberculosis*
Primary infection may occur in the lung, skin or gut
Miliary TB (bloodstream spread) is the most serious complication in childhood

Prevention

Bacille Calmette–Guérin (live attenuated virus) given intradermally to tuberculin-negative teenagers, and at birth to babies from high risk families

History

Prolonged fever
Malaise
Anorexia
Cough
Weight loss
Contact with infected adult*

NB *Signs and symptoms are variable

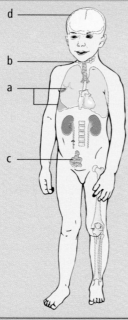

Confirmatory investigations

Demonstration of tuberculin sensitivity by Heaf or Mantoux testing
Chest X-ray evidence of pulmonary TB
Culture of gastric washings

Management

Even if asymptomatic, tuberculin-positive children require treatment
Active TB requires treatment over many months

Prognosis/complications

Postprimary TB may present as local or disseminated (miliary) disease affecting :
• bones
• joints — arthritis
• kidneys — haematuria, renal failure
• pericardium — constrictive pericarditis
• CNS — mental retardation, hydrocephalus
Morbidity and mortality is significant if TB is detected late

Physical examination

Signs depend on focus of infection:
• primary in lung — signs of bronchial obstruction, pleural effusion, etc. (a)
• primary in tonsils — cervical adenitis (b)
• primary in small bowel — malabsorption, peritonitis (c)
• miliary TB — meningitis, chest signs, hepatosplenomegaly (d)

BCG vaccination

BCG (bacille Calmette–Guérin) is a live attenuated virus strain of *Mycobacterium tuberculosis*, which is given intradermally. It causes formation of a papule that enlarges over a few weeks and may ulcerate. It heals over 6–8 weeks leaving a residual scar. In addition to being given to tuberculin-negative teenagers, it is given at birth to babies from high-risk families. In many parts of Britain, Asian babies are immunized in the first week of life.

GROWTH

Growth during childhood is discussed in some detail in Chapter 1. Monitoring of children's growth is an important part of child health surveillance. Normal growth reflects a child's well-being and any deviation may be indicative of adverse physical or psychosocial factors.

Normal growth

A baby's weight and length at birth are influenced by both intrauterine and genetic factors and so do not correlate well with parental heights. Over the next year or two the baby's growth adjusts, so that by the age of 2 years most children have attained their genetically destined centile. From the age of 2 years until the onset of puberty it is usual for a child to grow steadily along their centile with little deviation. During puberty it is normal for centiles to be crossed again until final height is achieved.

GROWTH AT A GLANCE

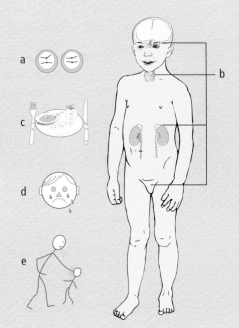

General

Growth reflects a child's well-being and deviation suggests abnormal physical or psychosocial factors. Between the age of 2 years and puberty, growth is usually steady along a centile

Factors that affect growth

- Genetics (**a**)
- Hormones (**b**)
- Nutrition (**c**)
- Illness (**d**)
- Psychosocial factors (**e**)

Growth standards

The 1993 Child Growth Standards are currently in use. Boys' and girls' charts exist, divided into three age groups. Centile lines range from the 99.6th to the 0.4th centile

Plotting a child's growth

Correction for gestational age must be made up to the age of 24 months

Growth monitoring

Benefits include:
- identification of endocrine conditions
- identification of other treatable conditions
- identification of eating disorders
- monitoring chronic diseases
- focus for discussion of health issues with parents
- access to children at risk
- public health issues

Guidelines for concern beyond the age of 2 years

Height or weight >99.6th or <0.4th centile
Crossing of centiles
Discrepancy between height and weight
Discrepancy with parental heights
Parental or professional concern

Growth monitoring

In the past, growth monitoring throughout childhood has been an important part of routine child care. It is still maintained elsewhere, but in Britain it has been pruned down so that it is principally carried out only in the younger years. Current recommendations for monitoring of growth are shown in Table 3.1. Growth monitoring has a number of benefits:

- *Identification of endocrine conditions.* Conditions leading to hormone excess or deficiencies profoundly affect growth, and may be missed if growth is not monitored (see p. 58).
- *Identification of other treatable conditions.* Although chronic illness usually presents with obvious signs and symptoms, some may only be detected by a fall off in growth (see p. 61)
- *Identification of eating disorders.* Growth monitoring can identify the child with an eating disorder, whether anorexia (see p. 351) or excessive eating (see p. 68).
- *Monitoring chronic diseases.* Chronic disease affects growth as a result of a number of factors. In some dis-

eases, such as diabetes, monitoring growth is an important part of management as it reflects adequacy of diabetic control.
- *Focus for discussion of health issues with parents.* Most parents are interested in their children's growth, particularly in the early years, and this can provide a good opportunity to discuss a variety of health issues with them.
- *Access to children at risk.* Children at risk may be identified through monitoring growth, which also serves to provide acceptable access to the family that might not otherwise welcome contact.
- *Public health issues.* Growth of a population reflects the population's health, and growth records can be an important source for epidemiological studies.

Guidelines for concern beyond the age of 2 years
In following children's growth, the following guidelines are recommended when concern should be aroused and an evaluation undertaken.
- *The short or tall child.* Height or weight beyond the dotted lines (>99.6th or <0.4th centiles, see Fig. 2.4) are outside the normal range and pathology is likely to be

found. Many children whose height or weight lies in the shaded areas are normal but an evaluation needs to be considered.

• *Crossing of centiles.* As a rule of thumb one should be concerned if two centile lines are crossed.

• *Discrepancy between height and weight.* There is a great deal of variation as regards leanness and obesity. The child who is very thin or overweight may have a problem.

• *Discrepancy with parental heights.* A child should be evaluated if there is a large discrepancy between the child's height centile and the midparental centile (an average of the parents' centiles). The child of tall parents who has a growth problem should not wait until he or she falls below the second centile to be evaluated.

• *Parental or professional concern.* A good clinical evaluation should be carried out in any child where the parents or other professionals are concerned about growth.

Common growth problems

Common problems identified through child health surveillance are shown in Table 3.4.

CHILD PROTECTION

In the course of child health surveillance, concerns often arise regarding the possibility that a child is the victim of neglect, non-accidental injury, or emotional or sexual abuse (see p. 95). In this circumstance, it is the duty of the professional (and indeed any individual) to report this to the authorities so that appropriate investigations can be made. The role of the child health service goes beyond the detection of these children and also includes the management of abuse and its prevention.

In a preventive role the child health service provides guidance and support to families, reducing the likelihood of children becoming victims of abuse and neglect. The health visitor is ideally positioned to follow children who are at risk. She is usually seen as being a non-threatening and supportive professional, who is a visitor to all homes. The social worker by contrast may be seen to be an imposition and may arouse antagonism.

When a child is found to be in need of child protection the health visitor, school nurse and community paediatrician have an important role in determining how the interests of the child are best met (p. 97). This involves close liaison with the family and other professionals. If the child is placed in care or on the Child Protection Register the child health service provides continuous surveillance and support to ensure that the needs of the child are met.

The role of the child health service in child protection

• Reporting suspected victims of abuse and neglect.
• Following children at risk for abuse and neglect. Health visitors are particularly well placed for this.
• Providing guidance to reduce the risk of abuse.
• Liaison with social services.
• Following children in care and on the child protection register.

Problems commonly detected or presenting in the course of child health surveillance

GROWTH PROBLEMS: SHORT STATURE

Given the social disadvantage of being short, especially for a man, it is not surprising that short stature commonly causes concern. In most short children height is simply a variant of normal, and delay in physical development (maturational delay) is often a factor. When a short child presents, it is important to exclude organic problems, particularly if a fall off in growth is observed over time. The causes of short stature are shown in Table 3.5.

The approach to the child with short stature

The most important aspect of the evaluation of the child with short stature is the history and physical examination, together with careful measurements of height. The purpose of the evaluation should not only be to discover underlying pathological conditions, but also to understand the impact that short stature has on the child.

Table 3.4 Problems seen in growth monitoring

Common problems
Short stature (see p. 56)
Failure to thrive (see p. 61)
Obesity (see p. 68)

Less common problems
Tall stature (see p. 61)
Fall-off in height (see p. 61)
Weight loss

History

The history needs to focus on symptoms suggestive of underlying conditions such as intracranial pathology, hormone deficiency, chronic illness and gastrointestinal symptoms.

Medical history A careful review of medical symptoms is needed, the most important to be elucidated are headache, diarrhoea and abdominal pain, constipation, cough, wheeze and fatigue. The presence of any chronic condition such as asthma, arthritis or diabetes is obviously relevant, as is any chronic medication.

Family history A child's growth cannot be interpreted without reference to parental and siblings' heights. A child's height normally falls on the centile between the parents' height centiles and if there is a disparity a cause should be sought. Enquiry into parental onset of puberty is important

as maturational delay is common and often familial. Most mothers can recall their age at menarche, and maturational delay is likely if it occurred after the age of 14 years. Onset of paternal puberty is harder to identify.

Birth history Low birthweight is significant. A child born small for gestational age (SGA) may have reduced growth potential particularly if height as well as weight is affected.

Psychosocial history Psychosocial factors can severely stunt a child's growth (see p. 61), and the physician must be alert to the possibility of emotional neglect and abuse. The assessment of any short child should also include an evaluation of any social or emotional difficulties resulting from their stature.

Physical examination

A very thorough examination is required focusing particularly on the following:
- *Pattern of growth*. Where possible previous growth measurements should be reviewed as they provide important clues to the aetiology of the condition. Fall-off in growth usually indicates a medical condition requiring treatment.
- *Anthropometric measures* (see p. 17). Careful measures of length (to age 24 months) or height and weight should be made and plotted on a growth chart (see p. 18).
- *General examination*. Signs of hypothyroidism, body disproportion, stigmata of Turner's syndrome (see below) and dysmorphism are particularly important to identify. Each organ system should be examined in turn, looking for evidence of occult disease.

Investigations

The clinical evaluation should guide the need for investigation. If a decrease in growth velocity has occurred, investigations are always required (Table 3.6).

Management of the child with short stature

The majority of short children will be found to have a physiological cause for their stature; either 'constitutional' or maturational delay. In this circumstance the family need reassurance that there is no underlying pathological problem. In addition it is important to address any psychosocial difficulties the child is having, and occasionally psychological counselling is required. These difficulties are uncommon before adolescence, but become particularly problematic for the teenage boy. The use of growth hormone in children with physiological short stature is controversial and probably has little effect on the child's final adult height.

Table 3.5 Causes of short stature

Physiological causes
Normal variant (often familial, also known as 'constitutional short stature')
Maturational delay (often familial)

Pathological causes
Endocrine
  Hypothyroidism
  Corticosteroid excess
  Growth hormone deficiency

Chronic illness
  Inflammatory bowel and coeliac disease, chronic renal failure may be
    occult

Genetic
  Turner's syndrome
  Other genetic syndromes
  Skeletal dysplasias

Intrauterine growth retardation

Psychosocial

Focal points
Evaluating short stature

- A good history and physical examination will identify most pathological causes of short stature

- The child's height must be related to the parents' heights

- Emotional and social consequences of the short stature should be identified

Table 3.6 Investigations in a child with short stature

Investigation	Relevance
Blood count and plasma viscosity or erythrocyte sedimentation rate	Inflammatory bowel disease
Urea and electrolytes	Chronic renal failure
Coeliac antibodies	Screening test for coeliac disease
Thyroxine and thyroid stimulating hormone	Hypothyroidism
Karyotype (in girls)	Turner's syndrome
Growth hormone tests	Hypopituitarism, growth hormone deficiency
X-ray of the wrist for bone age	Delayed bone age suggests maturational delay, hypothyroidism, growth hormone deficiency or corticosteroid excess. A prediction of adult height can be made from it

Physiological causes of short stature

Normal variant short stature

Stature is largely genetically determined, and short parents tend to have short children.

Clinical features The history and physical examination is normal, and the bone age is appropriate for age. Social difficulties are common in the adolescent years, particularly for boys.

Management and prognosis Reassurance is often all that is required. Occasionally children need psychological support in the adolescent years. There are social disadvantages to being short.

Maturational delay

Children with maturational delay are often called 'late developers' or 'late bloomers'. The biological clock operates more slowly than usual.

Clinical features Children are short and reach puberty late, their final height depending on their genetic constitution, which may be normal. A family history of delayed puberty and menarche is often obtained. The bone age is delayed.

Management and prognosis Most families simply require reassurance that final height will not be affected. Occasionally teenage boys find the social pressures to be so great that it is helpful to artificially trigger puberty early, thus causing

an early growth spurt. Treatment does not have an effect on final height.

Endocrine causes of short stature

Hypothyroidism

Hypothyroidism may be congenital (see p. 272) or acquired. Autoimmune thyroiditis (Hashimoto's syndrome) occurs particularly in girls.

Clinical features Thyroid deficiency has a profound effect on growth, and the presenting feature is often short stature. Other features include a fall-off in school performance, constipation, dry skin and delayed puberty. Investigations include a low T_4, high thyroid-stimulating hormone (TSH) and antithyroid antibodies.

Management Treatment is with thyroid hormone. Parents are often alarmed when their quiet, good child is transformed into a normal, active teenager.

Prognosis Treatment is lifelong, but the prognosis is good.

Corticosteroid excess

Cushing's syndrome and disease are extremely rare in childhood; growth suppression from exogenous steroids being much more common. In children requiring long-term high steroid therapy, the deleterious effects on growth can often be minimized by giving the steroids on alternate days.

Growth hormone deficiency

Growth hormone deficiency is a rare cause of short stature. It may occur secondary to lesions of the pituitary such as tumours or cranial irradiation. Growth hormone deficiency can be isolated or accompanied by deficiency of other pituitary hormones.

Clinical features Growth hormone deficiency causes poor growth, with a delay in bone age. This deficiency can be confirmed by growth hormone testing. Brain imaging is needed to identify any underlying pathology.

Management Growth hormone deficiency is treated with daily subcutaneous injections of synthetic growth hormone until the child stops growing. Underlying lesions, if any, need to be treated.

Prognosis As regards growth, the prognosis is dependent on the age at which growth hormone therapy was initiated;

ACQUIRED HYPOTHYROIDISM AT A GLANCE

Epidemiology

More common in girls than boys

Aetiology/pathophysiology

Autoimmune (Hashimoto's) thyroiditis (TSH deficiency very rare)

History

Constipation*
Fall-off in school performance*
Cold intolerance*

Physical examination

- Fall-off in growth or short stature (**a**)
- Dry skin and thin dry hair (**b**)
- Goitre (**c**)
- Slow relaxing reflexes (**d**)
- Bradycardia (**e**)
- Obesity* (**f**)
- Delayed puberty* (**g**)

NB *Signs and symptoms are variable

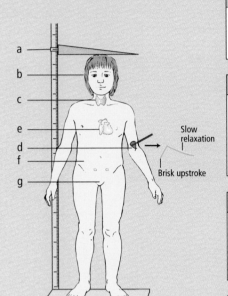

Slow relaxation
Brisk upstroke

Confirmatory investigations

Low T4
High TSH
Antithyroid antibodies

Differential diagnosis

Other causes of short stature
(see Table 3.5)
Other causes of fall-off in growth
(see Table 3.7)
Other causes of goitre

Management

Thyroxine replacement for life
Monitor growth and development
Monitor thyroid function tests
regularly

Prognosis

Good prognosis, provided there is
compliance with treatment

---

the younger the child the greater the chances that final height will be in the normal range. In secondary growth hormone deficiency the prognosis is related to the underlying lesion.

Chronic illness as a cause of short stature

Any chronic illness can lead to stunting of growth. However, chronic illnesses rarely present as short stature because the features of the illness are usually all too evident. Chronic conditions that may present with poor growth, in advance of other clinical features, include inflammatory bowel disease (see p. 167), coeliac disease (see p. 166) and chronic renal failure.

Genetic causes of short stature

Turner's syndrome

Turner's syndrome (gonadal dysgenesis) is an important cause of short stature and delayed puberty in girls. It is a genetic disorder caused by the absence of one X-chromosome. The resulting phenotype is female, with gonads which are merely streaks of fibrous tissue. Mosaicism is common. Intelligence is usually normal.

Clinical features (Fig. 3.8) As neonates, babies with Turner's syndrome often have marked webbing of the neck and lymphoedematous hands and feet. In childhood short stature is marked and the classic features of webbing of the neck, shield-shaped chest, wide-spaced nipples and a wide carrying angle, may or may not be evident. Some girls are only diagnosed in adolescence when puberty fails to occur.

Management During childhood, growth can be promoted by small doses of growth hormone and oestrogen. Puberty must be initiated and maintained by oestrogen therapy.

Prognosis Women with Turner's syndrome, despite treatment, are generally short. Recent advances in infertility treatment have resulted in a few women becoming pregnant through *in vitro* fertilization with donated ova.

TURNER'S SYNDROME AT A GLANCE

Epidemiology

One in 2500 female births

Aetiology/pathophysiology

45 XO karyotype leads to streak gonads (gonadal dysgenesis) and failure of oestrogen production
Mosaicism is common

Clinical features

- Short stature (**a**)
- Delayed puberty (**b**)
- Webbing of the neck (**c**)
- Shield-shaped chest, widely spaced nipples (**d**)
- Wide carrying angle (**e**)
Classic features are often absent*

Confirmatory investigations

Chromosome analysis
May be diagnosed at amniocentesis

NB *Signs and symptoms are variable

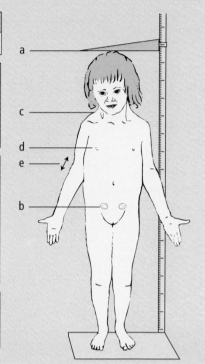

Differential diagnosis

Other causes of short stature (see Table 3.5)
Other causes of delayed puberty (see Table 11.6)

Management

Promotion of growth in childhood by low dose growth hormone and oestrogen therapy
Induction of puberty and maintenance with oestrogen replacement therapy

Associated problems

Coarctation of the aorta
Renal malformations

Prognosis

Generally remain short despite treatment
New advances provide some chance of fertility

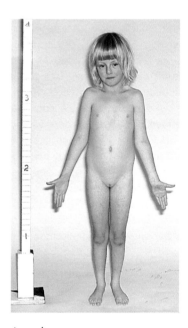

Fig. 3.8 Turner's syndrome.

Other genetic syndromes

Short stature is a common feature in many genetic syndromes. Dysmorphic features are usual and learning disability is common.

Skeletal dysplasias

The skeletal dysplasias are a group of disorders where body disproportion occurs resulting in shortened limbs. The commonest of these is achondroplasia which is inherited as an autosomal dominant trait.

Intrauterine growth retardation as a cause of short stature

Intrauterine growth retardation can result from a variety of causes (see p. 242). The impact on postnatal growth depends at which stage of the pregnancy the growth retardation occurred. If the insult occurred early in gestation, the baby is born not only underweight but also short and often with a small head. Many short newborns have a reduced growth potential and remain short throughout life. If catch-up growth occurs, it does so in the first 2 or 3 years.

Psychosocial causes of short stature

Adverse psychosocial factors can severely affect a child's growth. In the young child it is referred to as failure to thrive (see p. 61). The true incidence of psychosocial short stature is unknown, but it is likely that it is quite common. Children often have a growth spurt on being placed in foster care, even if growth has been apparently normal.

GROWTH PROBLEMS: PLATEAUING IN GROWTH

A less common problem than short stature is fall-off in growth. This cannot be identified on one measurement but is a pattern observed over time. If the child is from a tall family, he or she may not be short in relation to peers. Fall-off in growth is always worrying and merits investigation. Causes of fall off in growth are listed in Table 3.7.

The clinical approach and management is the same as that described in the previous section, but the chance of finding pathology is higher.

GROWTH PROBLEMS: TALL STATURE

Tall stature is only rarely pathological and is usually simply a variant of normal. Tall women often encounter social difficulties and tall girls may present for help. Obese children tend to be tall for their age but on the whole reach puberty early and so their final height is usually in the normal range.

Table 3.7 Causes of fall-off in growth

Endocrine
Hypothyroidism (see p. 58)
Corticosteroid excess (see p. 58)
Growth hormone deficiency (see p. 58)

Chronic illness (see p. 59)
Inflammatory bowel and coeliac disease, and chronic renal failure may be occult

Psychosocial causes (see p. 61)

Table 3.8 Causes of failure to thrive

Organic
Gastro-oesophageal reflux
Malabsorption
Chronic illness
Endocrine dysfunction

Genetic
Genetic constitution
Intrauterine growth retardation
Genetic syndromes

Environmental/psychosocial (non-organic)
Maternal depression/psychiatric disorder
Disturbed maternal–infant attachment
Eating difficulties
Neglect

GROWTH PROBLEMS: FAILURE TO THRIVE

The term failure to thrive implies both a failure to grow and a failure of emotional and developmental progress. It is usually used in reference to a toddler or baby, although it may also be used in connection with an older child. Because infants commonly cross centiles during the first 2 years of life (see pp. 1, 21), expertise is required to differentiate the normal infant from the one who is failing to thrive. If the baby is healthy and thriving in other respects, it is better to refer to the child as demonstrating growth or weight faltering.

The causes of failure to thrive are listed in Table 3.8. A child may fail to thrive for organic or psychosocial reasons. In the past children were classified as having organic (OFTT) or non-organic failure to thrive (NOFTT). In fact, children usually do not fall simply into one category or the other, but fail to thrive for a combination of reasons. It is important to identify all the factors involved rather than to classify the child into a category too simplistically.

There are no established criteria for defining failure to thrive. However, the following can act as guidelines as to when a clinical evaluation is advisable:
- weight below the 2nd centile;
- height below the 2nd centile;
- crossing down two centile channels for height or weight.

Approach to the child with failure to thrive

It is very distressing for the family when a young child fails to thrive and the evaluation needs to be carried out sensitively. The purpose of the evaluation is first to differentiate the child with a problem from those who are demonstrating normal growth faltering, and then to identify the contributing factors, whether organic or non-organic.

History

- *Nutritional history*. A good dietary history must be obtained, and it is helpful to ask the mother to keep a food diary for a few days, recording all that the baby has eaten. The nutritional history should include questions about feeding difficulties, which may have been present from birth but often become particularly problematic at weaning and in the toddler years. Eating difficulties may be the cause of the failure to thrive. However, eating difficulties may also result from the anxiety generated when a baby grows poorly because of other causes.
- *Review of symptoms*. Most organic conditions are identifiable by history. Diarrhoea, colic, vomiting, irritability, fatigue and chronic cough are the most important ones to elicit.
- *Past medical history*. The birth history is important. A low birth weight may indicate adverse prenatal conditions which affect growth potential. Recurrent illness of any nature may affect growth.
- *Developmental history*. A good evaluation is required for two reasons. First, failure to thrive can affect a baby's developmental progress and, secondly, the child who has neurodevelopmental problems often has associated eating difficulties which may limit nutritional intake.
- *Family history*. The child's growth must be related to that of other family members. Medical problems affecting other children in the family may suggest a diagnosis. A good social history should identify psychosocial problems that may be causing or at least contributing to the problem.

Physical examination

- *General observations*. The baby's appearance is important. The healthy small baby will look very different from the neglected or ill child. The latter is likely to look unclean and uncared for. The child who is malnourished for whatever reason will appear thin, with wasted buttocks, a protuberant abdomen and sparse hair. Observations must also extend to the mother and how she relates to the baby, which can provide valuable clues to maternal infant attachment difficulties.
- *Growth*. Growth measures must be plotted on a growth chart and compared with previous measurements. The pattern of growth can be very helpful in the diagnostic process (Fig. 3.9).
- *Physical examination*. A complete physical examination is needed to complement the history. Occasionally clinical signs alone can indicate a cause for the poor growth.

Investigations

There is good evidence that 'fishing' for a diagnosis by carrying out multiple investigations is a futile exercise. Investigations should only be carried out if clues to a problem are obtained on history and physical examination. The only exception is a blood count and ferritin level, as iron deficiency is extremely common in this group of children, and can affect both development and appetite. Other investigations which may be helpful, if clinically justified, are shown in Table 3.9.

Management

The ability to nurture a baby is perhaps the most basic attribute of parenting. When a child fails to thrive it usually causes extreme distress, anxiety and feelings of inadequacy. It is important therefore that a normal, healthy but small baby is not wrongly labelled as having a problem. On the other hand it is important that both organic and psychosocial problems are identified and addressed, as failure to thrive has important consequences on the child's developmental progress as well as growth. A thorough clinical evaluation, together with information from the health visitor can usually sort out the problem. Occasionally it may be helpful to admit the baby to hospital for observation.

Focal points
Evaluating failure to thrive

- Differentiate the baby who is failing to thrive from the normal baby who is crossing centiles

- Identify any symptoms and signs suggestive of organic conditions

- Only perform laboratory investigations if there are clinical leads in the history and physical examination

- Identify psychosocial problems that are affecting the baby's growth

---

Organic causes of failure to thrive

Gastro-oesophageal reflux (see p. 158)

Vomiting and possetting are common complaints in a baby, and usually do not deleteriously affect growth. However, occasionally reflux can cause failure to thrive, particularly if associated with oesophagitis which causes pain and anorexia.

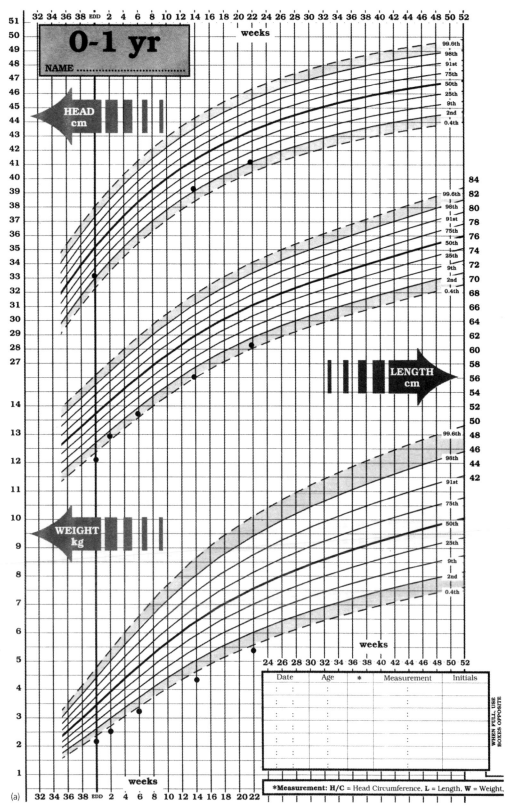

Fig. 3.9 Growth charts (a–d). (a) *Intrauterine growth retardation*. The growth of a baby who was born following intrauterine growth retardation, showing steady growth below the centile lines. © Child Growth Foundation. (*Continued on p. 64*)

other end of the spectrum is the neglected child who shows physical signs of poor care and emotional attachment. In this case the problem is often denied and compliance with intervention poor.

Management Management of failure to thrive must fit the problem. Most families can be helped by appropriate intervention, usually consisting of dietary advice and psychological support. Practical support can ease the stress, and nursery placement can be very helpful in this regard as well as helping to resolve eating difficulties. In those cases where neglect is the cause and the family are not amenable to help, social services must be involved (see pp. 56, 97).

Prognosis With appropriate intervention, the problem usually resolves or at least stabilizes. A few children need to be removed from their homes.

OBESITY

Obesity is increasing as a problem in childhood. As such it needs to be addressed from the angle of public health as well as a problem for the individual child. The vast majority of overweight children have nutritional obesity, and this diagnosis can be simply made on the basis of the clinical evaluation.

The importance of identifying the obese child is principally in order to provide support and advice and to attempt to prevent the complications of obesity later in life. Although there is a folk belief that obesity is caused by a child's 'glands', this is very rarely the case. Causes of obesity are given in Table 3.10.

NON-ORGANIC FAILURE TO THRIVE AT A GLANCE

Epidemiology

2% hospital admissions

Definition

Diagnosis is considered when height or weight below 2nd centile **or** cross down two centiles **and** organic causes have been excluded

Aetiology/pathophysiology

Psychosocial problems such as
• disturbed maternal–child attachment
• maternal depression/psychiatric disorder
• eating difficulties
• neglect

History

• Poor weight gain (a)
• Eating difficulties* (b)
• Inadequate diet* (c)
• Maternal anxiety/depression*

NB *Signs and symptoms are variable

Physical examination

• Fall-off in weight velocity (1)
• Fall-off in linear growth and head circumference* (2)
• Developmental delay* (3)
• Signs of malnutrition: thin child, wasted buttocks, thin hair* (4)
• Signs of neglect: dirty, unkempt, nappy rash, unusual reaction to strangers* (5)

Confirmatory investigations

Exclusion of organic causes of failure to thrive (see Table 3.9)
Iron status (iron deficiency is common)

Differential diagnosis

Organic causes of failure to thrive (see Table 3.8)

Management

Dietary advice
Psychological support
Social support (nursery placement particularly effective)
Referral to social services in some cases

Prognosis

With good early intervention, the process is likely to reverse
Without intervention the child is at severe risk for emotional and intellectual deficits and poor growth

The approach to the obese child

Weight alone is not a measure of obesity in childhood, but must be related to the child's height. The clinical evaluation should focus on excluding the rare endocrine causes of obesity. As all of these are accompanied by poor growth, they can be excluded on clinical grounds fairly easily. The evaluation should then assess those aspects of the child's life-style that predispose to obesity and any emotional and behavioural difficulties the child is having.

History

A detailed description of the child's diet and level of physical activity is required to form a basis for advice. Inquiry into any physical symptoms suggestive of organic conditions, such as hypothyrodism (see pp. 58, 227), should be made. As obesity is a familial condition (genetically and environmentally) a family history is important. The degree to which the child is affected or suffering from the problem must also be determined.

Physical examination

- *Growth*. In nutritional obesity the child is relatively tall. With pathological causes, the child is either short or demonstrates a fall off in height as the weight increases.
- *Signs of endocrinological problems*. In the child with poor growth, signs of hypothyroidism (goitre, developmental delay, slow return of deep tendon reflexes, bradycardia) and steroid excess (moon face, buffalo hump, striae, hypertension, bruising) should be sought.
- *Signs of dysmorphic syndromes*. Certain dysmorphic syndromes are characterized by obesity. These children are invariably short.

Investigations

Investigations are only required if the child is short or demonstrating a fall-off in height, in which case thyroid function tests and diurnal cortisol levels are indicated.

Causes of obesity

Nutritional obesity

The metabolic factors that predispose some individuals to becoming obese have yet to be determined. Certainly the correlation between nutrient intake and development of obesity is not simple.

Clinical features
The nutritionally obese child tends to be tall for his or her age, and tends to develop puberty early, so that final height is therefore not excessively tall. Boys' genitalia may appear deceptively small if buried in fat. Knock-knees are common. Obese children have a high incidence of emotional and behavioural difficulties.

Management

The diet In planning a diet basic nutritional needs must be met. Rapid decreases in weight should not be attempted and during the growing years maintenance of weight, while the child increases in height, is a reasonable goal (Fig. 3.10).

Physical activity The child should be encouraged to increase physical activity. He or she may be reluctant to participate in organized sports, but walking to school or swimming may be more acceptable.

Support Obese children are often the victims of teasing by peers and psychological disturbance is common. Even if weight control is not successful, continuous support is necessary to help these children cope with their condition.

Prognosis
Despite medical intervention, reduction of obesity once it is well established is difficult. Psychological difficulties may well persist into the adult years. Society deals harshly with

Table 3.10 Causes of obesity in childhood

Common
Nutritional
Rare
Hypothyroidism
Cushing's syndrome or disease
Various genetic syndromes

Focal points
Evaluating obesity

- Organic causes of obesity are accompanied by short stature or a fall-off in growth

- A clear picture of the child's life-style—nutrition and exercise should be obtained

- Psychosocial difficulties should be identified

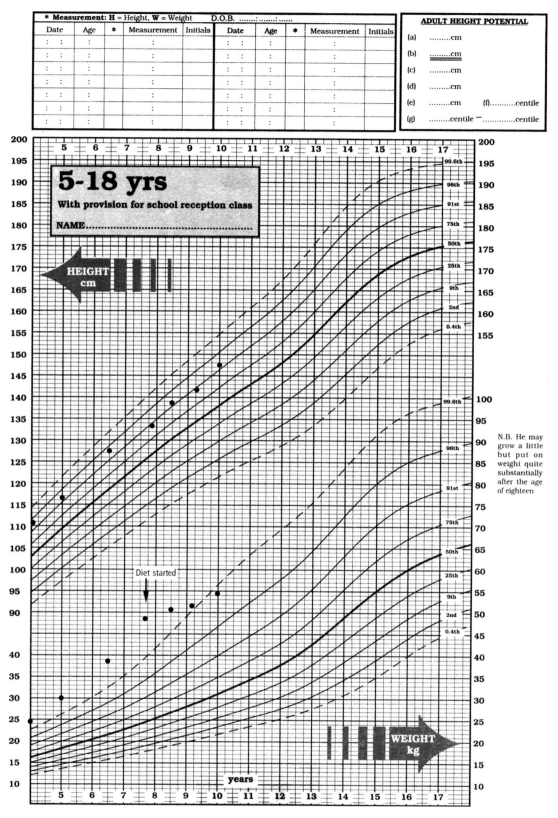

Fig. 3.10 Growth chart of an obese child. The goal of treatment is to reduce the rate of weight gain (but not actual weight loss) so that the child continues to grow. © Child Growth Foundation.

the obese and studies show that obesity is a handicap later in life.

In childhood the medical complications are few. Obese children are more susceptible to musculoskeletal strain and slipped capital femoral epiphyses (see p. 154). Rarely, insulin-resistant diabetes mellitus develops in childhood. As obese adults, the morbidity is significant with diabetes and hypertension common, leading to early mortality from ischaemic heart disease and strokes. Gallstones and certain cancers are also more prevalent.

Prevention

As in most conditions, prevention is better than cure. There is some evidence that breast-feeding in infancy is protective and promotion of good nutrition in the early years, when food habits are developing, is important. Physical activity needs to be encouraged in all children, not simply the obese. There is a need for these health issues to be addressed in school, particularly during adolescence when high intake of high fat foods and decrease in exercise is common. If intervention is provided early in the course of obesity, weight control is likely to be more successful.

THE LARGE HEAD

The head grows rapidly in the first 2 years of life and then slows down, but continues to grow throughout childhood. In the early years the sutures are open, and then fuse around the age of 6 years. Prior to fusion they can separate in response to raised intracranial pressure. The posterior fontanelle usually closes by 8 weeks of age, and the anterior by 12–18 months.

Head size is not directly proportional to body size, but large children are more likely to have large heads, and vice versa. As in body growth, it is not unusual for head circumference measurements to cross centiles in the first year. However, when this occurs clinical assessment is needed to exclude pathological causes.

A large head is usually a normal variant, and often is a

OBESITY AT A GLANCE

Epidemiology

2–3% of school-aged children

Definition

Clinically, no precise anthropometric definition used
Weight must be interpreted in relation to height

Aetiology

- Genetic factors (a)
- Excessive nutritional intake (b)
- Inadequate physical activity (c)

History

Excessive dietary intake*
Emotional/behavioural difficulties*

Physical examination

Excessive weight
Tall stature
Boys' genitalia apparently small
Genu valgus*

NB *Signs and symptoms are variable

Confirmatory investigations

None (endocrine tests only need to be considered if the child is short or a fall-off in growth is observed)

Differential diagnosis

Hypothyroidism, Cushing's **only** if obesity is associated with poor growth
Certain genetic syndromes if the child is short

Management

Dietary advice
Increased physical activity
Support

Prognosis/complications

Obese children/adolescents at high risk for adult obesity
High risk of psychological problems
Susceptible to slipped capital femoral epiphysis and musculoskeletal strain

familial feature. An unusually large head may indicate hydrocephalus, in which case evidence of raised intracranial pressure may be present. Large heads may also be a feature of certain genetic syndromes. The causes of a large or enlarging head are shown in Table 3.11.

Approach to the baby with a large head

History

- *Is the baby developing normally?* Abnormal developmental progress in a child with a large head is strongly indicative of pathology.
- *Are there symptoms of raised intracranial pressure?* The baby with hydrocephalus or subdural effusion is likely to be irritable and lethargic, have a poor appetite and vomit.

Physical examination

- *Growth measures.* The pattern of head growth is important. Crossing of centile lines is more concerning than steady growth of a large head. Length and weight indicate whether the head is disproportionately large (Fig. 3.11).
- *Signs of hydrocephalus.* The child with hydrocephalus has characteristic features (see below).
- *Development.* A developmental examination should accompany the developmental history.

Investigations

If raised intracranial pressure is suspected immediate investigation is required. If the anterior fontanelle is still open, a cranial ultrasound can be performed to detect hydrocephalus, effusions or haemorrhage. If the fontanelles are closed computer tomography (CT) or magnetic resonance imaging (MRI) scans are required to delineate underlying pathology.

Management

Frequent measurements of head circumference can generate anxiety, and should not be performed if the head size is considered to be a variant of normal. If pathology is suspected investigations should be carried out and the baby referred for neurosurgery.

Pathological causes of a large head

Hydrocephalus

Hydrocephalus may result from a congenital abnormality of the brain such as aqueductal stenosis, or acquired as a result of intracranial haemorrhage, infection or tumour. Premature babies with severe intracranial haemorrhage are particularly at risk. Hydrocephalus is commonly associated with neural tube anomalies and occurs in 80% of babies with spina bifida (see p. 237).

Clinical features The clinical features vary with the age of onset and the rate of rise of intracranial pressure. Irritability, lethargy, poor appetite and vomiting are common. In infants, accelerated head growth is the most prominent sign. The anterior fontanelle is wide open and bulging, the sutures separated and the scalp veins dilated. The forehead is broad and the eyes deviated down giving the 'setting sun' sign. Spasticity, clonus and brisk deep tendon reflexes are often demonstrable. In the older child the signs are more subtle, with headache and a deterioration in school performance.

Management Cranial ultrasound, CT and MRI scans provide information which determines the appropriate neurosurgical procedure. Most cases of hydrocephalus require extracranial shunts to drain the cerebral fluid away. Most shunts are ventriculoperitoneal, with ventriculoatrial shunts now rarely used. Complications of shunt placement include blockage and infection, and parents must be taught to recognize the features of raised intracranial pressure, which would suggest these problems. They need to seek help urgently if the child becomes lethargic or irritable or there is a change in personality.

Prognosis Children with hydrocephalus are at increased risk for a variety of developmental disabilities and learning

---

Focal points
Evaluating the large head

- An enlarging head is more concerning than a steadily growing large head

- Parental head size is helpful in deciding if this is a normal variant

- Developmental skills must be assessed

- Evidence of raised intracranial pressure indicates hydrocephalus or subdural collection of fluid

---

Table 3.11 Causes of a large or enlarging head

Normal variation (often familial)
Hydrocephalus
Subdural effusion or haematomas
Feature of certain dysmorphic syndromes

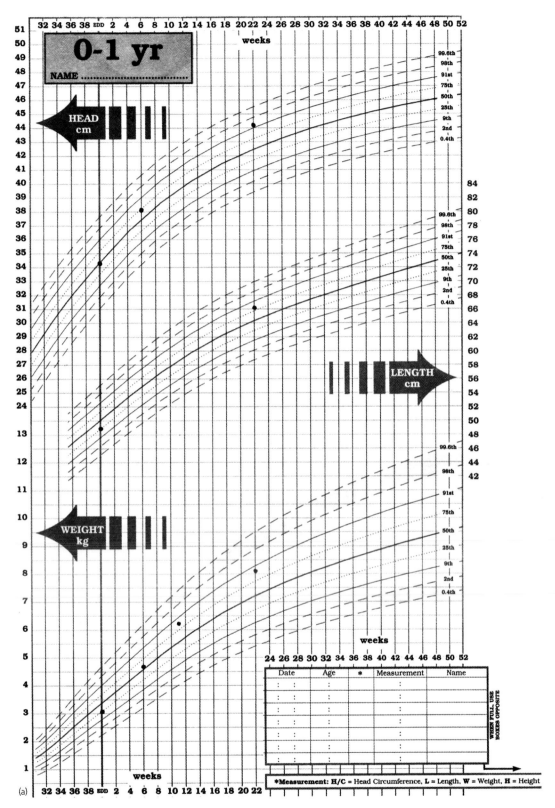

Fig. 3.11 (a) Normal increase in head circumference in a rapidly growing baby and (b) the development of hydrocephalus. © Child Growth Foundation. (*Continued on p. 74*)

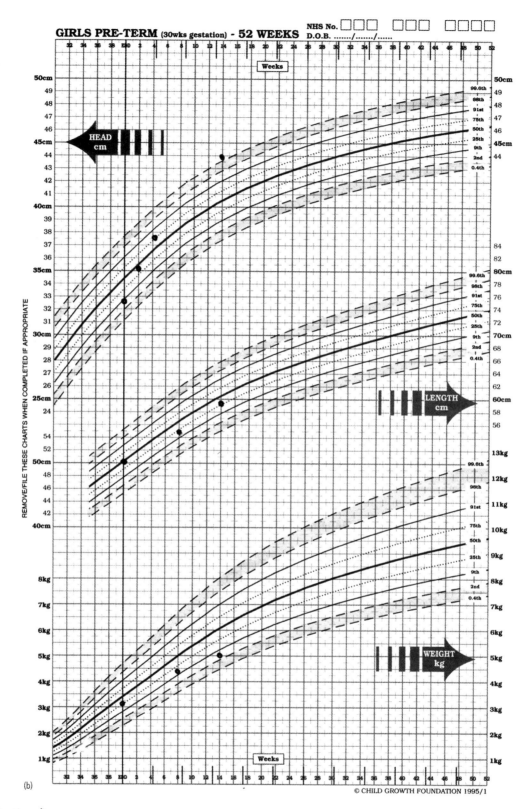

Fig. 3.11 (*Continued*)

difficulties, particularly as related to performance tasks and memory. Visual problems are also common. For these reasons it is important that they receive long-term follow-up.

Subdural effusions and haematomas

A subdural haematoma is a collection of bloody fluid under the dura. It results from rupture of the bridging veins that drain the cerebral cortex. Although any form of head trauma may produce subdural bleeding, the physically abused infant who is forcibly shaken is particularly susceptible to this injury (see p. 95). Subdural haematomas may be acute or chronic, in which case they may eventually be replaced by a subdural collection of fluid. Subdural haematomas can lead to blockage of cerebrospinal fluid flow and hydrocephalus.

Clinical features Although an enlarging head is a feature, the infant is more likely to present with fits, irritability, lethargy, vomiting and failure to thrive. Signs of raised intracranial pressure and retinal haemorrhages are common (Fig. 3.12). Diagnosis is made by radiological imaging.

Management Management is neurosurgical. All cases of subdural haematoma should be evaluated thoroughly for the possibility of abuse.

Prognosis The prognosis for recovery is variable and depends on the associated cerebral insult.

THE SMALL HEAD (MICROCEPHALY)

The head grows in response to brain growth. In most circumstances therefore small head size indicates limited brain growth. Very rarely poor head growth occurs as a result of premature fusion of cranial sutures (craniostenosis). The causes of microcephaly are shown in Table 3.12.

HYDROCEPHALUS AT A GLANCE

Epidemiology

Premature babies with intracranial haemorrhage
Common association with neural tube anomalies

Aetiology

Impaired circulation and absorption of CSF leads to increased intracranial pressure and expansion of the head
Causes include:
• Intracranial haemorrhage
• Infection
• Trauma
• Congenital aqueductal stenosis

History

Irritability
Lethargy
Poor appetite
Vomiting

NB *Signs and symptoms are variable

Physical examination

Accelerated head growth
Open, bulging fontanelle
Separated sutures
Dilated scalp veins
'Setting sun' eyes
'Cracked pot' sound on skull percussion
Transillumination of the skull*
Spasticity, clonus, brisk tendon reflexes*

Head circumference (cm) vs Age (weeks) graph showing 90%, 50%, 10% percentile curves, with Hydrocephalus and Normal large baby plots.

Confirmatory investigations

Cranial ultrasound
CT/MRI scan

Differential diagnosis

Subdural haematoma
Normal variation large head
Megalencephaly associated with some inborn errors of metabolism

Management

Extracranial, usually ventriculo-peritoneal, shunt
Long term follow-up

Prognosis/complications

At risk from developmental disability
Severe neurological damage if pressure is not relieved
Shunt is at risk for blockage and infection

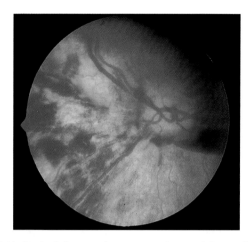

Fig. 3.12 Retinal haemorrhages seen in an infant who was admitted with fits and lethargy following a severe shaking injury.

Table 3.12 Causes of microcephaly or poor head growth

Normal variant (often familial)

Limited brain growth
Perinatal insult to the brain, e.g. hypoxic–ischaemic insult
Genetic syndromes usually associated with learning disability
Neurodegenerative conditions

Craniostenosis (very rare)

The approach to the child with a small head

History

• *Is the baby developing normally?* If a baby is developing normally it is unlikely that the head size is a cause for concern. If developmental delay is present the baby needs to be evaluated for perinatal insults or genetic syndromes.
• *Past medical history.* The perinatal history may throw light on factors such as infection, alcohol or hypoxic–ischaemic events which may have affected brain growth.

Physical examination

• *Growth measures.* Length and weight of the baby indicate whether the head size is disproportionately small. The pattern of head growth is important. Crossing of centile lines is more concerning than steady growth of a small head.
• *Parental head size.* Microcephaly in normal individuals is often familial.

• *Developmental skills.* The developmental history should be confirmed by examination.
• *Dysmorphic features.* Dysmorphic features would suggest the diagnosis of a genetic syndrome.

Investigations

A skull X-ray shows premature fusion of the sutures if craniostenosis is present. A karyotype and neurometabolic screen is indicated if a neurodegenerative or dysmorphic syndrome is suspected.

Management

Frequent measurements of head circumference can generate anxiety, and should not be continued once the head size is considered to be a normal variant. If developmental disability is suspected close follow-up is required (see Chapter 7).

Pathological causes of microcephaly

Cranial insults

A variety of insults to the developing brain can affect brain growth detrimentally and lead to microcephaly. These include:
• hypoxic–ischaemic encephalopathy (see p. 234);
• congenital infections (see p. 243);
• toxins, such as alcohol;
• malnutrition;
• meningitis.

Developmental disorders

Many dysmorphic syndromes are accompanied by microcephaly. The commonest of these is Down's syndrome.

Craniostenosis (craniosynostosis)

In this rare condition premature fusion of the sutures occurs. Very rarely all the sutures are involved, so restricting growth of the skull and as a consequence, growth of the brain. This results in a rise in intracranial pressure. The diagnosis is made on plain skull X-ray and urgent neurosurgical intervention is required.

VISUAL PROBLEMS

Refractive errors

As part of child health surveillance children's eyes are tested periodically to identify the common refractive errors—myopia, hypermetropia and astigmatism (Fig. 3.13). Refractive errors, if uncorrected, can cause an indifference to schoolwork and have a deleterious effect on educational progress.

Myopia

Myopia is infrequent in infants and preschool children, other than preterm infants and children of myopic parents. There is increased refractive power of the eye, so that light focuses short of the retina. The result is blurred vision for distant objects.

The incidence of myopia increases during the school years especially during the preteen and teen years. Concave lenses of appropriate strength are required, with changes in prescription required periodically, particularly during adolescence.

Hypermetropia

In hypermetropia refractive power is less than normal, resulting in normal vision over distance but greater accommodative effort required for close work. This may result in eyestrain, headaches and fatigue. Convex lenses are required to allow for comfort in focusing on near objects.

Astigmatism

Astigmatism is a distortion of vision that results from irregularities in the curvature of the cornea or irregularity of the lens. Cylindrical or spherocylindrical lenses are used to provide optical correction.

Squint (strabismus)

Squints are very common in childhood. They may be convergent, divergent or alternating. Some squints are manifest, but some may be latent and only appear with fatigue, illness and stress. The causes of squint are shown in Table 3.13.

Most squints in childhood are caused by a failure of binocular alignment of the eyes, the reason for which is unknown. More rarely a squint may be caused by an underlying ocular or refractive problem. Rarely, squints are a result of paralysis of the extraocular muscles in which case serious pathology may be the cause.

Irrespective of the cause, the image from the squinting eye is suppressed in the optical cortex so that diplopia is avoided. If the squint is left untreated, the visual pathways from the squinting eye become irreversibly suppressed and a permanent visual defect develops. This is known as amblyopia (see below).

Approach to the child with strabismus

In primary care the importance of the evaluation is to confirm the presence of a squint and to refer the child for early treatment before irreversible suppression of visual acuity occurs. Evaluation involves simple observation and the application of two relatively simple clinical techniques:

Table 3.13 Causes of squint

True strabismus
Non-paralytic strabismus
Failure of binocular alignment
Refractive errors
Ocular abnormalities, e.g. cataracts
Paralytic strabismus
'False strabismus'

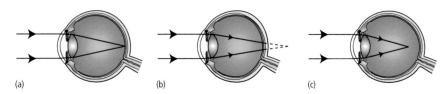

(a)   (b)   (c)

Fig. 3.13 Disorders of refraction: (a) normally focusing on the retina; (b) the hypermetropic eye focuses the object beyond the retina; and (c) the myopic eye focuses the object too short—the eye is too long.

the corneal light reflex test and the cover test. The latter is particularly important if a squint is latent. These are described in detail on pp. 26–27.

Management

All fixed squints, and any squint persisting beyond 5 or 6 months of age, need to be referred for ophthalmological evaluation. There are two goals of treatment:

1 To achieve the best possible vision in each eye. This is accomplished by correcting any underlying defect by surgery for a cataract, prescribing glasses for refractive errors and treating amblyopia by occlusion therapy.

2 To achieve the best possible ocular alignment. In many cases surgery is required and is particularly important in congenital strabismus. It needs to be carried out at the earliest possible age to give the child the best opportunity for developing normal visual pathways.

Types of strabismus

Paralytic strabismus

Paralytic strabismus is caused by weakness or paralysis of the extraocular muscles. The squint is fixed and characteristically worsens on gazing in the direction of the affected muscle. Paralytic strabismus may be congenital or acquired and, if the latter, is an ominous sign of serious pathology.

Non-paralytic strabismus

Non-paralytic strabismus is the more common type. The problem is one of malalignment of the eyes and no defect is present in the extra-ocular muscles themselves. The squint may be apparent (manifest) or latent, in which case it is only detected if fatigued or on clinical examination. The underlying causes of non-paralytic strabismus include failure to develop binocular vision at the normal time and, more rarely, underlying ocular defects such as cataracts or high refractive errors.

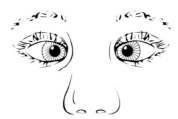

Fig. 3.14 Pseudosquint or false strabismus. A wide nasal bridge and epicanthic folds give the appearance of a squint, but the corneal light reflex test is normal.

'False' strabismus

Some children, particularly if they have prominent epicanthal folds and broad, flat nasal bridges, give the appearance of being cross-eyed (Fig. 3.14). The corneal light reflex and cover test are, however, normal.

Disorders of vision

Amblyopia

Amblyopia can be defined as subnormal visual acuity in one or both eyes despite the correction of any refractive error, and is familiarly known as 'lazy eye'.

Under normal conditions the development of visual acuity proceeds rapidly in infancy. However, if interference in the formation of a clear retinal image occurs during this critical period, irreversible suppression of the visual pathway on that side develops. Examples of interference include cataracts and strabismus, where the child tunes out the image of the deviating eye to avoid diplopia (see above).

Treatment of amblyopia includes:

• Providing the clearest possible retinal image, for example by removing the cataract or by prescribing glasses.

• Stimulation or forced use of the amblyopic eye. This is achieved by occlusion therapy or 'patching'. Covering glasses is not very satisfactory and the best results are obtained by adhesive eye patches. Treatment can be trying and must be closely supervised or amblyopia can develop in the patched eye.

THE TEETH

Dental caries

The development of dental caries is dependent on the inter-relationship between the tooth surface, dietary carbohydrates and oral bacteria. The bacteria break down carbohydrates to form organic acids which demineralize the surface of the tooth. The important factor governing the process of decay is the frequency of carbohydrate consumption rather than the actual quantity of carbohydrates consumed. There has been a decrease in incidence in recent years because of the use of fluorides.

Clinical features Caries start in the pits and fissures of the teeth, and then affect the contact surfaces between the teeth. In severe cases caries affect the tooth close to the gums. An important form in young children is known as baby bottle caries (Fig. 3.15), which results from sleeping with a bottle.

AMBLYOPIA AT A GLANCE

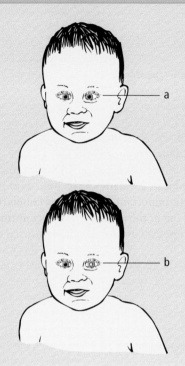

Epidemiology

Common
2–3 year olds are most susceptible

Aetiology/pathophysiology

Suppression of vision in one eye develops
- As a result of malalignment of the eyes (**a**)
- Or rarely, cataracts or high refractive error (**b**)

History

Parental report of squint*

NB *Signs and symptoms are variable

Physical examination

Squint may be latent or manifest
Cover test

Confirmatory investigations

Orthoptic evaluation

Management

Patching good eye to force use of amblyopic eye
Early treatment essential

Prognosis/complications

If left untreated, suppression of the visual pathways causes permanent visual impairment in the amblyopic eye
Surgery may be needed to correct the squint

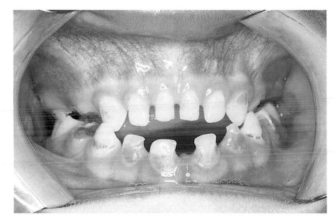

Fig. 3.15 Severe dental caries in a 2-year-old child who was given milk and juice by propping the bottle in the cot during night feeds.

Management Most teeth can be salvaged and treated conservatively. Children under the age of 3 years and those with learning difficulties need to be restrained, sedated or given general anaesthesia in order for treatment to be given. If teeth are severely affected and extraction required, there is a risk that impaction or malocclusion of the permanent teeth will occur.

Prognosis Dental caries left untreated cause pain and infection, sepsis and facial cellulitis if bacterial invasion extends into the bone. If this occurs in a deciduous tooth, the development of the underlying permanent tooth may be disrupted.

Prevention The most effective preventive measure is fluoridation of communal water supplies. In fluoride deficient areas fluoride supplements are advised, and topical fluoride agents are sometimes used by dentists. Healthy eating and dental hygiene are important aspects of health promotion. Children should be encouraged to clean their teeth regularly from babyhood, although they are unlikely to be effective at this before the age of 8 years. As the frequency of carbohydrate ingestion determines the development of caries, between-meal carbohydrate snacks should be avoided. To prevent baby bottle caries infants should be weaned from the bottle by the age of 1 year, and bedtime bottles should contain only water.

Teething

Teething is blamed for a variety of ills. Certainly, as teeth erupt inflammation and sensitivity of the gums can occur together with irritability and increased drooling. However, there is no evidence that systemic disturbances such as fever, facial rashes and diarrhoea result from teething.

HEART MURMURS

Heart murmurs are very common in childhood, being present in some 50% of children, particularly between the ages of 3 and 7 years. The commoner causes of cardiac murmurs are shown in Table 3.14.

The vast majority of these murmurs are not associated with significant haemodynamic abnormalities and are referred to as functional or innocent. It is important to learn to distinguish the innocent murmur clinically from the murmur associated with cardiac disease.

The approach to the child with a murmur

The key factor in the clinical evaluation is the recognition of the innocent murmur, so saving the child from unnecessary investigations and the family from anxiety. With experience, the various pathological murmurs can be differentiated on clinical grounds. If a murmur is suspected to be pathological, signs and symptoms of cardiac failure should be sought.

History

• *Does the baby or child have symptoms of heart failure?* Fatigue is the most important symptom of cardiac failure. Questions should focus around feeding in a baby, as the baby in failure can take only small volumes of milk, becomes short of breath on sucking and often perspires. The older child tires on walking and may become breathless too.

• *Have the parents noticed cyanosis?* This would be an unusual finding in most children identified as having a cardiac murmur.
• *Is there a family history of congenital heart disease?* There is a higher risk of heart defects in siblings of children with congenital heart disease. This question also helps in understanding the level of anxiety which may occur if a murmur is detected.

Physical examination

The cardiac examination is discussed in more detail in Chapter 2 and the salient points highlighted here:
• *The murmur.* If a murmur is heard it is important to decide from the quality and site of the sound whether it is likely to be pathological in nature (Table 3.15). It is important to listen for radiation of the murmur over the praecordium, the back and the neck, and to listen with the child both sitting and lying, as some innocent murmurs lose their intensity in changing position.
• *Growth.* Failure to thrive and poor growth are important signs of cardiac failure in childhood, and are also important in monitoring medical management.
• *Vital signs.* Tachycardia is a sign of cardiac failure. The character of the pulse can give a clue to cardiac pathology. Palpation of the femoral pulses is particularly important as in coarctation of the aorta they are absent or weak, and delayed when compared with the radial pulse. Blood pressure should be measured, and if coarctation is

Table 3.14 Common cardiac murmurs

Innocent murmurs
Systolic ejection murmur
Venous hum
Vibratory murmur
Pathological murmurs
Ventricular septal defect
Atrial septal defect
Aortic stenosis
Coarctation of the aorta
Pulmonary valve stenosis
*Patent ductus arteriosus (p. 249)
*(Fallot's tetralogy, p. 255)

* These conditions do not usually present with cardiac murmurs in childhood and are covered elsewhere.

> **Focal points**
> **Evaluating cardiac murmurs**
>
> • Learn to identify the innocent murmur
>
> • Look for signs and symptoms of heart failure, including failure to thrive

Table 3.15 Characteristics of innocent and pathological murmurs

Innocent	Pathological
Systolic	Pansystolic or diastolic
Musical quality	Harsh or long
No radiation	The presence of a thrill, radiation or cardiac
Varies in intensity with posture and respiration	symptoms indicate a pathological murmur
Asymptomatic	
Normal peripheral pulses	

suspected this should be carried out in both the arms and legs.

• *Other signs of heart failure.* Tachypnoea, hepatomegaly and crepitations in the lungs are the major clinical manifestations of cardiac failure in childhood. Peripheral oedema is rare.

• *Cyanosis.* Cyanosis is an unlikely accompaniment to a child presenting with a cardiac murmur.

Investigations

Investigations are required only if the murmur is thought to be pathological in nature. A chest X-ray provides information about cardiac size and shape, and pulmonary vascularity. The electrocardiograph (ECG) gives further information about ventricular and atrial hypertrophy. Echocardiography is important in evaluating cardiac structure and performance, gradients across stenotic valves and the direction of flow across a shunt. Cardiac catheterization is now rarely required for diagnosis.

Management

The lack of significance of an innocent murmur must be discussed with the parents. Full reassurance must be given so that lingering doubts do not generate anxiety and overprotectiveness. It is helpful to describe that the murmur is simply a 'noise' and does not indicate the presence of a cardiac defect. In general no investigations are required. If a murmur is considered to be pathological referral to a cardiologist is required.

Innocent (functional) murmurs

These murmurs are commonly heard in children and have no clinical significance. Figure 3.16 indicates the sites on auscultation these murmurs can best be heard.

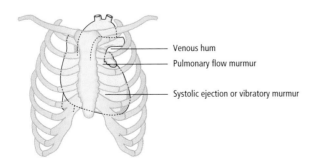

Fig. 3.16 Site of innocent cardiac murmurs.

Venous hum
Pulmonary flow murmur
Systolic ejection or vibratory murmur

Systolic ejection murmur

This is a short systolic murmur occurring during ejection and heard along the left sternal edge or at the apex. It is musical in character, frequently sounding like the vibration of a tuning fork. It varies in intensity when the child changes from lying to sitting and is intensified by fever, excitement or exercise.

Pulmonary flow murmur

This murmur is caused by rapid flow of blood across a normal pulmonary valve. It is a brief, high pitched, blowing murmur, best heard in the second left intercostal space, with the child lying down.

Venous hum

A venous hum is caused by flow through the systemic great veins. It is a blowing, continuous murmur heard at the base of the heart just below the clavicles, sounding like a soft hum during both systole and diastole. It varies with positioning of the head and disappears when the child lies down.

Pathological murmurs: defects causing a left to right shunt

The commonest defects occur between the two sides of the heart at the level of the ventricles or atria. The hole allows shunting of blood from the left to the right side of the heart. If the hole is large and allows a considerable volume of blood to be shunted, an added burden is imposed on the heart and hypertrophy, dilatation and failure result. A large heart with a prominent pulmonary artery and increased vascular markings are seen on chest X-ray and signs of ventricular hypertrophy on the ECG.

Atrial septal defect (Fig. 3.17)

As the murmur is soft, it may not be detected until the child starts school.

Clinical features The systolic murmur, which is heard in the second left interspace, is caused by high flow across the normal pulmonary valve and not by flow across the defect. Characteristically the second heart sound is widely split and is 'fixed' (does not vary with respiration). Occasionally the child may experience breathlessness, tiredness on exertion or recurrent chest infections.

Management If the defect is moderate or large, closure is carried out at open heart surgery.

Prognosis The prognosis following surgery is good. If untreated, cardiac symptoms usually develop in the third decade of life or later.

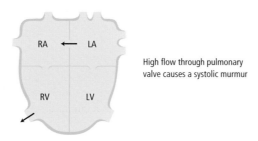

High flow through pulmonary valve causes a systolic murmur

Fig. 3.17 Atrial septal defect.

Ventricular septal defect (Fig. 3.18)

This is the commonest of all congenital heart lesions.

Clinical features The clinical features depend on the size of the defect. If it is small the child is asymptomatic. A larger defect causes breathlessness on feeding and crying, failure to thrive and recurrent chest infections. On auscultation a harsh pansystolic murmur is heard at the lower left sternal border. In large defects the heart is enlarged clinically, a thrill is present and the murmur radiates over the whole chest. The child may have signs of congestive heart failure and be severely ill. Cardiac failure does not occur immediately following birth as the pulmonary vascular resistance is initially high, inhibiting a left to right shunt. There is no correlation between the loudness of the murmur and the size of the shunt.

VENTRICULAR SEPTAL DEFECT (VSD) AT A GLANCE

Epidemiology

Commonest congenital heart lesion

Aetiology/pathophysiology

Clinical features depend on the size of the VSD
There is no correlation between loudness of murmur and size of shunt

Presentation

Murmur usually detected at routine examination

History

Most asymptomatic
Breathlessness on feeding and crying*
Failure to thrive*
Recurrent chest infections*

Physical examination

• Harsh pansystolic murmur at lower left sternal border
• Clinically enlarged heart*
• Parasternal thrill*
• Radiation of murmur over whole chest*
• Signs of congestive heart failure*

NB *Signs and symptoms are variable

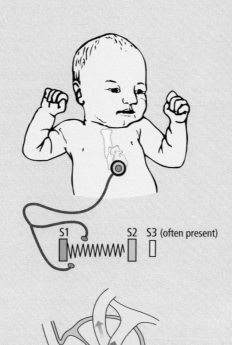

S1   S2   S3 (often present)

Investigations

Small defect: normal chest X-ray and ECG
Large defect: cardiomegaly and large pulmonary arteries on X-ray, biventricular hypertrophy on ECG
Echocardiography confirms the diagnosis

Differential diagnosis

See Distinguishing Features box p. 84
See Table 3.15

Management

Reassurance for small defects
Treatment of cardiac failure if present
Surgery if medical management fails
Antibiotic prophylaxis for infective endocarditis (see p. 338)

Prognosis/complications

Small defects tend to close spontaneously
Excellent prognosis for larger defects after surgery
Increased pulmonary blood flow through an uncorrected large VSD causes pulmonary hypertension (cor pulmonale) with reduced life-span

Investigations If the defect is small, the chest X-ray and ECG are normal. The child with a large defect will have cardiomegaly and large pulmonary arteries on X-ray and demonstrate biventricular hypertrophy on ECG. Echocardiography confirms the diagnosis.

Management Small defects usually close spontaneously and the parents can be reassured of their benign nature. Initial management of large defects is medical, and aimed at control of the cardiac failure. If the child does not respond then surgical treatment is required. Antibiotic prophylaxis is needed in any child with a ventricular septal defect as there is an increased risk of infective endocarditis (see p. 222).

Prognosis and complications Small defects tend to close spontaneously, or may remain the same size but become insignificant as the child grows. The prognosis for larger defects after surgery is excellent. If a large ventricular septal defect is uncorrected, pulmonary hypertension can result from the increased pulmonary blood flow, making the defect inoperable and reducing the child's life-span (cor pulmonale).

Pathological murmurs: obstructive lesions

Obstructive lesions occasionally occur at the pulmonary and aortic valves and along the aorta, causing hypertrophy in the chamber of the heart proximal to the lesion. If the obstruction is severe heart failure may develop.

Aortic stenosis (Fig. 3.19)

Aortic stenosis may occur in isolation or in combination with other heart defects.

Clinical features In most cases aortic stenosis is identified by discovery of a heart murmur on routine examination, although heart failure may develop in infancy in severe cases. Some older children may become symptomatic, experiencing faintness or dizziness on exertion. The systolic ejection murmur is heard at the right upper sternal border and radiates to the neck and down the left sternal border. The murmur may be preceded by an ejection click and the aortic second sound is soft and delayed. The peripheral pulse is of small volume and the blood pressure may be low. A thrill may be palpable at the lower left sternal border and in the suprasternal notch over the carotid arteries.

Investigations The chest X-ray may show a prominent left ventricle and prominence of the ascending aorta. Left ventricular hypertrophy is found on ECG. Echocardiography is useful in evaluating the exact site and severity of the obstruction.

Management If the stenosis is severe it is relieved by balloon valvuloplasty—a catheter tip is passed through the aortic valve from the femoral artery and a balloon inflated to widen the stenosed valve. If unsuccessful, open heart surgery is required. Infective endocarditis is a risk and prophylaxis is required for all children.

Prognosis Children with aortic stenosis are at risk for sudden death and so this is the one congenital heart lesion in which strenuous activity should be avoided. If surgery is carried out in childhood, reoperation is often required at a later date.

Coarctation of the aorta (Fig. 3.20)

This is a localized constriction of the aorta usually occurring at the origin of the ductus arteriosus. Arterial blood bypasses the obstruction reaching the lower half of the body through collateral vessels which enlarge. The left ventricle hypertrophies to overcome the obstruction and heart failure may result.

In severe cases the baby may present with collapse at the end of the first week of life when the ductus arteriosus (through which systemic blood flow has been maintained closes) (p. 249).

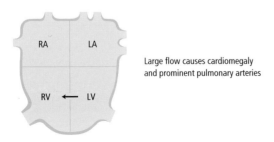

Large flow causes cardiomegaly and prominent pulmonary arteries

Fig. 3.18 Ventricular septal defect.

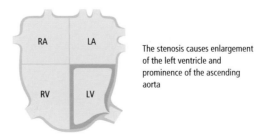

The stenosis causes enlargement of the left ventricle and prominence of the ascending aorta

Fig. 3.19 Aortic stenosis.

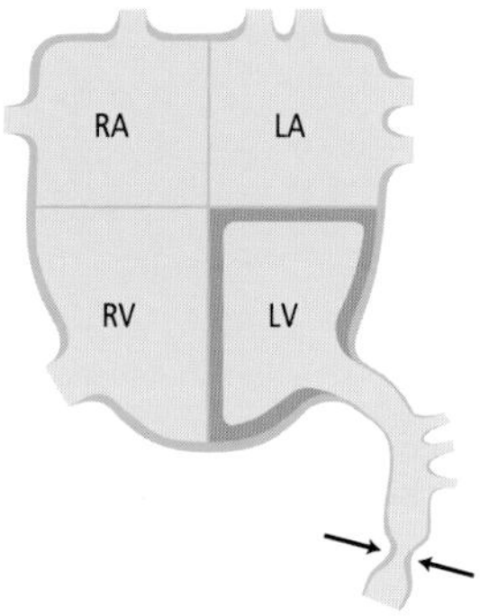

The left ventricle hypertrophies to overcome the obstruction

Constriction of the aorta causes reduced BP to the lower half of the body (absent femoral pulses). As vessels to the arms are above the constriction, brachial blood pressure is high

Fig. 3.20 Coarctation of the aorta.

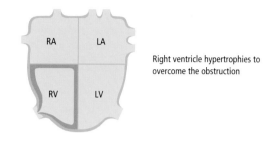

Right ventricle hypertrophies to overcome the obstruction

Fig. 3.21 Pulmonary stenosis.

Clinical features The systolic murmur is usually heard over the left side of the chest especially at the back. The cardinal sign of coarctation is disparity in the pulses and blood pressure of the arms and legs. The right brachial and radial pulses are normal, but the femoral pulses are absent or weak and delayed. Hypertension is found in the arms, but not when measured in the legs.

Investigations The left ventricle may be prominent on X-ray, and rib notching may be seen where enlarged intercostal arteries have eroded the underside of the ribs. An ECG may show left ventricular hypertrophy.

Management Surgery to resect the narrowed section of the aorta is required as soon as the diagnosis is made.

Prognosis and complications Following surgery, narrowing may recur at the resected site and surgery is then required again. If the coarctation is left untreated complications related to hypertension develop with death commonly occurring between the ages of 20 and 40 years.

Pulmonary stenosis (Fig. 3.21)

In this condition the pulmonary valve is thickened and stenosed, and the right ventricle hypertrophies to overcome the obstruction.

Clinical features A short ejection systolic murmur is heard over the upper part of the left chest anteriorly and is conducted to the back. It is usually preceded by an ejection click. With mild or moderate stenosis there are usually no symptoms, and the heart is of a normal size. In more severe stenosis a systolic thrill is palpable in the pulmonary area.

Investigations On chest X-ray, dilatation of the pulmonary artery is seen beyond the stenosis and, if severe, an enlarged right atrium and ventricle. The ECG shows right axis deviation, right atrial and ventricular hypertrophy.

Management The extent of the stenosis can be demonstrated by echocardiography and cardiac catheterization. If severe, balloon valvuloplasty is performed.

Prognosis Surgery is generally successful and further procedures are rarely required.

Distinguishing features Pathological cardiac murmurs

	Characteristics of the murmur	Associated clinical features
Ventricular septal defect	Loud harsh pansystolic murmur at lower left sternal border, radiating all over the chest	If severe: heart failure, failure to thrive and recurrent chest infections
Atrial septal defect	Soft systolic murmur in second left intercostal space, wide fixed splitting of the second sound	
Aortic stenosis	Systolic ejection murmur at right upper sternal border, radiating to the neck and down the left sternal border	Dizziness and loss of consciousness in a minority of older children
Coarctation	Systolic murmur over the left side of the chest especially at the back	Absent or delayed weak femoral pulses Hypertension
Pulmonary stenosis	Systolic ejection murmur over the upper part of left chest anteriorly and conducted to the back, usually preceded by an ejection click	

Table 3.16 Causes of scrotal swellings

Hydrocoele
Inguinal hernia
Testicular torsion

Focal points
Evaluating scrotal swellings

- Enquire if the swelling is intermittent
- Palpate the swelling to determine the pathology
- Transilluminate the scrotum

GENITALIA: SCROTAL SWELLINGS

A swelling in the scrotum may present because of parental concern, or may be an incidental finding identified in the course of child health surveillance. The causes are shown in Table 3.16.

Approach to the child with a scrotal swelling

Careful clinical evaluation should differentiate the various causes of scrotal swelling.

History

- *Characteristics.* An inguinal hernia characteristically causes intermittent swelling, particularly when intra-abdominal pressure is increased as in crying or straining. Hernias (unless incarcerated) and hydrocoeles are painless, although parents may think a hernial swelling is painful as it tends to occur when the baby cries. Testicular torsion in contrast is acutely painful. Hydrocoeles are often present at birth and show little variation in size over time.

Physical examination

- *Observation.* The boy with testicular torsion is obviously in acute pain. The swelling caused by an inguinal hernia extends up into the groin, whereas the hydrocoele usually does not.
- *Palpation.* On palpation the inguinal hernia can be felt to reach up to the inguinal region, and can usually be reduced through the inguinal ring. The testis is palpable apart from the hernial swelling. A hydrocoele in contrast does not usually extend up into the groin and the testis cannot be palpated through the fluid. Neither are usually tender, although the hernia is if it becomes incarcerated. A testicular torsion is

so tender that palpation is not possible. Reduction of an inguinal or inguinoscrotal mass, whether spontaneously or by manipulation is diagnostic of a hernia.
- *Transillumination.* When a torch is held to the scrotum, a hydrocoele transilluminates, whereas a hernia does not.

Investigations

The differentiation between these conditions is clinical. No investigations are indicated.

Causes of scrotal swellings

Hydrocoele

A hydrocoele is an accumulation of fluid in the tunica vaginalis. Hydrocoeles do not fluctuate in size, unless they communicate with the peritoneal cavity. Most hydrocoeles resolve by the age of 1 year, but occasionally large ones persist and require surgical treatment. Rarely, the development of a hydrocoele in an older boy is indicative of malignancy.

Inguinal hernia (see At A Glance Box, p. 86)

Inguinal hernias in childhood are indirect. They are far more common in boys and result from persistent patency of the processus vaginalis which normally closes at birth (see Figs 3.22 & 3.23). They are particularly common in premature infants.

Clinical features A swelling is evident in the groin which may extend down into the scrotum. It tends to be most obvious when intra-abdominal pressure is raised as a result of crying, straining or coughing and often disappears when the baby or child is relaxed and lying down. A hernia is usually not painful unless incarcerated, in which case signs of intestinal obstruction may occur. The observation of an inguinal or inguinoscrotal mass that reduces spontaneously or on manipulation is diagnostic of a hernia.

Management Management of a hernia is surgical. Rarely, if a hernia is incarcerated and irreducible, this must be carried out as an emergency. More commonly the hernia can be gently reduced by the doctor or parent (relaxing the child in a warm bath or with a drink can help). Surgery can then be carried out as an elective procedure.

Testicular torsion

Testicular torsion usually occurs below the age of 6 years. The testes in young boys are unusually mobile and torsion

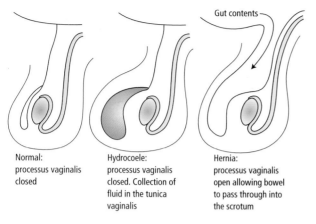

Normal:
processus vaginalis
closed

Hydrocoele:
processus vaginalis
closed. Collection of
fluid in the tunica
vaginalis

Hernia:
processus vaginalis
open allowing bowel
to pass through into
the scrotum

Fig. 3.22 Anatomical development of an inguinal hernia and hydrocoele.

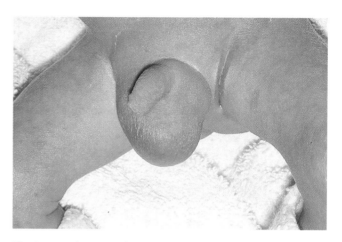

Fig. 3.23 Right inguinal hernia.

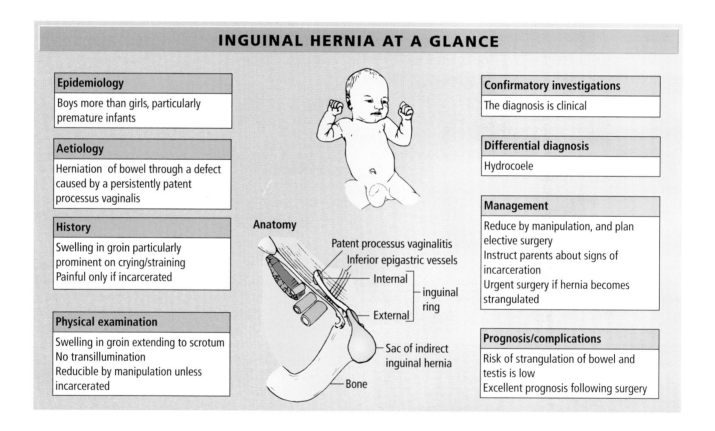

INGUINAL HERNIA AT A GLANCE

Epidemiology

Boys more than girls, particularly premature infants

Aetiology

Herniation of bowel through a defect caused by a persistently patent processus vaginalis

History

Swelling in groin particularly prominent on crying/straining
Painful only if incarcerated

Physical examination

Swelling in groin extending to scrotum
No transillumination
Reducible by manipulation unless incarcerated

Anatomy

Patent processus vaginalitis
Inferior epigastric vessels
Internal
External
inguinal ring
Sac of indirect inguinal hernia
Bone

Confirmatory investigations

The diagnosis is clinical

Differential diagnosis

Hydrocoele

Management

Reduce by manipulation, and plan elective surgery
Instruct parents about signs of incarceration
Urgent surgery if hernia becomes strangulated

Prognosis/complications

Risk of strangulation of bowel and testis is low
Excellent prognosis following surgery

---

results when the testis rotates on the spermatic cord. Prompt diagnosis and treatment is required for the testis to survive.

Clinical features The boy presents with acute pain and swelling of the scrotum. On examination the scrotum looks tender and swollen and examination is resisted.

Management and prognosis Prompt surgical exploration is required to untwist and fix the testis to the scrotum. If this takes place within 6 hours, the majority of gonads survive. The contralateral testis must also be fixed as it is also prone to torsion.

GENITALIA: SWELLINGS IN THE GROIN

The causes of groin swelling are shown in Table 3.17.

Distinguishing features
Scrotal swellings

	Hernia	Hydrocoele	Torsion
Usual age	Infants, particularly premature	Babies	Boys under 6 years
Pain	No (unless incarcerated)	No	Intense
Extends to groin	Yes	Usually not	No
Transilluminates	No	Yes	No

Table 3.17 Causes of swelling in the groin

Inguinal hernia
Inguinal lymphadenopathy
Ectopic testis

Approach to the child with a lump in the groin

Like scrotal swellings, lumps in the groin are distinguishable clinically. The features of inguinal hernias are described in the previous section. In contrast, the inguinal lymph node has a firm consistency with clear borders. It may be tender, and the responsible infected lesion may be evident on the legs. Obviously, if an enlarged lymph gland is found, the child must be fully examined for more generalized lymphadenopathy and hepatosplenomegaly. Rarely the lump may be an ectopic testis and the scrotum should be examined for the presence of both testes. Small shotty inguinal nodes are very common in young children, and are related to the degree of minor trauma the legs incur at this age. They are of no significance.

GENITALIA: ABSENT TESTES

Cryptorchidism (undescended testes) is an important condition to be identified in babies and is screened for during child health surveillance, as there is a risk of infertility and malignancy if they are left uncorrected. Causes of impalpable testes are shown in Table 3.18.

Approach to the child with impalpable testes

The commonest reason for a testis or testes to be impalpable is an exaggerated cremasteric reflex which retracts the testes high into the scrotum. Retractile testes can be brought down by careful palpation when the child is relaxed in a warm

Table 3.18 Causes of absence of testes in the scrotum

Undescended or ectopic testes
Retractile testes
True testicular absence

Focal points
Evaluating impalpable testes

- Examine the child in a warm room with warm hands

- Scrotal examination is facilitated if the child is in a squatting or crossed leg position

room, and scrotal examination is facilitated if the child is in a squatting or crossed leg position. Often more than one examination is required to establish whether the testis is truly absent from the scrotum.

Management

Undescended testes may descend into the scrotum spontaneously before the age of 1 year. Beyond that age, if the testes cannot be palpated and brought down into the scrotum, referral to a paediatric surgeon is required. Surgery should be carried out before the age of 2 years to minimize the risk of complications.

Causes of impalpable testes

Undescended and ectopic testes

Undescended and ectopic testes can only be differentiated from each other at operation, and both conditions are referred to as cryptorchidism. Testes usually descend from their fetal intra-abdominal position through the processus vaginalis and into the scrotum during the seventh month of gestation (see Fig. 3.22). The undescended testicle is found along the normal path of descent and the processus vaginalis is usually patent. If bilateral, the diagnosis of hypopituitarism should be considered. The ectopic testis is one that has completed its descent through the inguinal canal, but lands up at the wrong destination, usually in the groin.

Clinical features The distinction between retractile testes and cryptorchidism is discussed above. One or both testes may be affected. Undescended testes are more common in

CRYPTORCHIDISM (UNDESCENDED/ECTOPIC TESTES) AT A GLANCE

Epidemiology

1–2% boys

Aetiology

Incomplete or maldescent of the testis during gestation
Hypopituitarism may cause bilateral cryptorchidism

History

Asymptomatic

Physical examination

Examine with child relaxed in a warm room
Testis impalpable, or high in inguinal region or scrotum
Inguinal hernia*

NB *Signs and symptoms are variable

Embryology of testicular descent

(a) **In utero**

Testis (under peritoneum)
Gubernaculum testis
Pubic symphysis
Processus vaginalis
Scrotal swelling
Rectum

(b) **At birth**

Pubic symphysis
Tunica vaginalis
Gubernaculum testis

Confirmatory investigations

Usually a clinical diagnosis
Ultrasound may help in locating the testis
Hormonal testing if testes impalpable bilaterally

Differential diagnosis

Retractile testes

Management

Orchidopexy before 2 years old

Prognosis/complications

There is a risk of malignancy in the undescended testis, and infertility in adulthood if left uncorrected

---

premature babies than in term babies, and are often accompanied by an inguinal hernia.

Management and prognosis Surgery should be performed before the age of 2 years as by this age the number of germ cells in undescended testes is already reduced and the risk of infertility increased whether the cryptorchidism is unilateral or bilateral. There is also an increased risk of testicular tumour occurring in the third and fourth decade if surgery is delayed.

Absent testes

Approximately 20% of non-palpable testes are absent. In most cases this is presumed to be a result of a vascular accident. If absent bilaterally, intersex must be considered and the chromosomal sex confirmed.

OTHER GENITAL FINDINGS

Irretractable prepuce

In the majority of boys the prepuce becomes retractable by the age of 3 years. Inability to retract before this age is not pathological.

True phimosis (the inability to retract the prepuce) can be congenital or a sequel to inflammation, and requires surgery.

Labial adhesions

The labia majora are sometimes found to be adherent in young girls who are still in nappies. The adhesions probably develop as a result of irritation secondary to nappy rash. There is no need for the labia to be forcibly separated as the adhesions resolve in later childhood.

MUSCULOSKELETAL PROBLEMS: CONCERNS ABOUT GAIT

In the course of child health surveillance parents often raise concerns about the shape of their child's legs or their gait. The causes for these concerns are shown in Table 3.19. They are rarely of significance and reassurance is usually all that is required.

The approach to the child with an odd gait

The child should be observed walking independently and without a nappy, trousers, socks or shoes, and then on standing still, from in front and from behind. All the joints should be examined lying down, and deep tendon reflexes elicited.

Causes of odd gaits

Flat feet

Most babies have flat feet, the arch gradually developing through childhood. Flat feet in childhood are painless and need no therapy.

Intoeing

Intoeing may occur as a result of rotation of the leg at the hip (femoral anteversion), at the tibia (medial tibial torsion) or in the foot (metatarsus adductus) (Fig. 3.24). The diagnosis is made clinically. The only condition which requires orthopaedic intervention is metatarsus adductus, as buying shoes is problematic if the feet are curved. Otherwise intoeing usually resolves by 4 or 5 years of age.

Bow legs and knock-knees

During the first 2 years the legs are naturally bowed in shape. During the third and fourth year a physiological knock-knee pattern emerges, which straightens by the age of 10 years, although may persist in the obese. Only rarely nowadays are bow legs indicative of rickets or other pathology.

Toewalking

Some children start to walk on their toes. This is usually a normal variant, but is occasionally a sign of cerebral palsy, which can be determined by neurological examination of the legs.

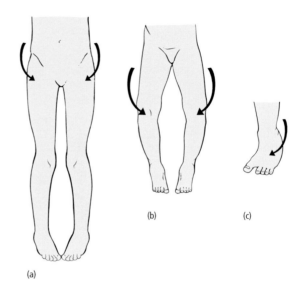

Fig. 3.24 Types of intoeing: (a) femoral anteversion; (b) tibial torsion; and (c) metatarsus adductus.

Congenital dislocation of the hip

This is usually detected through screening before the child starts to walk, but should be considered if there is a limp (see p. 239).

Cerebral palsy

Occasionally mild forms of cerebral palsy present with an abnormal hemiplegic or diplegic gait (see pp. 22, 277). The diagnosis is made clinically by the finding of spasticity, increased deep tendon reflexes and an extensor plantar response in affected legs.

MUSCULOSKELETAL PROBLEMS: SCOLIOSIS (CURVATURE OF THE SPINE)

Scoliosis (see p. 38) is common in teenage girls and is usually idiopathic. If severe, it can produce life-threatening cardiorespiratory compromise. It is detected clinically by observing the back from behind and asking the patient to bend forward (see Fig. 2.33).

Minor curves are treated with a thoracolumbosacral orthosis which usually prevents progression. Severe scoliosis may require surgery.

PALLOR AND ANAEMIA

Anaemia is usually detected when a blood count is performed routinely or on investigating another problem. It

Table 3.19 Causes of abnormal gait

Common
Flat feet
Intoeing
Bow legs and knock-knees
Toe walking
Rare but important
Congenital dislocation of the hip
Cerebral palsy

may also be suspected if a child is noted to look pale. Causes of anaemia are shown in Table 3.20.

Anaemia arising as a consequence of iron deficiency is very common in the childhood years, as it is difficult to sustain iron stores in the face of rapid growth and an inadequate intake of iron-rich foods which is common in toddlers. If a child fails to respond to iron therapy other causes of microcytic hypochromic anaemia must be considered, namely lead poisoning and thalassaemia trait.

If a child is ill, more serious causes of anaemia must be considered. Chronic infection and chronic renal failure give a normochromic normocytic picture. The haemoglobinopathies have characteristic clinical features. The commonest malignancy is leukaemia, which can usually be suspected on the peripheral blood count.

The approach to the child with anaemia

Haemoglobin levels vary during childhood (p. 357) and blood counts should be interpreted accordingly. The neonate starts life with a polycythaemic picture, and a physiological fall occurs in the first years.

In adulthood, anaemia should always be investigated before treatment is initiated. In childhood, nutritional iron deficiency is so common that it is customary to give first a therapeutic trial of iron, and only to investigate further if the response to iron treatment is inadequate.

If a child fails to respond to iron, and the picture is one of microcytic hypochromic anaemia, thalassaemia trait and lead toxicity should be considered, and haemoglobin electrophoresis and testing for lead carried out (Fig. 12.1, p. 358). If the child is ill, then investigations should not be delayed (see Table 3.21).

Table 3.20 Causes of pallor/anaemia in childhood

Common causes (all hypochromic microcytic)
Iron deficiency anaemia
Lead poisoning
Thalassaemia trait
Less common causes
Haemolysis, e.g. thalassaemia major, sickle cell anaemia
Chronic infection
Chronic renal failure
Malignancy

Causes of anaemia in childhood

Iron deficiency anaemia

In the early childhood years the demand for iron is high in order to keep up with the rapid growth that occurs at this time. Babies and children compound this by commonly having a poor intake of iron-rich foods. The combination of these two factors results in a high prevalence of iron deficiency. Blood loss may also exacerbate low iron stores, an important cause being chronic blood loss induced by exposure to a heat-labile protein in whole cow's milk. The incidence of iron deficiency anaemia can be as high as 50% in some populations, depending on dietary and social habits.

Clinical features Pallor is the most important clue to iron deficiency. If the haemoglobin level falls significantly, irritability and anorexia occur. Iron deficiency may also have a detrimental effect on neurological and intellectual functioning. A number of reports suggest that iron deficiency, even in the absence of anaemia, affects attention span, alertness and learning.

Investigations The initial finding in iron deficiency is a low ferritin level reflecting inadequate iron stores. As the deficiency progresses the red blood cells become smaller and the haemoglobin content decreases. With increasing severity the red blood cells become deformed and misshapen and present characteristic microcytosis, hypochromia and poikilocytosis.

Table 3.21 Possible investigations in the child with anaemia who is ill or unresponsive to iron treatment

Investigation	Relevance
Full blood count	Degree of anaemia
	Type of anaemia (microcytic, hypochromic, etc)
	Presence of bizarre cells
	Presence of blast cells
Ferritin	Low in iron deficiency
Lead level	High in lead toxicity
Haemoglobin electrophoresis	Abnormal in haemoglobinopathies (e.g. thalassaemia)
Urea and electrolytes	Abnormal in renal failure
Blood and urine culture	Chronic infection
Bone marrow aspiration	Presence of leukaemic cells

IRON DEFICIENCY ANAEMIA AT A GLANCE

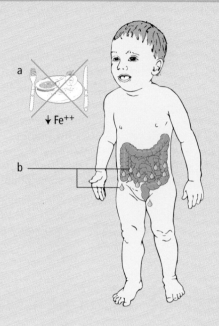

Epidemiology

Common
Up to 50% toddlers in some populations

Aetiology

- Inadequate iron intake in diet (**a**)
- Occult blood loss from gut in bottlefed babies (**b**)

History

Asymptomatic
Irritability and anorexia if severe*

Physical examination

Pallor*

NB *Signs and symptoms are variable

Confirmatory investigations

Low Hb, low MCV on FBC (see p. 357)
Low ferritin

Differential diagnosis

Thalassaemia trait
Lead toxicity

Management

Iron supplements for 2–3 months
No need to investigate for cause of anaemia unless failure to respond to treatment
Dietary advice about iron-rich foods

Prognosis/complications

Behavioural and intellectual deficits if uncorrected

Management The treatment is iron salts given orally over 2–3 months so that iron stores are adequately built up. Parents should be advised to limit the consumption of milk to 1 pint daily in order to reduce blood loss and encourage the consumption of more iron-rich foods. The haemoglobin level starts to increase within 1 week of starting treatment. Failure to do so suggests non-compliance or an incorrect diagnosis.

Prevention Breast milk is somewhat protective against the development of iron deficiency as, although it has a relatively low iron content, the iron is absorbed more efficiently because of the iron-binding protein lactoferrin. As unmodified cow's milk can cause subtle chronic intestinal blood loss it should not be given during the first year of life. Tea is also inadvisable as it reduces the absorption of iron. In many countries screening for anaemia is carried out routinely in the first year of life.

Lead poisoning

Lead affects many enzyme systems but particularly those involved in haem synthesis. The main sources of lead poisoning used to be lead paint and water from lead pipes. More recently there has been concern regarding inhalation of atmospheric lead from car exhaust fumes.

Clinical features Symptoms are usually subtle and non-specific consisting of irritability, anorexia and decreased play activity. Colic may be present and pica (the chronic ingestion of non-nutrient substances) is a feature of lead poisoning. Acute encephalopathy with vomiting, ataxia and seizures is now rare.

Investigations The blood picture is one of hypochromic microcytic anaemia. High lead levels confirm the diagnosis. X-ray of the abdomen may demonstrate radiopaque flecks if foreign matter containing lead was recently ingested. X-ray of the long bones may show bands of increased density at the growing ends of the bone (leadlines).

Management Treatment is directed at removing lead from the body. This is achieved by using lead chelating agents which increase lead excretion. The source of lead must be identified and removed.

Prognosis Chronic lead exposure has a detrimental effect on intellectual development. Severe lead poisoning carries a high mortality and survivors are often neurologically handicapped.

Thalassaemia

The thalassaemias are a heterogeneous group of heritable hypochromic anaemias of varying degrees of severity. The underlying genetic defect results in a suppression of haemoglobin polypeptide chain synthesis. Beta thalassaemia is the commonest form, and affects individuals from Asian and Mediterranean backgrounds.

Clinical features Heterozygous beta thalassaemia produces a mild anaemia, known as thalassaemia trait. Homozygous thalassaemia results in a severe haemolytic anaemia, where compensatory bone marrow hyperplasia produces a characteristic overgrowth of the facial and skull bones. The treatment of repeated blood transfusions causes haemosiderosis with cardiomyopathy, diabetes and skin pigmentation.

Investigations A hypochromic, microcytic anaemia is found in thalassaemia trait, which may be confused with iron deficiency. Precise diagnosis of the type of thalassaemia can be made by haemoglobin electrophoresis.

Management Thalassaemia trait requires no treatment. In thalassemia major blood transfusions are given on a regular basis to maintain haemoglobin levels. Haemosiderosis is an inevitable consequence, but can be minimized by the use of continuous subcutaneous infusions of the chelating agent desferrioxamine.

Sickle cell anaemia

Sickle cell anaemia is the commonest of the haemoglobinopathies, and principally occurs in black populations. The homozygous condition is referred to as sickle cell

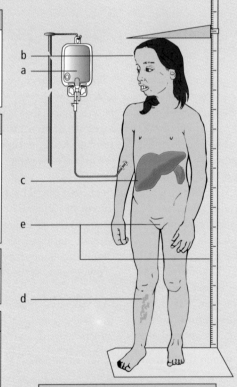

THALASSAEMIA MAJOR AT A GLANCE

Epidemiology

Beta thalassaemia is the commonest form
In the UK it is seen predominantly in children of Greek Cypriot or Bangladeshi origin

Aetiology/pathophysiology

A genetic defect of globin chain synthesis causing ineffective erythropoiesis in the bone marrow and premature destruction of circulating red blood cells by the spleen
Clinical features are related to haemosiderosis caused by treatment

History

Anaemia and jaundice from babyhood
Family history of thalassaemia

Physical examination

- Anaemia (**a**)
- Maxillary overgrowth, frontal bossing (**b**)
- Hepatosplenomegaly (**c**)
- Skin pigmentation due to haemosiderosis (**d**)
- Short stature and delayed puberty (**e**)

NB *Signs and symptoms are variable

Confirmatory investigations

Hypochromic microcytic anaemia
High HbF and HbA$_2$ on haemoglobin electrophoresis
Antenatal diagnosis is available

Differential diagnosis

Thalassaemia major: other causes of severe haemolytic anaemia
Thalassaemia minor: iron deficiency, lead toxicity

Management

Regular blood transfusions to maintain haemoglobin levels
Continuous subcutaneous desferrioxamine to chelate and excrete iron overload
Genetic counselling for family

Prognosis/complications

Without treatment life expectancy is only a few years
Haemosiderosis caused by frequent blood transfusions leads to cardiomyopathy, cirrhosis, diabetes and endocrinopathies
Thalassaemia minor (the heterozygous carrier state) is asymptomatic, and detected by a hypochromic microcytic blood film, and high HbF and HbA$_2$ on electrophoresis

SICKLE CELL ANAEMIA AT A GLANCE

Epidemiology

Commonest haemoglobinopathy
Predominantly seen in black
Americans, Africans, Afro-Caribbeans

Pathogenesis

Genetic mutation of the Hb chain
results in unstable haemoglobin (HbS)
When deoxygenated, HbS causes
sickling of red cells which occlude the
microcirculation
Crises are precipitated by dehydration,
hypoxia, acidosis

History

Recurrent acute painful crises
affecting any organ

Physical examination

Chronic anaemia
Flow murmur
• Jaundice* (a)
• Chronic leg ulcers* (b)
• Dactylitis (c)
• Splenomegaly in young child only (d)
• Haematuria* (e)

Confirmatory investigations

Low haemoglobin, sickle cells on smear
HbS and absent HbA on haemoglobin
electrophoresis
Abnormal liver function tests

NB *Signs and symptoms are variable

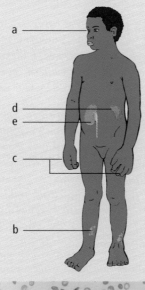

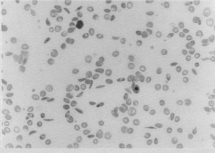

Differential diagnosis

Leukaemia
Arthritis

Complications

Chronic haemolysis
Recurrent painful crises due to
ischaemic occlusions
Aplastic crises
Sequestration crises causing
circulatory collapse
Pneumococcal infection due to
asplenism
Osteomyelitis
Renal damage with reduced ability to
concentrate urine
Gallstones
Heart failure from chronic anaemia

Management

Analgesics, antibiotics, warmth, fluids
during crises
Blood transfusion if Hb falls markedly
during an aplastic, sequestration or
haemolytic crisis
Maintenance of immunizations
Penicillin prophylaxis to prevent
pneumococcal infection
Genetic counselling for family

Prognosis

High mortality from sepsis under age
3 years
85% survive to age 20 years
Heterozygous state is asymptomatic
(unless in very low oxygen tensions as
with GA or high altitude)

---

anaemia, and the heterozygous condition as sickle cell trait. The underlying genetic defect is a substitution of one of the amino-acid sequences in the globin chain, causing an unstable haemoglobin (HbS). When haemoglobin S is deoxygenated, it forms highly structured polymers which cause brittle, spiny red cells. The clinical manifestations of the disease are caused by ischaemic changes, which result from masses of sickled cells occluding blood vessels.

Clinical features Sickle cell anaemia is a serious disease, characterized by chronic haemolytic anaemia. Children experience recurrent, acute, painful crises which can be precipitated by dehydration, hypoxia or acidosis. Painful swelling of the hands and feet is a common early presenta-

tion. Repeated splenic infarctions tend to occur in the early years, eventually leaving the child asplenic and susceptible to serious infections. Renal damage leads to a reduced ability to concentrate urine, making dehydration a severe problem. Sickle cell trait is asymptomatic other than in conditions of low oxygen tensions such as occur at high altitude or under general anaesthesia.

Investigations The peripheral blood smear in the homozygote state typically contains target cells, poikilocytes and irreversibly sickled cells. Diagnosis is made by haemoglobin electrophoresis, which may also be used for screening in susceptible populations.

Management Treatment is largely symptomatic with analgesics, antibiotics, warmth and adequate fluids during crises. Immunization status must be maintained and daily penicillin given in asplenic individuals.

Prognosis Neonatal screening programmes to identify babies with sickle cell anaemia can reduce morbidity and mortality by providing prophylactic measures.

Leukaemia (see also p. 340)

Leukaemia is characterized by a malignant proliferation of white cell precursors which occupy the bone marrow. These blast cells may also circulate in the blood and deposit in various tissues. The commonest leukaemia in childhood is acute lymphatic leukaemia (ALL), in which the blast cells resemble primitive precursors of lymphoid origin. It can occur at any age but the peak incidence is 5 years.

Clinical features The onset is usually insidious with anorexia, irritability and lethargy. As the bone marrow fails, pallor, bleeding and fever occur. Bone pain may be an important presenting complaint. Rarely, signs of increasing intracranial pressure such as headache and vomiting indicate meningeal involvement. On examination petechiae or mucous membrane bleeding may be present, and lymphadenopathy and splenomegaly may be found.

Investigations Most patients have an elevated white cell count, anaemia and thrombocytopenia on the peripheral blood smear. Blast cells may also be seen. The definitive diagnosis is made on examination of the bone marrow which is replaced by leukaemic lymphoblasts.

Management The basic components of treatment include induction chemotherapy which is given until the child no longer shows leukaemic cells, prophylactic treatment to the central nervous system and a continuation of systemic treatment for 2–3 years. The child needs to be followed closely for relapse and, if this occurs, intensive retreatment is required. The management of the child with cancer is covered in Chapter 10.

Prognosis The prognosis varies with the type of ALL. In some forms a cure rate of more than 75% is achieved. The prognosis is less favourable if the child is less than 2 or more than 10 years of age.

LEUKAEMIA AT A GLANCE

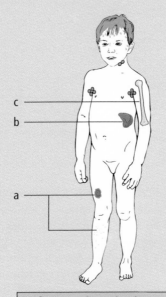

Epidemiology

Commonest childhood malignancy
80% childhood leukaemias are acute lymphoblastic leukaemia (ALL)

Aetiology

Malignant proliferation of white cell precursors

History

Insidious onset
Anorexia, irritability, lethargy
Fever
Bone pain*
Mucous membrane bleeding*

Physical examination

Pallor
• Petechiae, bruising* (a)
• Lymphadenopathy, splenomegaly* (b)
• Bone tenderness* (c)

NB *Signs and symptoms are variable

Confirmatory investigations

Peripheral blood: high white cell count, anaemia, thrombocytopenia, blast cells
Bone marrow: replaced by leukaemic lymphoblasts

Differential diagnosis

Chronic infection
Bleeding diatheses
Other causes of lymphadenopathy
Other tumours infiltrating the bone marrow

Management

Chemotherapy to induce remission
Ongoing less intense chemotherapy for 2 years
Prophylaxis (chemotherapy/radiation) to the CNS
Close monitoring and treatment of relapses
Psychosocial support

Prognosis

Depends on the leukaemia. In favourable presentations of ALL 75% are cured. There is a less favourable outcome of <2 years or >10 years

ABUSE AND NEGLECT

During the course of child health surveillance children may be identified as being the victims of neglect or abuse. This may emerge on finding characteristic physical signs at a routine examination, or witnessing abnormal behaviour on the part of the child. The older child may take the opportunity of a routine contact with a doctor or nurse to disclose abuse. Types of child abuse are shown in Table 3.22.

Approach to the child where abuse is suspected

The clinical evaluation of a child who is the victim or suspected victim of abuse or neglect requires skill. Enough time must be allowed so the evaluation is not rushed, and the setting private to ensure confidentiality. The doctor's attitude is important as it is vital to gain both the child's and, where possible, the family's trust. There is no place for the doctor to be accusatory in any way.

The evaluation must be thorough, including a full history and physical examination, or important clues may be missed. If injuries are present it is important to decide whether they were incurred accidentally or could have been inflicted.

It is important to contact other professionals such as social workers, the GP and the school, who may throw light on the child's home circumstances.

History

• *How was the injury incurred?* The most important part of the history is the explanation given for any injuries found, which helps determine whether the lesions are likely to have occurred non-accidentally. Characteristically, in non-accidental injury the explanation given does not match the

Characteristics of non-accidental injury
• Injuries in very young children
• Explanations which do not match the appearance of the injury and sound unconvincing
• Multiple types and age of injury
• Injuries which are 'classic' in site or character
• Delay in presentation
• Things the child may communicate during the evaluation

Table 3.22 Types of child abuse

Physical neglect
Emotional abuse
Non-accidental injury
Sexual abuse
Non-organic failure to thrive (see p. 67)

appearance of the injury and often sounds unconvincing. There is often a delay before medical advice is sought. It is suspicious if young, not yet mobile infants get injured. The child may communicate details which conflict with the parental explanation.

• *Past medical history.* A history of previous injuries is obviously relevant.

• *Developmental history and behaviour.* A child's psychosocial development can be severely affected by neglect and abuse, and an assessment can also be useful to serve as a baseline for the future.

• *Social history and family history.* In order to gain a complete picture a full social history is required. It is important to know who is in the home, and who other than the mother is responsible for caring for the child. Child abuse is more likely to occur in unstable homes where there are changes of partner. Other professionals such as health visitors and nursery nurses can often provide important details about the family.

Physical examination

A thorough physical examination with the child completely undressed is always mandatory.

1 *General appearance.* The appearance of the child must be noted. The child may show signs of neglect, such as an unkempt dirty appearance, sores and untreated nappy rash. The child's reaction to the examiner is important. The child who has experienced prolonged abuse may have a 'frozen

Focal points Evaluating child abuse
• Evaluations should be conducted in privacy and the child's trust gained
• Helpful information can be obtained from other health professionals and social services
• If injuries are present, indications that they have been inflicted must be sought in the history and physical appearance
• A thorough examination, including growth and general appearance must be made to identify other injuries, failure to thrive and signs of neglect
• Comprehensive clear notes must be made and where necessary photographs taken as they may be required for evidence

watchful' appearance; appear motionless, with an expressionless face and wary eyes. The neglected child may be abnormally affectionate to strangers as if seeking any human contact.

2 *Growth.* Abused and neglected children commonly fail to thrive. Height, length, weight and head circumference need to be measured, plotted and compared with previous measurements.

3 *Injuries.* The child should be examined for signs of injury. Many injuries incurred non-accidentally have a characteristic appearance, and multiple injuries at different sites and of different ages are particularly suspicious.

- *Bruises.* Multiple bruises are commonly found on the legs of any toddler, but bruises at other sites may be suspicious. The age of the bruises can be estimated from the colour and may help in refuting an implausible explanation. The pattern of the bruise may indicate how it was acquired (Fig. 3.25a–d).
- *Burns and scalds.* When a toddler accidentally scalds him- or herself the scald is usually irregular and asymmetrical in shape with additional splash marks. Inflicted scalds are classically symmetrical and may cause a doughnut-shaped lesion on the buttocks, which are centrally spared where the bottom of the bath protects the skin from contact with the hot water (Fig. 3.25c). Inflicted cigarette burns cause deep circular ulcers (Fig. 3.25e) as compared with superficial lesions seen with accidental burns.
- *Bites.* Lesions are found in the shape of a dental impression. These can be used forensically to identify the perpetrator (Fig. 3.25g).
- *Hidden head injuries.* The fundi should be examined for retinal haemorrhages (p. 76) as they may occur when a baby is shaken and indicate the presence of subdural haematomas (see p. 75).
- *Bone injuries* (Fig. 3.26). Clinical evidence of fractures may be found.

4 *Signs of sexual abuse.* If the child discloses sexual abuse or is suspected of being a victim, examination of the genitalia and anus is required. Signs of sexual abuse may be overt such as bruising and tears, or may be more subtle, and the absence of physical signs does not in any way refute the possibility that a child has been sexually abused. The examination should only be carried out by an experienced paediatrician in a setting where the child's privacy can be respected.

Investigations

Table 3.23 shows the investigations which may be helpful in children suspected of being victims of abuse. If suspicious injuries are found, photographs should be taken so that they are available for future consultation and evidence in court.

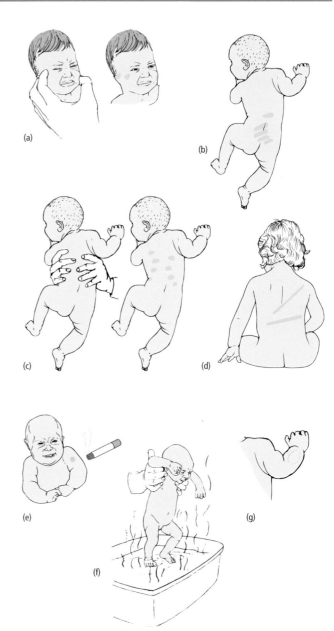

Fig. 3.25 Skin lesions indicative of non-accidental injury: (a) facial squeeze, (b) slap marks, (c) grip marks, (d) stick marks, (e) cigarette burns, (f) scalding, and (g) bite marks.

As the implications of non-accidental injury are so serious, rare medical causes of excessive bruising or fragile bones must be ruled out. A full blood count, bleeding time and clotting screen will identify a haematological cause for bruising. In the case of fractures, osteogenesis imperfecta (brittle bone disease) may be considered and can usually be ruled out on clinical evaluation.

In any child suspected of being a victim of abuse or neglect a skeletal survey (X-ray of the entire body) should be requested to determine whether there have been previous

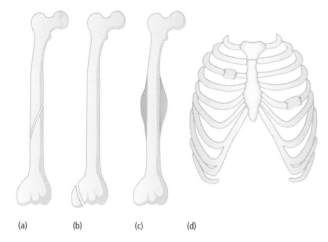

Fig. 3.26 Types of fractures associated with non-accidental injury: (a) spiral fractures, (b) metaphyseal chips, (c) periosteal bleeds, and (d) callus around ribs.

Clinical features of physical abuse

- Physical neglect

- Failure to thrive

- Bruises

- Fractures

- Burns and scalds

- Bites

- Ligature marks

Table 3.23 Investigations in suspected child abuse

Investigation	Relevance
Photographs	Useful for further consultation and evidence in court
Full blood count, bleeding time, prothrombin time and partial thromboplastin time	To rule out thrombocytopenia or other haematological disorder as a cause for excessive bruising
Skeletal survey (X-rays)	Characteristic fractures and fractures at various stages of healing may be found in non-accidental injury
Pregnancy test and cultures for sexually transmitted disease	In children suspected of sexual abuse the finding of sexually transmitted disease is strong corroborative evidence (and needs treating)

unreported injuries. Fractures that have been inflicted often have a characteristic appearance and tend to occur through the growthplate as this is the most vulnerable part of growing bones. Spiral fractures are particularly likely to result from violent inflicted trauma. When multiple fractures are found they are often seen to be at different stages of healing.

The child who has disclosed sexual abuse needs to be investigated for sexually transmitted diseases, and forensic samples taken. A pregnancy test is needed in the postpubertal girl who has been raped.

Management

Where there is any suspicion that a child has suffered abuse or neglect, the child should be referred immediately for the specialist opinion of a paediatrician experienced in child protection work. If he or she concludes that the child has been abused or is at risk of abuse the social services department is immediately informed.

If the child is deemed to be in danger, or further assessment is required, he or she needs to be admitted to a place of safety, usually a hospital ward or a social services institution until a fuller inquiry can be made. An emergency care order can be obtained from court if the family resists admission or investigation.

The social work team usually take the lead in planning the strategy for management. Initial policy is worked out at a case conference, attended by all professionals involved and the parents. Many children are allowed home, initially under supervision and with appropriate support. Occasionally it is necessary to take the child away from the parents. This is generally a difficult decision and requires a court order. The child may be placed with another member of the family, in foster care or, in the case of an older child, a group home.

For the child returned to his or her home, support must be provided. This may be in the form of placement in a social service day nursery, or voluntary and self-help groups may be available to help the parents overcome their difficulties. Social services departments keep a record, the Child Protection Register, of children who have been abused or neglected, so that professionals can readily determine if a child or others in the family are known to be at risk.

Types of abuse and neglect

Physical abuse (non-accidental injury)

Parents who abuse their children come from all ethnic and socioeconomic groups. In most cases the abuser is a related caretaker or male friend of the mother. Most have neither psychotic nor criminal personalities, but tend to be unhappy, lonely, angry adults under stress, who have often themselves experienced physical abuse as children. The event often coincides with the loss of a job or a home, marital strife or physical exhaustion.

Clinical features Injuries may range in severity from minor bruises to fatal subdural haematomas. Characteristic injuries are shown in Fig. 3.25.

Management The injuries, if severe, require medical attention. The general management of abused children is discussed above.

Prognosis About 5% of abused children who are returned to their parents without intervention are killed and 25%

seriously injured. Children with repeated injury to the central nervous system may develop brain damage with learning disabilities or epilepsy. Abused children are commonly fearful, aggressive and hyperactive, and many go on to become delinquent, violent and the next generation of abusers.

Munchausen by proxy

In this bizarre form of abuse the carer fabricates the child's symptoms or signs. The child is likely to become subject to extensive hospitalization and investigations, and may be in actual physical danger (as when apnoea is fabricated by suffocation). The diagnosis is difficult to make, but must be suspected if the presentation is unusual and incongruous, and if symptoms and signs emerge in the parent's presence alone.

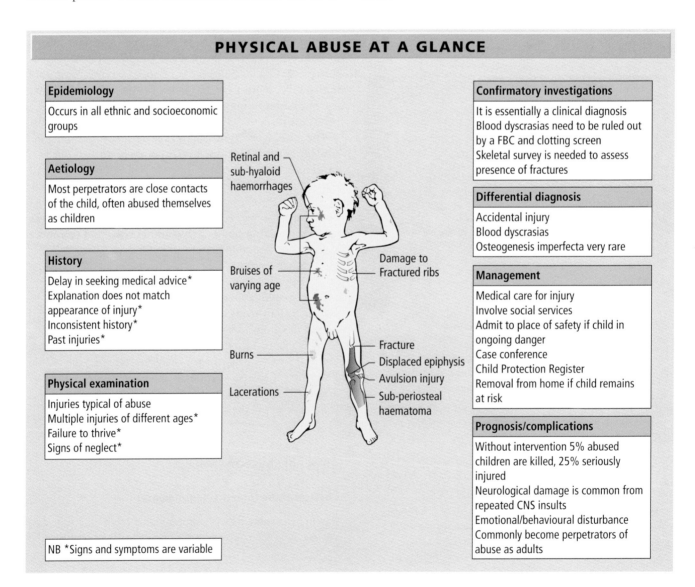

PHYSICAL ABUSE AT A GLANCE

Epidemiology

Occurs in all ethnic and socioeconomic groups

Aetiology

Most perpetrators are close contacts of the child, often abused themselves as children

History

Delay in seeking medical advice*
Explanation does not match appearance of injury*
Inconsistent history*
Past injuries*

Physical examination

Injuries typical of abuse
Multiple injuries of different ages*
Failure to thrive*
Signs of neglect*

NB *Signs and symptoms are variable

Retinal and sub-hyaloid haemorrhages

Bruises of varying age

Burns

Lacerations

Damage to
Fractured ribs

Fracture
Displaced epiphysis
Avulsion injury
Sub-periosteal haematoma

Confirmatory investigations

It is essentially a clinical diagnosis
Blood dyscrasias need to be ruled out by a FBC and clotting screen
Skeletal survey is needed to assess presence of fractures

Differential diagnosis

Accidental injury
Blood dyscrasias
Osteogenesis imperfecta very rare

Management

Medical care for injury
Involve social services
Admit to place of safety if child in ongoing danger
Case conference
Child Protection Register
Removal from home if child remains at risk

Prognosis/complications

Without intervention 5% abused children are killed, 25% seriously injured
Neurological damage is common from repeated CNS insults
Emotional/behavioural disturbance
Commonly become perpetrators of abuse as adults

Emotional abuse

Emotional abuse can be defined as the frequent rejection, scapegoating, isolation or terrorizing of a child by caretakers. It is usually very difficult to prove, and has long-term emotional and developmental consequences for the child.

Sexual abuse

Sexual abuse may take the form of inappropriate touching, forced exposure to sexual acts, vaginal, oral or rectal intercourse and sexual assault. Secrecy is often enforced by the offender, who is usually male and a family member or acquaintance of the family, but rarely a stranger.

Clinical features Sexual abuse may come to light if disclosure is made as a result of genital infections or trauma, or if a child exhibits inappropriate sexual behaviour. Signs of trauma may be evident in the mouth, anus or genitalia, but absence of signs is common and less than half of the victims have any substantiating physical evidence.

Management Particularly sensitive and skilled management is required and should only be undertaken by those experienced in the work. All victims require psychological support, and the offender too may be amenable to help.

Prognosis With intervention most incest victims can lead normal adult lives. Without intervention they are likely to become seriously disturbed and grow up unable to form close relationships. Victims commonly enter abusive relationships with men later in life and often need psychiatric help.

Non-organic failure to thrive

A proportion of young children who fail to thrive (see p. 67) do so as a result of neglect, the principal factor being inadequate nutrition. The mother is commonly deprived and unloved herself and often is clinically depressed.

Clinical features The child looks malnourished and uncared for, and immunizations are often not up to date. Delays in development are common, and signs of physical abuse may be seen. When admitted to hospital these babies often show rapid weight gain.

Management If the problem is clearly one of neglect, child protection procedures must be initiated.

Prognosis Without detection and intervention a small proportion of these children die from starvation. With intervention, catch-up growth may occur, but brain growth may be jeopardized and emotional and educational problems are common.

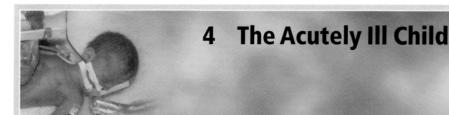

4 The Acutely Ill Child

Introduction, 100
Presentation of acute illness, 100
The febrile child, 101
Common infections causing fever in
   childhood, 103
Dehydration, 116

Causes of dehydration, 119
Acute wheeze, 119
Causes of wheeze, 122
Stridor, 126
Causes of stridor, 128
Jaundice, 128

Causes of jaundice, 131
Acute abdominal pain, 132
Causes of acute abdominal pain, 135
The generalized convulsion, 138
Causes of generalized convulsions, 140

Christopher Robin
Had wheezles
And sneezles,
They bundled him
Into
His Bed.
. . . They examined his chest
For a rash,
And the rest
Of his body for swellings and lumps.

Now We are Six
A.A. Milne

Introduction

Every child from time to time becomes suddenly unwell and exhibits acute symptoms. These symptoms are usually mild, self-limiting and may not cause particular anxiety to parents. Fever is the commonest symptom of acute illness in childhood and is often accompanied by malaise and irritability. This chapter discusses commoner acute symptoms of childhood and diseases which cause them.

It is usually the primary care doctor who first sees the child with acute symptoms and who must decide whether the child should be referred to hospital or whether it is safe to leave the child at home. It is important for the doctor to be able to recognize the ill child. This is more difficult in young babies as they often show very few specific symptoms or signs of serious infection. It is necessary to approach acute symptoms in babies in a very careful and methodical manner in order to detect those with serious illness or those with progressive signs suggestive of severe illness.

Pathophysiology

In paediatrics a variety of factors predispose children to develop acute illness (Table 4.1). The commonest cause of

acute illness in children is infection. Predisposition to infectious disease is dependent on a number of factors:

1 *Age*. Newborn babies are particularly prone to infection. This is usually bacterial and acquired either from mother (perinatal) or carers (nosocomial). Beyond the newborn period, infectious diseases are usually acquired through contact with other children, and the age at which a child starts nursery or playgroup is commonly the time at which they have 'one infection after another'. Second and subsequent children are more likely to contract illnesses from their older siblings than first-born babies who meet other children less regularly.

2 *Immunity*. This may be passive or active. (a) *Passive immunity*. Babies are born with passive immunity acquired from the maternal transfusion of IgG which occurs in the last 3 months of pregnancy. Premature infants miss out on this transfer and are more prone to infection. The maternally acquired IgG protects babies against certain types of infection for 3–6 months and serious infectious diseases are very uncommon in this time. (b) *Active immunity*. This is based on Ig mediated memory of infectious agents acquired through contact with these agents. This is the basis of immunization. Natural immunity is also mediated through polymorphonuclear leucocytes, complement, lysozyme and interferon.

3 *Immunodeficiency* The immune response may be impaired by prematurity, malnourishment, drugs (steroids in particular), malignant disease and its management and, rarely, an inherited or acquired abnormality in their immune function. AIDS is still a very rare cause of immune deficiency in childhood and congenital immune deficiency disorders are also rare.

Presentation of acute illness

Presentation of acute illness depends to an extent on the age of the child. Babies and young children obviously cannot

Table 4.1 Factors predisposing to the development of severe and acute illness in children

Factor	Risk group
Age	Neonates
	Infants <1 year
Impaired immune function	Premature infants
	Steroid treatment
	Malignancy
	Immune deficiency (AIDS)
Malnutrition	e.g. Malabsorption
Chronic disease	e.g. Cystic fibrosis
Immunization status	
Exposure to infectious agents	Children in hospital
	Institutionalized children

Table 4.2 Features to look for in determining whether a baby in the first 6 months of life is acutely ill. (From Baby Check*)

Symptom	Particular features to consider
Vomiting	Regular vomiting
	Bile stained vomiting
Fluid intake	Reduction of one-third on normal 24 hour volume
Urine output	Fewer wet nappies than expected
Blood in stool	Frank blood in stool
Drowsiness	Abnormally drowsy most of time
Abnormal cry	High pitched
Floppiness	Persistent and generalized
Alertness	Less watchful of mother
	Less interested in environment
Wheeze	Expiratory
Recession	Deep indrawing of intercostal or subcostal area
Pallor	
Cyanosis of periphery	
Skin perfusion	Is there a significant delay in reperfusion of big toe after squeezing?
Swelling in groin	Is there an inguinal hernia?
Rash on trunk	Generalized?
Pyrexia	Rectal temperature >38.3°C

verbalize their distress. The older the child the more specific the symptom will be and the greater the ability to describe the site of any pain. Physical signs may also vary with age, for example signs such as Kernig's or neck stiffness are specific in older children, but in very young children meningitis is not associated with Kernig's sign and neck stiffness may not occur at all or occur very late in the illness.

For these reasons, assessing whether a baby of 6 months of age or less is significantly ill may be difficult and attempts have been made to develop easily applied rating scores to evaluate how ill a baby is. The Baby Check* is designed to be used by parents and depends on symptoms and signs over the previous 24 hours as well as examination findings. Each item is given a score and the total score can be read off from a scale to indicate whether the baby is mildly, moderately or seriously ill. The major features of the

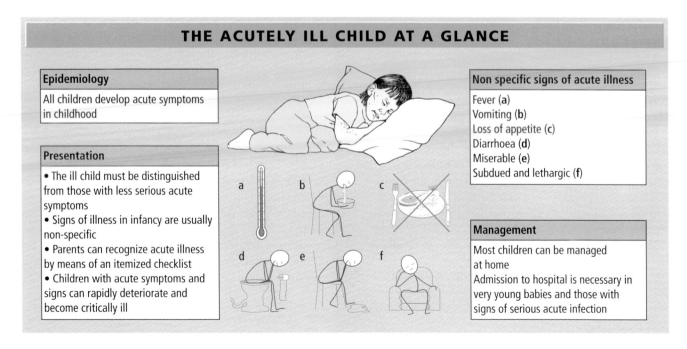

THE ACUTELY ILL CHILD AT A GLANCE

Epidemiology

All children develop acute symptoms in childhood

Presentation

• The ill child must be distinguished from those with less serious acute symptoms
• Signs of illness in infancy are usually non-specific
• Parents can recognize acute illness by means of an itemized checklist
• Children with acute symptoms and signs can rapidly deteriorate and become critically ill

Non specific signs of acute illness

Fever (**a**)
Vomiting (**b**)
Loss of appetite (**c**)
Diarrhoea (**d**)
Miserable (**e**)
Subdued and lethargic (**f**)

Management

Most children can be managed at home
Admission to hospital is necessary in very young babies and those with signs of serious acute infection

* C.J. Morley, A.J. Thornton, T.J. Cole, P.H. Hewson & M.A. Fowler. Baby check: a scoring system to grade the severity of acute systemic illness in babies under 6 months old. *Archives of Disease in Childhood* 1991, **66**, 100–6.

Table 4.3 Signs of acute and potentially severe illness in older children

Symptom	Features
Toxicity	This includes a high fever with marked facial flushing and confusion
	Hallucinations may occur with high fever
Severe pain	Associated with pallor, tachycardia, immobility or writhing
Change in conscious level	This is always significant of severe illness
Shortness of breath	Causing difficulty in speaking
Dehydration	See p. 116
'Going off their feet'	Any acute difficulty in walking or unsteadiness of gait

Table 4.4 Common causes of acute fever in childhood

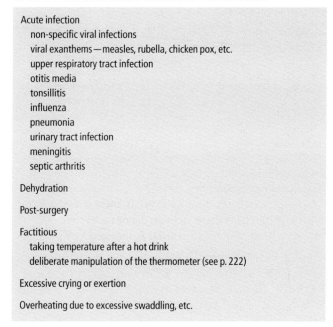

Acute infection
  non-specific viral infections
  viral exanthems—measles, rubella, chicken pox, etc.
  upper respiratory tract infection
  otitis media
  tonsillitis
  influenza
  pneumonia
  urinary tract infection
  meningitis
  septic arthritis

Dehydration

Post-surgery

Factitious
  taking temperature after a hot drink
  deliberate manipulation of the thermometer (see p. 222)

Excessive crying or exertion

Overheating due to excessive swaddling, etc.

Baby Check are shown in Table 4.2. The signs of acute and potentially severe illness in older children are shown in Table 4.3.

A child may become critically ill very rapidly and it is essential to recognize symptoms or signs including:
- shock (see p. 303 for definition);
- coma;
- acute cyanosis;
- profound apnoea;
- major trauma;
- progressive purpuric rash (see p. 198).

Critically ill children must be rushed to hospital for resuscitation and supportive care without delay. The problem of the critically ill child is described in Chapter 9.

THE FEBRILE CHILD

A fever is a temperature above 37.0°C. Fever is a very common symptom in children, but the height of the fever does not correlate with the severity of the illness. High fever occurs in many non-serious conditions.

Fever is the body's response to pyrogens. These usually arise as a result of infection, but may occur because of chronic inflammation or an immune response. Pyrogens have an effect on the brain nuclei responsible for temperature control. The body's response to fever is to lose heat by skin vasodilatation. This causes the flush that is often seen in feverish children.

There are very many causes of acute fever in childhood. The commoner causes are listed in Table 4.4.

Pyrexia of unexplained origin is a condition where there has been prolonged or intermittent fever unexplained by physical examination and investigations. This is discussed in more detail on p. 220.

The approach to the child with a fever

The diagnosis of fever is usually made by a parent detecting that a child feels hot and is confirmed by taking the child's temperature.

Taking the temperature

In children old enough to cooperate, temperature is measured by placing the bulb of the thermometer under the tongue for 1 minute. In younger children the thermometer is placed in the axilla and the arm held down by the child's side for 3–5 minutes. Axillary temperatures are 0.5°C lower than oral or rectal temperatures. Core body temperature is normally 37.5°C and is measured by inserting a suitable thermometer in the rectum. This is the most convenient method in infants or unconscious children.

Disposable plastic strip chemical thermometers are widely available. These are most reliable if placed in the axilla for 3 minutes, but have been shown to register slightly higher temperatures than the mercury in glass thermometers. The commercially available plastic strip thermometer that is placed on the child's forehead is not a reliable way of measuring temperature but may be used at home to indicate to parents that a child needs treatment (see Febrile convulsions, pp. 140–1).

History

The following points should be elicited.
- *Character of fever.* Duration and whether it occurs at particular times of the day.
- *Pain.* Has the child complained of earache, difficulty in

swallowing (dysphagia), dysuria or frequency? Excessive crying in an infant may be a feature of pain.

• *General features*. Enquire about the child's appetite, whether there has been malaise and how long it has lasted.

• *Associated symptoms*. These are non-specific of any particular type of infection and include vomiting, coryza, cough and rash.

Examination

A full physical examination is required in all children with fever. Leave the examination of throat and ears to the end as this often upsets young children.

• *General*. Does the child look ill? Is there a rash? Is the child dehydrated? Is there tachycardia or tachypnoea?

• *Throat*. Determine if the throat is infected or the tonsils inflamed or have an exudate.

• *Ears*. Examine the tympanic membranes. Are they red and/or bulging?

• *Chest*. Are there signs of respiratory distress? Auscultate for crepitations.

• *Central nervous system*. Is the child orientated? Is the child floppy? In older children assess for the presence of neck stiffness or Kernig's sign.

Investigations

In young babies there may be few or no localizing signs of infection and investigations are mandatory in these cases to elicit the cause of the fever (Table 4.5).

At any age urinary tract infection (UTI) should be suspected as the cause of fever. The only way to confirm or exclude this is by microbiological culture of the urine and this should be done if no other focus of infection can be found.

Management

Fever, an unpleasant symptom, should be treated when the temperature exceeds 38.5°C or if the child is uncomfortable with a fever below that level.

Fever is treated by a number of methods.

• Undress the child. Many parents' reaction to a fever is to wrap the child with blankets. This must be strongly discouraged.

• Antipyretics of which paracetamol (Calpol) is most widely used. Aspirin should not be given to children because of its association with the development of severe liver disease (Reye's syndrome).

• Sponging or tepid baths. Heat loss is encouraged by wetting the skin to allow vasodilatation and evaporative heat loss. Tepid water should be used rather than cold, which causes vasoconstriction and may increase body temperature.

Early and effective treatment of fever is particularly important in children prone to febrile convulsions (p. 140).

Table 4.5 Investigations which may be indicated in a child with fever (these are always required in an infant <8 weeks old)

Investigation	Significance
Full blood count	Elevated white cell count with increased granulocytes suggests bacterial infection
Throat swab	Isolation of beta-haemolytic streptococcus requires treatment with penicillin
Rectal swab for culture	Identification of gastrointestinal pathogen
Blood cultures	Isolation indicates probable septicaemia Multiple organisms suggest contamination
Lumbar puncture	See p. 109 and also Table 12.9, p. 361
Chest X-ray	Consolidation (generalized or focal) indicates pneumonia
Urine analysis and culture	$>10^5$ pure growth of organisms, with white cells, red cells and protein present, indicates infection (pp. 111, 361)

Focal points
Evaluation of the febrile child

• Confirm presence of fever

• Assess whether child requires hospital admission

• Examine for focal signs of infection

• If a child is acutely ill, re-evaluate when fever settles

• Admit and investigate babies below 8 weeks of age

Principles of management
The febrile child

• Determine the cause of the fever

• In young babies a full infection screen is necessary

• Investigations may be necessary in older children if the site of infection not obvious

• Start antibiotics only where clinically indicated

• Take measures to reduce temperature

COMMON INFECTIONS CAUSING FEVER IN CHILDHOOD

Upper respiratory tract infection

Upper respiratory tract infection (URTI) is very common in young children, particularly when they first start playgroup and later as 4–5-year-olds when they start school. They are exposed to a large number of viral organisms for the first time for which they have no immunity. The mother often describes her child as having 'one cold after another', but mothers (and doctors) should understand that frequent mild infections in these young children are common and benign.

The main cause of URTI is either coryza or acute pharyngitis. The commonest cause of coryza is a rhinovirus, but a number of other viruses can produce similar symptoms. Acute pharyngitis is a very common viral infection.

Clinical features Coryza presents with running nose (rhinitis) and sneezing. Fever is variable. After a few days the child's nose becomes blocked with consequent mouth breathing. Upper respiratory tract infection is commonly associated with cough for which the child may unnecessarily receive repeated courses of antibiotics.

On physical examination purulent mucus is visible in the nares or running down the upper lip. The tympanic membranes may be infected. In acute pharyngitis the pharynx, the soft palate and the tonsillar fauces are inflamed and swollen. There is often cervical lymphadenopathy.

Investigation is unnecessary unless the child has a tonsillar exudate when a throat swab for culture may be taken.

Management Treatment is symptomatic. In infants, nasal obstruction may be a particular problem as young babies are obligate nose breathers and cannot breathe through their mouths. Either saline or 0.5% ephedrine nasal drops immediately before feeds is helpful. Ephedrine should not be used for more than a few days at a time because of the risk of mucosal hypertrophy.

Fever in older children is treated with antipyretics and nasal obstruction may be relieved by a decongestant. Antibiotics are not indicated for uncomplicated URTI.

Tonsillitis

Tonsillitis is usually caused by a viral infection, particularly in young children. In children over 5 years, the commonest bacterial organism is the group A beta-haemolytic streptococcus.

Clinical features The child is feverish and may complain of a sore throat. In younger children, pain may not be localized to the throat but they may complain of abdominal pain probably because of mesenteric adenitis.

On examination the tonsils are enlarged and inflamed. It is important to recognize that the tonsils normally enlarge rapidly from birth to reach maximum size by 4–5 years and then get smaller. Normal tonsillar enlargement should not be confused with enlargement caused by infection.

Acute follicular tonsillitis is usually due to bacterial tonsillitis when associated with a white exudate (Fig. 4.1). The white exudate must be differentiated from the creamy material which may be visible in the tonsillar crypts and does not necessarily indicate infection. Exudate on the tonsil must also make the doctor rule out infectious mononucleosis and diphtheria, although the latter is very rare as a result of immunization.

Cervical lymphadenopathy occurs in most children with bacterial tonsillitis (see Fig. 2.23, p. 30). In particular, the jugulodigastric nodes, palpated just below the angle of the jaw, are enlarged and painful.

Throat swab should be performed where there is the clinical possibility of bacterial infection (exudate, systemic illness, frequent recurrences and tender cervical lymphadenopathy).

Management Symptomatic treatment with saline gargles and paracetamol is helpful. Most cases of tonsillitis in young children do not require antibiotics, but these are indicated in children with exudate and systemic symptoms.

Streptococcal tonsillitis should be treated with benzyl penicillin for 10 days. Tonsillectomy is only rarely indicated even in recurrent tonsillitis.

Prognosis Some complications are given below.
• Otitis media.
• Chronic tonsillitis. Upper airway obstruction and sleep apnoea is an important complication of chronically enlarged tonsils and this requires tonsillectomy.
• Peritonsillar abscess (quinsy).

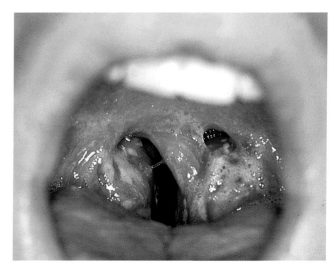

Fig. 4.1 Exudate in acute follicular tonsillitis.

TONSILLITIS AT A GLANCE

Epidemiology

Common, except under 24 months

Aetiology

Beta-haemolytic Strep, Group A
Viral

History

Sore throat, dysphagia
Fever
Abdominal pain

Physical examination

Large inflamed tonsils with exudate
Cervical lymphadenopathy

NB *Signs and symptoms are variable

Confirmatory investigations

Throat swab grows beta-haemolytic
Strep, Group A

Differential diagnosis

Viral pharyngitis
Infectious mononucleosis

Management

Antipyretics for fever
Gargles
Penicillin for 10 days

Prognosis/complications

Recurrent tonsillitis ⎤
Otitis media   ⎦ Most common
Peritonsillar abscess (rare but serious)
Acute glomerulonephritis (certain
strains of Strep only)

• Post-streptococcal allergic disorders, e.g. acute glomerulonephritis (p. 189).

Otitis media

This is an extremely common childhood disorder and occurs most frequently in the first 7 years of life. It may occur in the neonate. The commonest infecting organisms are *Streptococcus pneumoniae*, *Haemophilus influenzae* and viruses.

Otitis media is especially common in conditions associated with eustachian tube dysfunction because fluid cannot drain from the middle ear. Eustachian tube dysfunction occurs in the following situations.
1 The common cold.
2 Obstruction caused by adenoidal hypertrophy.
3 Functional disorders:
   • cleft palate;
   • Down's syndrome.

Clinical features Presentation is with fever, painful ear and hearing loss. It is usually preceded by an URTI. In younger children, anorexia, vomiting and diarrhoea may be the presenting features and there may be no obvious symptoms pointing to the ear as the source of infection. For this reason routine aural examination (p. 28) should be performed on all febrile children. Examination of the ear reveals the tympanic membrane to be inflamed and bulging, with loss of the light reflex (see Fig. 2.21).

Perforation of the tympanic membrane may occur spontaneously and on examination the perforation may be obscured by pus in the auditory meatus. There are no specific investigations. The diagnosis is made on otoscopic findings.

Management All children with a clinical diagnosis of otitis media should be treated with ampicillin as the antibiotic of choice. Children should be re-evaluated 2 weeks after starting treatment. If the ear is abnormal at that time, further examination should be undertaken 4 weeks later. Persistent abnormality may indicate serous otitis media (see below).

Prognosis Most cases of otitis media resolve satisfactorily even if perforation has occurred. Complications may occur and include:
• secretory otitis media;
• conductive deafness (p. 284);
• mastoiditis (p. 229).

Secretory otitis media and glue ear

During episodes of otitis media, inflammation develops

OTITIS MEDIA AT A GLANCE

Epidemiology

Common, especially as a complication of URTI

Aetiology

Viral
Haemophilus infuenzae
Streptococcus pneumonia

History

Ear pain and hearing loss (older child)
Irritability (younger child)
Fever*
URTI symptoms

Physical examination

Bulging inflamed tympanic membrane

NB *Signs and symptoms are variable

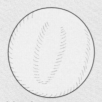

(a) Bulging tympanic membrane (acute otitis media)

(b) Retracted tympanic membrane (glue ear)

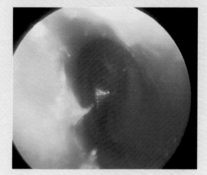

Confirmatory investigations

None

Differential diagnosis

URTI
Secretory otitis media

Management

Oral antibiotics in all cases as no cultures available to confirm organism

Complications

Perforated ear drum with discharge (generally heals well)
Chronic secretory otitis media with or without conductive hearing loss
Mastoiditis

---

within the middle ear. Antibiotics eradicate the infection and the inflammatory fluid drains through the eustachian tube. Repeated episodes of acute secretory otitis media may lead to inadequate drainage of the inflammatory fluid because of eustachian tube dysfunction. This leads to thickening of the fluid leaving a thick, glue-like exudate which causes progressive immobility of the ossicles with conductive hearing impairment (p. 284).

The treatment of deafness resulting from glue ear is drainage of the middle ear structures by placing a very small plastic drainage tube (a grommet) through the tympanic membrane. This allows aeration of the middle ear structures with breakdown of the glue-like material. Eventually the grommet drops out and the tympanic membrane heals spontaneously. All children with a history of recurrent otitis media should have a hearing assessment to detect mild or moderate conductive hearing loss.

Non-specific viral infections

Febrile illnesses of a non-specific nature are caused by a number of viruses of which the influenza virus is one. These viruses are spread by droplet from the upper respiratory tract of affected children and adults.

Clinical features Children usually present with a brief but acute illness with fever, malaise, chills, headache, cough and myalgia. An erythematous rash is a relatively common symptom. The term 'influenza' is often used to describe these symptoms.

There are no specific physical signs on examination. It is rarely necessary to undertake a viral screen to identify the causative agent.

Management Treatment is symptomatic with antipyretics. Antibiotics are only necessary if there is evidence of secondary bacterial infection.

Prognosis Some children are particularly susceptible to viral infections such as those who have cystic fibrosis, congenital heart disease or those who are immunosuppressed. These children should receive regular influenza immunization.

Pneumonia

Pneumonia is caused by a wide range of viral and bacterial organisms (Table 4.6). *Streptococcus pneumoniae* often causes lobar pneumonia.

Predisposing factors to acute pneumonia should always be considered in children who present with pneumonia. These include:
- congenital abnormality of the bronchi;
- inhaled foreign body;

Table 4.6 The commoner organisms causing pneumonia

Bacterial
Streptococcus pneumoniae (especially in younger children)
Mycoplasma pneumoniae (more insidious onset)
Haemophilus influenza (uncommon in Britain)
Group B beta-haemolytic streptococcus (only in the newborn)

Viral
Respiratory syncytial virus
Influenza viruses
Parainfluenza
Adenovirus
Coxsackie viruses

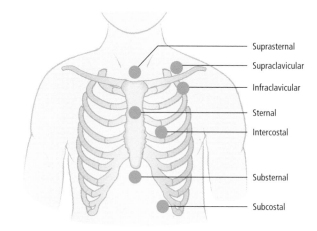

Fig. 4.2 Sites of recession.

PNEUMONIA AT A GLANCE

Aetiology

Viral (particularly RSV in infants)
Strep. pneumoniae at all ages
Mycoplasma pneumoniae at school age
Staphylococcus aureus, Haemophilus influenzae uncommon

History

Fever
Cough
Respiratory distress
Shoulder tip/abdominal pain*
Sputum production in older child*

Physical examination

Tachypnoea
Nasal flaring
Intercostal/subcostal regression
Grunting in infants
Meningism*

Confirmatory investigations

Chest X-ray: focal consolidation suggests bacterial cause; diffuse consolidation suggests viral
Blood count: leucocytosis and shift to left if bacterial
Blood culture
Cold agglutinins in older child for mycoplasma

NB *Signs and symptoms are variable

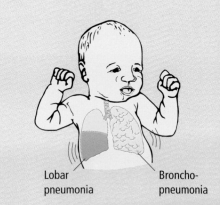

Lobar pneumonia   Broncho-pneumonia

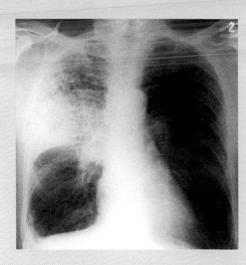

Differential diagnosis

URTI
Bronchiolitis
Acute bronchitis
Asthma
Non-specific viral infection
Inhaled foreign body

Management

Appropriate antibiotic (based on appearance of chest X-ray); often amoxicillin or IV penicillin if acutely ill
Antipyretics
Repeat chest X-ray 1 month post-treatment
Cough syrup unnecessary

Prognosis/complications

Complete recovery usual
Rare complications include:
• lung abscess
• empyema
• pneumothorax
• septicaemia
• bronchiectasis

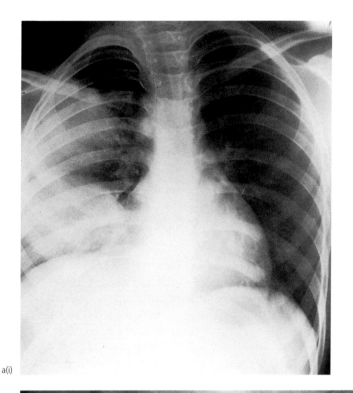

a(i)

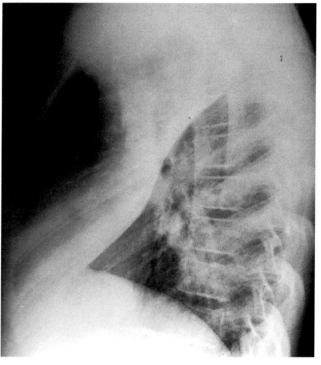

a(ii)

(b)

Fig. 4.3 (a[i]) Chest X-ray of a boy presenting with fever and cough. Consolidation of the right upper and middle lobes are seen. (a[ii]) The lateral film shows the consolidation clearly delineated posteriorly by the oblique fissure. (b) X-ray of a child with viral pneumonia. Diffuse shadowing is seen throughout the lung fields.

- persistent lobar collapse;
- chronic aspiration;
- large left to right intracardiac shunt;
- immunocompromise.

Clinical features The child with acute pneumonia presents with a short history of fever, cough and signs of respiratory distress. These signs include tachypnoea, nasal flaring, intercostal and subcostal recession (Fig. 4.2). Grunting is a common feature in infants. Meningismus may be present and shoulder tip or abdominal pain can divert attention from the correct diagnosis.

Clinical signs include dullness to percussion indicating underlying consolidation. Crepitations are commonly heard. In young children, in contrast to adults, focal signs may not correlate with the anatomical site of infection seen on the X-ray.

Diagnosis is made by X-ray and may show focal (confined to a lobe) or diffuse changes (Fig. 4.3). Sputum (obtained in older, cooperative children) and blood cultures should be taken which may isolate the infecting organism. Cold agglutinins are present in the serum in cases of *Mycoplasma pneumoniae*.

Management Antibiotics should be used in all cases of pneumonia. If the child is acutely ill then intravenous penicillin is given, alternatively oral amoxycillin is appropriate in a less ill child. A repeat chest X-ray should be obtained 1 month after stopping treatment to ensure that the X-ray changes have fully resolved.

Prognosis Complications of pneumonia include:
• lung abscess (rare, but may follow staphylococcus infection);
• empyema (infected pleural effusion);
• pneumothorax;
• septicaemia with infective foci elsewhere;
• bronchiectasis (following pertussis or measles in malnourished children);
• pleural effusion.

Meningitis

Meningitis is a common and serious illness in childhood. It is commonest in the neonatal period (p. 256), but even excluding neonatal meningitis, one in 200 children develop this condition in the first 10 years of life. Meningitis is caused by either viral or bacterial infection invading the membranes overlying the brain and spinal cord. Bacterial infections usually remain confined to the meninges, but viruses may invade the underlying brain causing meningoencephalitis. The viral and bacterial organisms commonly causing meningitis are shown in Table 4.7.

Clinical features Viral meningitis is usually preceded by pharyngitis or gastrointestinal upset. The child then develops fever, headache and neck stiffness. The classical features of head retraction as seen in adults are late features of meningitis in children. Neck stiffness is not a reliable sign in infants, and the diagnosis must be considered in any irritable febrile child.

In bacterial meningitis, drowsiness is an early feature; the

Table 4.7 Causes of meningitis outside of the neonatal period

Viral causes
Mumps virus
Coxsackie viruses
ECHO virus
Herpes simplex
Poliomyelitis (only in developing countries)

Bacterial causes
Haemophilus influenza type B (commoner in younger children)
Neisseria meningitidis (commonest cause in UK)
Streptococcus pneumoniae
Tuberculous meningitis (rare in UK)

infant has a vacant expression with staring eyes and, in severe cases, may present with coma. A reduction in the normal level of consciousness is always a serious sign, but this rarely occurs in viral meningitis. The cry is often high pitched ('meningeal'). Convulsions are common in infants and may be the presenting feature, although a history of the child being off colour and refusing feeds for a few hours is often obtained.

On examination the child looks ill and a squint of acute onset is common. Petechial haemorrhages may be present in the early stages of meningococcal disease (pp. 114, 198). Papilloedema is rarely seen in children and Kernig's sign, although present in older children, is often absent or a late sign in infancy. A bulging fontanelle in infants is a late sign.

The differential diagnosis of meningitis includes:
• septicaemia and other forms of severe infection;
• other causes of raised intracranial pressure (p. 151);
• meningismus — neck stiffness as a result of tonsillitis, otitis media, pneumonia and pyelonephritis.

Diagnosis Distinction between bacterial and viral meningitis cannot reliably be made clinically and the diagnosis of meningitis is made by lumbar puncture and examination of the cerebrospinal fluid (CSF). The one contraindication to lumbar puncture is the clinical suspicion of raised intracranial pressure (papilloedema is present) because of the risk of coning (see below).

The appearance of the CSF gives important clues as to the cause of the meningitis. The fluid is often cloudy in bacterial meningitis. Microscopy is essential to count and identify the cells. In some cases of fulminating bacterial meningitis there may be few, or no cells at all, but the fluid is teeming with bacteria. Organisms can be best identified by Gram's stain and this should be a routine part of the CSF examination. The fluid must be cultured to confirm the type of infecting organism.

The CSF findings usually allow the distinction between

viral or bacterial meningitis (p. 361). If the child has been treated with antibiotics in the few days prior to admission no organisms may grow, despite the cell count suggesting a bacterial cause. This is referred to as partially treated meningitis and these children should be treated as if they had bacterial meningitis.

Coning This refers to the herniation of the brainstem and/or the cerebellar structures through the foramen magnum. It occurs following a lumbar puncture when there is a release of spinal fluid with consequent production of differential pressure between the intracranial structures and the intraspinal compartment. The contents of the posterior intracranial fossa are squeezed into the upper spinal canal. This causes very acute and severe brainstem neurological signs with paralysis and respiratory inhibition which may be irreversible.

Management Viral meningitis is usually self-limiting and requires no specific treatment. Herpes simplex meningoen-cephalitis, a very rare condition, is treated with the antiviral agent acyclovir.

Treatment of bacterial meningitis is directed towards antimicrobial sterilization of the CSF and avoidance or treatment of complications. If the organism is identified on Gram's stain then the choice of antibiotics is straightforward (Table 4.8). In children with partially treated meningitis identification of the causative organism may be impossible. In these cases intravenous cefotaxime should be used for 14 days. Steroids (dexamethasone) given at the time of diagnosis reduces meningeal inflammation with fewer risks of complications in *Haemophilus influenzae* meningitis.

Meningococcal meningitis is associated with a high carrier rate of *Neisseria meningitidis* in the nasopharynx of contacts, and prophylactic rifampicin should be given for 2 days to all household contacts to reduce the risk of cross infection. Rifampicin is also given to the infected child at the end of the course of intravenous antibiotics. Meningococcal septicaemia is discussed on p. 114.

MENINGITIS AT A GLANCE

Epidemiology

0.5% children <10 years
Neonates are particularly prone to meningitis

Causal factors

Bacterial and viral meningitis are equally common
After the neonatal period the following bacteria are responsible:
- *Haemophilus influenzae* type B
- *Neisseria meningitidis*
- *Streptococcus pneumoniae*

NB *Signs and symptoms are variable

Mother first notices child is unwell/ irritable

Drowsy/fits/ purpuric rash

Level of consciousness (%)
100
80
60
40
20
0
−2 0 2 4 6 ... 16 ... 24
Time (hr)

RIP

Coma

Rapid progression of bacterial meningitis in a baby

Presentation

Classical symptoms include fever, drowsiness, headaches, bulging fontanelle and convulsions
Kernig's sign seen in older children
In early stages and in infants symptoms and signs are often non-specific
Neck stiffness is a late sign in infants

Differential diagnosis

Lumbar puncture is essential to make diagnosis in any suspected cases
Viral and bacterial causes distinguished on CSF findings

Management

See Principles of Therapeutics Box
p. 111

Prognosis

Excellent in viral cases
Deafness is the commonest sequela
In bacterial meningitis, 10% sustain severe neurological damage

Table 4.8 First-line antibiotics for bacterial meningitis

Bacteria	Antibiotic
Haemophilus	Ampicillin
Neisseria meningitidis	Benzyl penicillin
Pneumococcus	Benzyl penicillin
Uncertain bacterium	Cefotaxime

Principles of therapeutics
Meningitis

- For viral meningitis no specific treatment is required. Supportive care is required

- If lumbar puncture suggests a bacterial cause, use appropriate intravenous antibiotics (see Table 12.9, p. 362)

- If partially treated meningitis, give intravenous cefotaxime

- Steroids reduce complication rate in bacterial meningitis

- Give rifampicin to all close contacts of meningococcal meningitis cases

Complications and prognosis Viral meningitis carries a good prognosis in the majority of cases. Sensorineural hearing impairment (p. 284) is the commonest long-term complication of mumps meningitis. Herpes meningoencephalitis is very rare and is associated with high mortality and morbidity rates.

The prognosis of bacterial meningitis depends on the delay between onset and the start of effective treatment. Important complications of bacterial meningitis include:
- hydrocephalus;
- subdural effusion;
- acute adrenal failure;
- deafness;
- major deficit (cerebral palsy and/or learning difficulties in 10%).

Neonatal meningitis (p. 256) carries a worse prognosis than bacterial meningitis in older children.

Urinary tract infection

Acute urinary tract infection is the commonest bacterial infection in childhood and occurs in 3% of girls and 1% of boys. *Escherichia coli* is the causative organism in 90% of cases. A clear diagnosis of UTI is important as it may be the first sign of a congenital anomaly of the urinary tract or vesicoureteric reflux (VUR) which, if untreated, may lead to renal failure.

Clinical features Symptoms are often non-specific and include fever, irritability, vomiting and diarrhoea. In the neonate prolonged jaundice, apnoea, weight loss and collapse may be the presenting signs. Older children are more likely to present with more specific symptoms including dysuria, frequency, bed-wetting and loin pain. Dysuria and frequency as isolated symptoms are very common and are often not caused by UTI, but this must always be excluded. Clinically it may be impossible to differentiate between cystitis and pyelonephritis in young children as both may present with fever.

Diagnosis UTI can only be reliably diagnosed by identifying a pure growth of bacteria in a urine specimen. Unfortunately, the collection of uncontaminated urine may be difficult. In older, cooperative and continent children a mid-stream urine sample is the most reliable method. An alternative in younger children is a clean catch specimen. Stimulation by tickling or gently pressing on the suprapubic region may encourage the passage of urine. A bag specimen of urine is often taken in babies, but even with careful cleansing of the genital region, bacterial contamination often occurs. If there is a doubt as to whether organisms in the urine are the result of contamination then a suprapubic aspirate is necessary.

The growth of >100 000 colony-forming units in a fresh urine specimen indicates UTI. Any organisms present in a suprapubic specimen indicate UTI (see also p. 361).

Management The principles of management can be summarized as:
- copious fluid intake;
- analgesia appropriate to the degree of pain;
- antibiotics.

Trimethoprim is the first line antibiotic and it should be continued in full dose for 7 days and then as a prophylactic, once daily dose until investigations are complete (see below).

In the neonate, or if the child is acutely ill, intravenous antibiotics are necessary. A follow-up specimen of urine should be tested for the presence of infection 3–5 days after completing the course of antibiotics.

Advice should be given to the parents to reduce the risk of further UTIs. This advice is summarized in Table 5.30.

All children should be carefully investigated following their first proven UTI. A guideline to investigations is shown in Fig. 4.4. The first line investigation is an ultrasound scan and a DMSA radioisotope scan to detect renal scarring. If renal scarring is present, a micturating cystourethrogram (MCUG) should be performed to detect the presence of VUR (see below). If significant reflux is present then long-term prophylactic antibiotics should be prescribed. If the reflux is severe, surgical reimplantation of the ureters should be considered.

URINARY TRACT INFECTION AT A GLANCE

Epidemiology

3% of girls, 1% boys

Aetiology

Escherichia coli causative organism in 90%

History

Non-specific symptoms in infants
Fever*
Dysuria
Frequency
Enuresis
Abdominal/loin pain

Physical examination

Often normal

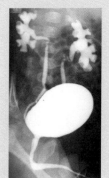

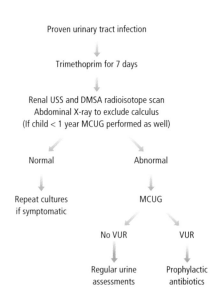

NB *Signs and symptoms are variable

Confirmatory investigations

• Clean urine for culture (bag urine in babies; though suprapubic aspiration sometimes necessary)
• >10^5 colony-forming units on culture (any number if suprapubic specimen)
• Pyuria and haematuria usual on microscopy
• Dipstick may show haematuria and proteinuria

Differential diagnosis

Any febrile illness in babies
Poor perineal hygiene in older girls

Management

Rapid sterilization of urine with antibiotics (IV in neonate or ill child)
Encourage fluid intake
Investigation of renal structure and VUR (see Principles of Management Box p. 113)
Regular urine culture for 12 months after first infection

Prognosis/complications

10–20% develop hypertension if scarring of the kidney occurs
Chronic renal failure very rare

It is recommended that all infants less than 1 year old with proven UTI should have an MCUG as part of the initial investigation screen because VUR is most likely to lead to renal damage in young children. If scarring or reflux is present then prophylactic antibiotics should be given.

Micturating cystourethrography is an unpleasant procedure as it requires the child's bladder to be catheterized and should only be carried out if the child is on prophylactic trimethoprim. It is the investigation of choice to visualize bladder neck outflow obstruction and VUR. MCUG should not be performed immediately after a UTI as the acute infection can cause transient ureteric reflux.

Persistent proteinuria in the presence of sterile urine suggests renal compromise, possibly as the result of the UTI. If present, biochemical assessment of renal function (creatinine clearance) should be regularly performed.

Prognosis Recurrence of UTI occurs in 50% of girls within 5 years. The follow-up of children with a proven UTI is

Proven urinary tract infection
↓
Trimethoprim for 7 days
↓
Renal USS and DMSA radioisotope scan
Abdominal X-ray to exclude calculus
(If child < 1 year MCUG performed as well)
↙   ↘
Normal   Abnormal
↓   ↓
Repeat cultures   MCUG
if symptomatic   ↙   ↘
No VUR   VUR
↓   ↓
Regular urine   Prophylactic
assessments   antibiotics

Fig. 4.4 Investigation of a child with UTI. If VUR is found then prophylacytic antibiotics should be given.

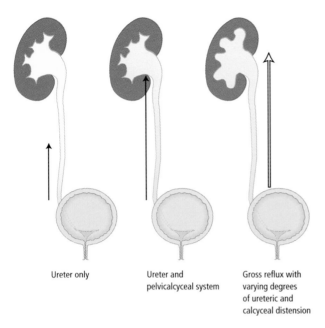

Ureter only

Ureter and
pelvicalyceal system

Gross reflux with
varying degrees
of ureteric and
calyceal distension

Fig. 4.5 Grading severity of VUR detected by MCUG examination. For clarity only one side has been shown.

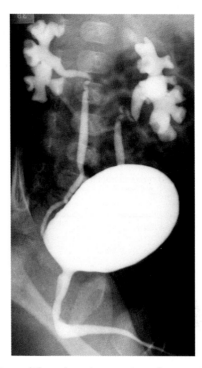

Fig. 4.6 Gross bilateral vesicoureteric reflux as the child is micturating.

summarized in the flow diagram (see Fig. 4.4). Provided the surveillance for urinary tract reinfection is effective, the prognosis is good for renal function.

Permanent renal damage as a result of UTI is rare in children but in infants, infection, particularly in the presence of vesicoureteric reflux, may cause permanent renal scarring with loss of function. Renal scarring is associated with hypertension in adult life and, rarely, chronic renal failure. Chronic pyelonephritis is usually a result of untreated reflux.

Principles of management
Urinary tract infection

- Sterilize urine with appropriate antibiotic

- Check that urine is sterile 3 days after cessation of antibiotic

- Investigate renal structure with ultrasound

- Investigate for VUR (see Fig. 4.4)

- If VUR, long-term prophylactic antibiotics and regular culture of urine for recurrent UTI

- If severe VUR, consider surgical reimplantation

- If renal scarring, long-term follow-up for hypertension

Vesicoureteric reflux

Vesicoureteric reflux refers to reflux of urine from the bladder up the ureter on micturition. It is found in 30% of children who present with UTI and its importance lies in the risk of renal scarring (reflux nephropathy), and this occurs in young children.

Clinical features The diagnosis of VUR is by investigation following UTI. There are no specific clinical features of VUR. It may be suspected in a fetus found to have dilated renal pelvices or scarring on antenatal ultrasound screening. VUR is diagnosed on MCUG investigation and graded as shown in Figs 4.5. & 4.6.

Management The majority of children with VUR tend to have less severe reflux as they get older. Therefore mild degrees tend to resolve spontaneously and only require long-term prophylactic antibiotics with careful surveillance for normal renal growth. Long-term prophylactic trimethoprim or nitrofurantoin is recommended. Children with grade 3 reflux require very close surveillance and may require surgical reimplantation of the ureter into the bladder, particularly if repeated UTI occurs on prophylactic treatment.

Prognosis More than half of children with severe VUR have renal scars. Renal scarring carries a 10–20% risk of

VESICOURETERIC REFLUX AT A GLANCE

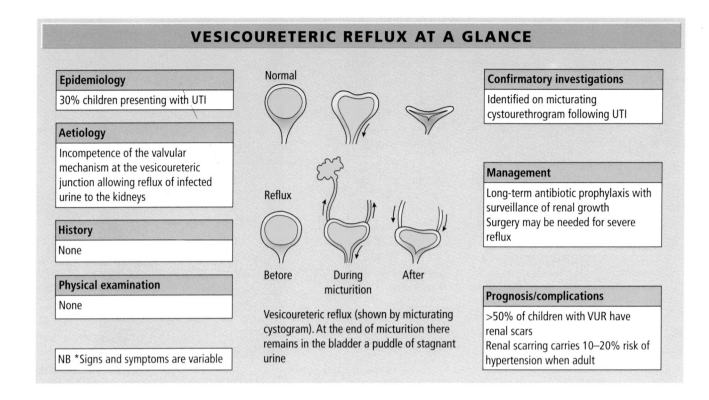

Epidemiology

30% children presenting with UTI

Aetiology

Incompetence of the valvular mechanism at the vesicoureteric junction allowing reflux of infected urine to the kidneys

History

None

Physical examination

None

NB *Signs and symptoms are variable

Normal

Reflux

Before   During   After
                micturition

Vesicoureteric reflux (shown by micturating cystogram). At the end of micturition there remains in the bladder a puddle of stagnant urine

Confirmatory investigations

Identified on micturating cystourethrogram following UTI

Management

Long-term antibiotic prophylaxis with surveillance of renal growth
Surgery may be needed for severe reflux

Prognosis/complications

>50% of children with VUR have renal scars
Renal scarring carries 10–20% risk of hypertension when adult

---

hypertension in adult life and less commonly chronic renal failure.

Meningococcal septicaemia

This condition presents insidiously and may rapidly become severe and life-threatening. *Neisseria meningitidis* most commonly causes meningitis, but in some cases septicaemia is the predominant presenting condition.

Clinical features There is often a short coryzal prodrome followed by fever, malaise and the development of a petechial/purpuric rash. The skin lesions do not blanche on pressure which is the hallmark of petechiae/purpuric lesions. The purpura may enlarge rapidly as the child deteriorates (see Fig. 5.17, p. 198). Signs of meningitis may be present.

Meningococcal septicaemia is often fulminant with rapid deterioration, disseminated intravascular coagulopathy and shock. Death may occur within a few hours of presentation caused by shock and adrenal failure (Waterhouse–Friderichsen syndrome).

Management As the course so often is fulminant, treatment must be started on the basis of strong clinical suspicion rather than awaiting the result of investigations. Any ill child seen at home with petechial or purpuric lesions should be given penicillin immediately. This should preferably be given intravenously, but intramuscular injection is acceptable. If it is possible to take blood cultures prior to giving antibiotics this is preferable, but may not be feasible. The child must be rushed to hospital as quickly as possible.

Management in hospital consists of antibiotics (intravenous benzyl penicillin) and intensive care directed towards supporting the circulation. Shock is a common and severe feature and massive volumes of plasma may be necessary to reverse this. Mortality is high.

The meningococcus colonizes the upper respiratory tract of asymptomatic children and close contacts of children with meningococcal infection are at increased risk of infection. Family members and children who have been in close

Principles of therapeutics
Meningococcal septicaemia

- Give IM or IV penicillin as soon as diagnosis suspected

- Arrange rapid admission to hospital

- Treat shock with intravenous fluids

- Treat all close contacts with rifampicin

MENINGOCOCCAL SEPTICAEMIA AT A GLANCE

Epidemiology

5 in 10 000 children <10 years

Aetiology

Neisseria meningitidis

History

Fever
Malaise

Physical examination

Ill child → shock
Petechial/purpuric rash
Meningeal signs*

NB *Signs and symptoms are variable

Confirmatory investigations

Immediate parenteral penicillin must be given on suspicion of diagnosis even if cultures not taken
Organism grown from blood, CSF or petechiae

Differential diagnosis

Septicaemia/meningitis caused by other organisms
Other causes of shock

Management

See Principles of Therapeutics Box

Prognosis/complications

High mortality in meningococcal septicaemia with shock
Good prognosis for meningococcal meningitis +/− septicaemia

contact in nurseries and school should be given a 2-day course of prophylactic rifampicin.

Prognosis Mortality is high in children who present with meningococcal septicaemia and some die before reaching hospital. Even with rapid antibiotic treatment death may occur as a result of irreversible shock.

If the child survives, the prognosis for intact recovery is good. Only a relatively small proportion of those with meningococcal septicaemia will have long-term sequelae.

Septic arthritis

Infection usually affects the larger weight-bearing joints such as hip, knee and ankle. The commonest organism is a staphylococcus, but *Haemophilus influenzae* may also cause infection. These organisms are blood-borne.

Clinical features Children present with fever and a hot, tender, swollen joint. Movement of the joint is very painful. In the neonate the child is usually very ill and holds the limb immobile which is described as 'pseudo-paralysis'.

The diagnosis is confirmed by identifying the organism in blood culture or from a joint aspiration.

Management Treatment involves intravenous antibiotics, and local instillation of antibiotic into the affected joint may

be beneficial. As soon as pain has subsided, a full range of joint mobility should be encouraged with physiotherapy.

Prognosis With early and effective treatment the prognosis

Distinguishing features
Causes of acute fever

	Clinical features	Investigations
Tonsillitis	Tonsillar redness +/− exudate	Throat swab
Otitis media	Bulging and red tympanic membrane	
Pneumonia	Respiratory distress Dullness to percussion	Chest X-ray
Meningitis	Neck stiffness* +/− change in conscious level	Lumbar puncture
Urinary tract infection	Dysuria, frequency	Urine microscopy and culture
Meningococcal disease	Shock, purpura	Blood cultures
Septic arthritis	Swollen painful joint	Aspiration of joint

* This sign is usually not present in young infants.

is very good. If the diagnosis is delayed then destruction of the joint may occur. This is most likely in the neonate.

DEHYDRATION

Water is the major constituent of the human body and a reduction in body water by more than 5% represents a significant dehydration. Eighty per cent of an infant's body weight is made up of water and this proportion falls to about 65% by 3 years. As such a large proportion of the young child is water, loss of body fluids is poorly sustained and dehydration occurs much more readily in infants than in older children and adults. In addition, the physiological mechanisms to prevent excessive fluid losses are less efficient in infants thereby further predisposing them to dehydration.

Pathophysiology

Body water is distributed between the cells (intracellular) and the extracellular compartments. The extracellular compartments can be further divided into the intravascular and extravascular (interstitial) spaces separated by the capillary endothelium. Dehydration may occur as the result of depletion of fluid from any of these compartments. Acute loss of fluid from the intravascular compartment may be associated with shock (see p. 303).

The clinical signs of dehydration also depend on the concentration of electrolytes in the intracellular and extracellular compartments. Sodium and bicarbonate are the major ions within the extracellular compartment and potassium is the major intracellular cation.

Normal body fluid is maintained by a balance between intake and output and depends on the following:
• fluid intake;
• urine volume;
• stool volume;
• sweating;
• insensible loss (water vapour in breath).

Dehydration occurs where the losses exceed the input. The commoner causes of dehydration are shown in Table 4.9. Gastroenteritis is the commonest cause of excessive fluid loss. Sodium may be lost in the same proportion as water and this is called isonatraemic (isotonic) dehydration. Sometimes rather more sodium than water is lost and this is referred to as hyponatraemic dehydration. More rarely, less sodium than water is lost or a relative excess of sodium is replaced causing hypernatraemic dehydration.

The approach to the dehydrated child

The purpose of the clinical evaluation is to determine the

Table 4.9 Commoner causes of dehydration

	Site of loss	Cause
Excess losses	Stool	Gastroenteritis
	Urine	Diabetes mellitus
	Vomiting	Pyloric stenosis
	Sweat	High fever
		Cystic fibrosis
		Hot climate
	Other body fluids	Acute surgical losses
		Fluid loss from burns
Decreased intake	Inability to drink	Stomatitis
		Tonsillitis

severity of the dehydration and to identify its cause. Assessing the extent of fluid loss is principally by clinical history and physical examination. When the assessment ends the doctor should be able to determine if the child has:
• mild dehydration   <5% losses
• moderate dehydration   5–10% losses
• severe dehydration   >10% losses.
  These are detailed in Table 4.10.

History

• *Causes of dehydration.* Enquire about diarrhoea, vomiting or excessive drinking (polydipsia is a common symptom in acute onset diabetes, see pp. 184, 325). Is the vomiting projectile (pyloric stenosis)?
• *Severity of dehydration.* Enquire into how many loose stools and how long the diarrhoea has persisted. Is the child passing less urine, and how many wet nappies have there been in last 24 hours? If the child has been vomiting, enquire how often and for how long.

Physical examination

This should assess both the severity of the dehydration and its most likely cause.
• *Causes of dehydration.* A thorough examination should identify foci of infection or other causes of dehydration. These include ears, throat, chest and abdomen. Particular attention should be paid to detecting a pyloric 'tumour' if vomiting has been a feature in a young infant.
• *Severity of dehydration* (Fig. 4.7). The following specific features should be examined to assess the severity of the dehydration:
  • dryness of the mucous membranes of the mouth;
  • mental state;
  • skin turgor;

Table 4.10 Clinical features in estimating the severity of dehydration

Clinical feature	Mild	Moderate	Severe
Mucosa of mouth	Dry	Dry	Dry
Reported urine output	Normal (at least × 3 in 24 hours)	Reduced in last 24 hours	No urine in last 12 hours
Mental state	Normal	Lethargic or stuporose	Irritable
Pulse	Normal	Tachycardic	Tachycardic
Blood pressure	Normal	Normal	Low
Capillary refilling	Normal	Slow	Very slow
Fontanelle	Normal	Sunken	Very sunken
Skin and eye turgor	Normal	Reduced	Very reduced
Percentage dehydrated	**<5%**	**5–10%**	**>10%**

Mild	Moderate	Severe
Dry mouth	Lethargy	Reduced level of consciousness
	Inelastic skin	Mottled skin
	Sunken fontanelle	Poor skin perfusion
	Sunken eyes	Deeply sunken eyes and fontanelle
	Tachycardia	Doughy skin

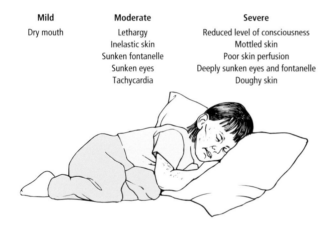

Fig. 4.7 Severity of dehydration.

- fontanelle;
- eye turgor;
- skin perfusion;
- pulse rate and character.

In mild dehydration the only physical sign may be a dry mouth. In moderate dehydration the child is lethargic, with inelastic skin, a sunken fontanelle and sunken eyes. The pulse may be fast, but is usually of normal volume and when the skin is blanched by finger pressure there may be some delay in refilling. Eye turgor may be a useful sign. Normal eye turgor can be assessed by pressing on the doctor's own eyeball through closed lids. The turgor of the child's eye can be compared to the examiner's own and in a moderately or severely dehydrated child the eyeball is soft.

In severe dehydration the child may be very confused and only semi-conscious. The skin is mottled and there is no refilling when blanched. The fontanelle and eyes are deeply sunken and the eye turgor is poor. When the skin is pinched between the examiner's finger and thumb it remains in a pinched position for some time. The pulse is thready and fast.

- *Weight.* Weighing the child is extremely important. Acute water loss can be estimated from the difference between actual weight and a recent weight made before dehydration occurred (1 g of body weight is roughly equivalent to 1 mL of water). Even if a recent weight is not available, regular weighing (twice daily in the acute situation) will allow accurate management of fluid replacement.

Investigations

- *Plasma electrolytes and blood pH estimate.* Serum sodium, potassium, chloride and bicarbonate should be measured. Sodium may be lost differentially leading to hyper- or hyponatraemia and the management differs depending on the type (see below). Bicarbonate may be lost as a result of diarrhoea causing a metabolic acidosis. If excessive vomiting occurs, excessive H^+ is lost which may cause an initial metabolic alkalosis (see Pyloric stenosis, p. 159). Disturbances in acid–base balance are discussed on p. 358.
- *Urine assessment.* Urine should be assessed for specific gravity or osmolality. Urinary electrolytes should also be measured. An assessment of urinary volume over a known period of time is helpful, but difficult to collect. Treatment must not be delayed for urine output to be measured.

Determining type of dehydration

Isotonic dehydration   This is the commonest form of dehydration. There are equal losses of sodium and water so that the serum sodium is normal. These children show physical signs commensurate with the degree of fluid loss.

Hyponatraemic dehydration   This is defined as dehydration with serum sodium <130 mmol/L. There is excess Na+ loss compared with fluid. The child is lethargic and the skin is dry and inelastic. The cause is usually replacement of fluid losses with hypotonic solutions such as water or fizzy drinks.

Hypernatraemic dehydration   This is defined as dehydration with serum Na+ >150 mmol/L. It may be caused by severe and acute water loss, but most commonly by a mother giving concentrated formula feeds in incorrectly measured-out scoops of powdered milk. The child characteristically appears to be very hungry, but has fewer clinical signs of dehydration. The skin feels doughy. Metabolic acidosis is a common feature of this condition.

Management

Mild (<5%) dehydration secondary to gastroenteritis may be treated at home by oral hydration therapy (see below). More severe dehydration (5–10%) requires hospital admission and intravenous rehydration. The management of the dehydrated child requires frequent reassessment of fluid balance. This involves maintaining an accurate input–output chart, regular weighings twice daily and frequent measurements of serum electrolytes.

The principles of rehydration are simple and require three calculations:

1 an estimate of the acute fluid loss;
2 an estimate of maintenance fluid requirements;
3 an estimate of on-going losses.

These three estimates are summed to represent the volume of fluid to be replaced over the next 24 hours.

Estimate of acute fluid loss The difference between actual weight and a recent normal weight is a good approximate method of estimating acute water loss. If the normal weight is unknown then a clinical assessment of dehydration must be made. If the child is thought to be 10% dehydrated clinically the estimate of fluid loss is:

$$\text{deficit (mL)} = (\text{actual weight in grams} \times 110\%) - \text{actual weight.}$$

Estimate of maintenance requirements Maintenance water and sodium intake depends on the age of the child and is summarized in Table 4.11.

Estimate of on-going losses If possible, on-going losses must be carefully measured on an hourly basis and added to the fluid regimen every 4–6 hours.

Rehydration protocol

The rate of rehydration depends on the type of dehydration. Rehydration should take place in three phases (Table 4.12). If shock is not present, rehydration starts with phase 2. If the child is not vomiting and is assessed to have mild to moderate dehydration, oral rehydration therapy should be attempted.

Dehydration should be corrected over 24 hours with one-

Table 4.11 Maintenance requirements of water and sodium at different ages

Age (months)	Water (m/kg/24 hours)	Sodium (mmol/L/kg/day)
0–6	150	2.5
6–12	120	2.5
12–24	100	2.5
>24	80	2.0

Table 4.12 The three phases of rehydration management

Phase 1

If a dehydrated child is in shock, treatment is urgent with rapid infusion of colloid over the first 30–60 minutes and frequent measurements of blood pressure. If the child is acidotic sodium bicarbonate should be given to half replace the estimated bicarbonate deficit

Phase 2

Over the next/first 4 hours the child should be given 10 mL/kg/hour of 0.5 N saline whilst awaiting the serum sodium result. The total fluid requirement over the next 24 hours (deficit + maintenance + on-going losses) should be calculated and this should be given as 0.18 N saline in 4% dextrose over the next 24 hour period. Once urine output is established potassium replacement should also be given

Example: A 15 kg boy who is estimated to be 10% dehydrated:
Expected weight = 15 × 110% = 16.5 kg
24 hour maintenance = 16.5 × 110 mL = 1815 mL
Deficit = 1.5 kg = 1500 mL
On-going losses (estimated) = 1000 mL
Total fluids over the next 24 hour = 4315 mL
Hourly requirement = 180 mL

Phase 3

Monitor electrolytes and weight. Start maintenance fluids alone if deficit is corrected and there are no further on-going fluid losses

half of the fluids given in the first 8 hours. Hypernatraemic dehydration should be corrected more slowly over 48 hours to avoid rapid shifts of water within the brain and resulting cerebral oedema.

Oral rehydration therapy

Children with mild to moderate dehydration who are not vomiting may be rehydrated orally as they can continue to absorb water and electrolytes through the bowel wall. Absorption is aided by glucose or sucrose sugars and commercially available oral rehydration solutions (e.g. Dioralyte, Rehidrat) are widely used. These are dispensed as oral solutions, effervescent tablets or powders and are reconstituted with freshly boiled and cooled water. Breast-feeding should be maintained while using these solutions.

DEHYDRATION AT A GLANCE

Epidemiology

Infants are the most vulnerable

Aetiology

Gastroenteritis is the commonest cause

Physical examination

- Excessive losses — vomiting, diarrhoea
- Inadequate replacement of fluids
- Lethargic
- ↓ level of consciousness (**a**)
- Sunken fontanelle and eyes (**b**)
- Dry mucous membranes (**c**)
- ↓ blood pressure (**d**)
- Tachypnoea (**e**)
- Oliguria (**f**)
- Reduced skin turgor (**g**)
- Cold (shut down) peripheries (**h**)
- Tachycardia (**i**)

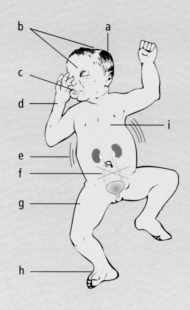

Confirmatory investigations

Examination findings and body weight
Estimate severity of dehydration
Serum and urinary electrolytes
Determine whether iso-, hypo- or hypernatraemic

Management

Replace deficit and on-going losses and give maintenance fluids (see Principles of Management Box, below)

Prognosis

Good
Convulsions most likely in hypernatraemic dehydration

Principles of management Dehydration

- Assess the severity of fluid loss (<5%, 5–10%, >10%)

- Assess whether dehydration is iso-, hypo-, or hypernatraemic

- Estimate on-going losses and maintenance fluid needs

- Replace estimated fluid loss, on-going losses and maintenance needs over 24–48 hours

- Determine the cause of dehydration and treat if necessary

If the baby is bottlefed, normal milk feed can be given once the diarrhoea has settled. Regrading onto formula milk feeds is no longer recommended. Recurrence of diarrhoea on refeeding is most likely to be caused by lactase deficiency and if >0.5% reducing substances are found in the stool, a lactose-free milk should be used.

Causes of dehydration

The major causes of dehydration are as follows and each are discussed elsewhere in the book.

- Gastroenteritis (p. 162).
- Pyloric stenosis (p. 159).
- Diabetes mellitus (pp. 184, 325).
- Tonsillitis (p. 104).

ACUTE WHEEZE

Noisy breathing is a common symptom in children which may be caused by partial obstruction of either the upper or lower airway. The upper airway comprises the nose, pharynx, larynx and extrathoracic portion of the trachea. The lower airway comprises intrathoracic trachea, bronchi and bronchioles. Partial obstruction of the upper airway causes an inspiratory noise (stridor) and of the lower airway an expiratory wheeze. In many cases noises can be heard both on inspiration and expiration and it requires concentration to determine the phase of breathing in which the predominant noise occurs.

Transmitted noises are derived from the upper airway and are heard when auscultating the chest. This may make interpretation of intrathoracic noises more difficult. It is often helpful to hold the bell of the stethoscope to the child's throat and listen to the upper airway noise. These noises can then be mentally subtracted from the noises heard when auscultating the chest to determine the intrathoracic signs.

Wheeze is a very common symptom in childhood. A wheeze is a prolonged musical note heard mainly on expiration and originating from the intrathoracic airways. It is usually fairly easily distinguished from stridor (p. 126) which is an inspiratory upper airway noise. On auscultation a wheeze is referred to as a rhonchus.

Acute wheezing is common in both infants and older children. It is estimated that 20% of all children will wheeze at some time in the first 5 years of life. Children (particularly under 3 years of age) are particularly prone to wheezing as bronchospasm, mucosal oedema and secretions have a greater impact in narrowing their relatively smaller airways.

The first episode of wheezing may cause great parental anxiety and, if there is a family history of asthma, the first episode of wheeze may cause the parents to jump to the conclusion that their child also has asthma.

This section considers the causes of an acute wheezing disorder. The management of children with chronic wheezing such as occurs in asthma is discussed in Chapter 10.

Pathophysiology

Wheeze is caused by partial obstruction of the intrathoracic airways and is a result of intrinsic or extrinsic factors (Fig. 4.8). Bronchi have a layer of smooth muscle within the wall of the tube. Various factors may cause the muscle to spasm thereby narrowing the tube. This process is reversible. Intrinsic factors are related to bronchial hyperreactivity with acute narrowing of the bronchi and bronchioles and are mediated through histamine release as part of the inflammatory response. The commonest causes are allergy and infection. Extrinsic causes of airway narrowing include the presence of a foreign body and mucus oversecretion as a result of infection. Therefore infection may cause

wheeze from both constriction of the tube's muscle wall as the result of intrinsic release of vasoconstrictive substances and from the production of mucus as a result of the infectious agent.

Airway hyperreactivity may be inherited and be present life-long although bronchospasm and wheeze may only occur at certain times of life. Hyperreactivity may also be stimulated by outside factors such as infection or air pollutants (e.g. sulphur dioxide). Wheeziness is particularly common in babies. The tendency to wheeze may not persist outside of infancy and may be acquired as a result of viral (respiratory syncytial virus) or bacterial (pertussis) infection.

Table 4.13 lists the commoner causes of acute wheeze.

The approach to the wheezing child

The clinical evaluation is important to determine the degree to which the wheezing is affecting the child and to identify conditions other than asthma which may present with wheezing.

History

If the child is young or acutely distressed the history must be taken from the parents. The specific questions that are important in determining a diagnosis are listed here and summarized in Table 4.14.
- *The acute episode.* Was there a triggering event? Asthma is often precipitated by trigger factors such as acute emotion, physical exercise or going out on a cold morning. Infection is an important trigger for asthma, but may cause wheezing in its own right (see Bronchiolitis, p. 124). Enquire whether cold symptoms preceded the wheezing. Asthma is often triggered by exposure to allergens such as house-dust mite, pet hair, grass pollens and irritants such as tobacco smoke.
- *Severity of the episode.* How incapacitated was the child during the wheezing episode? Enquire whether the child was able to feed normally and whether it interfered with play and activity. Severe wheeze and breathlessness may be associated with inability to talk.

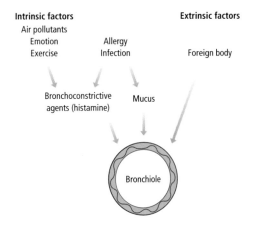

Fig. 4.8 Intrinsic and extrinsic factors causing wheeze in childhood.

Table 4.13 Commoner causes of acute wheeze

Asthma
Bronchiolitis and other viral agents
Air pollutants (e.g. sulphur dioxide)
Aspiration of food or a foreign body
Cystic fibrosis
Sequelae of chronic lung disease (bronchopulmonary dysplasia)
Cardiac failure

- *Family history.* Asthma is suggested by a family history of *atopy*. This refers to a predisposition to asthma, eczema or hay fever.
- *History of choking.* Aspiration of food or a foreign body is most likely in a toddler who is mobile and puts everything he or she finds in his or her mouth. A recent history of choking should be enquired about.
- *Apnoea.* Bronchiolitis and other viral infections cause wheezing in infants and may be associated with apnoea and quite severe respiratory distress.

Physical examination

- *Assessment of growth.* The child's height and weight should be plotted on a centile chart. Growth failure does not occur in asthma unless it is very severe; poor growth suggests a condition such as cystic fibrosis.
- *Signs of respiratory distress on observation.* These include shortness of breath (dyspnoea), cyanosis and recession with use of accessory muscles. Features of severe respiratory distress include inability to talk in an older child, cyanosis, confusion, restlessness and drowsiness and any of these symptoms demands rapid assessment and investigation (see below).

Signs of chronic lung disease such as barrel chest and clubbing must be sought. Clubbing is suggestive of chronic suppurative lung disease and rarely occurs in chronic asthma.

- *Chest signs.* Physical examination of the chest may elicit signs which help confirm the diagnosis (Table 4.15). On auscultation, the presence of widespread crepitations with rhonchi suggest infection, particularly bronchiolitis in infants. A localized distribution of rhonchi suggests aspiration of a foreign body.

Wheezing may be a sign of cardiac failure in a child with congenital heart disease. Listen for murmurs, clinically assess heart size (p. 33) and examine the upper abdomen for hepatomegaly.

- *Peak flow.* This should be part of the assessment of any wheezing or breathless child. The assessment of peak flow is discussed on p. 321.

Investigations

Many children with acute wheeze will be seen in the home and with careful history and examination will not require further investigations. Particular features that suggest the need for investigations are the onset of wheeze in a very young child, asymmetrical signs on examination and failure to thrive. The child who is acutely ill should be investigated with a full blood count, and chest X-ray (Table 4.15). In a child with recurrent episodes of acute wheeze, particularly where this is thought to be caused by asthma, repeated chest X-rays are not warranted.

Cyanosis indicates the need for measurement of arterial blood gases, and oxygen therapy can then by monitored by transcutaneous oxygen measurement and additional oxygen titrated against oxygen saturation.

The child who shows severe signs of respiratory distress will also need careful assessment for respiratory failure. Arterial blood gas measurement is the main way to determine whether the child is in respiratory failure which may require respiratory support (see p. 300).

Table 4.14 Features in the history of children presenting with acute wheeze

Feature from history	Possible diagnosis
Cough preceding wheeze	Asthma
	Infection
	Foreign body
Aspiration	Foreign body
? eating peanuts	
? recent episode of choking	
Family history of atopy	Asthma
Recent URTI	Asthma
	Infection
Trigger factors:	Asthma
exercise-induced wheeze	
emotion-induced wheeze	
cold weather-induced wheeze	
Apnoea in infants	Bronchiolitis

Table 4.15 Signs on examination and findings on investigation of the wheezy child and their significance

	Asthma	Foreign body	Bronchiolitis
Distribution of rhonchi	Widespread	Focal	Widespread
Crepitations	Variable	Focal	Widespread
Percussion noise	Increased	Focal dullness with increased resonance if compensatory emphysema	Variable
Full blood count	Usually normal	Normal	Increased lymphocytes
Chest X-ray	Overinflated	Segmental collapse and compensatory emphysema	Overinflation Consolidation

Management

Children with acute onset of wheeze and their parents may be very frightened by the symptom and reassurance is necessary after appropriate assessment. Specific management depends on the cause of the wheeze.

Immediate management is directed towards assessing whether the child is in actual or incipient respiratory failure when respiratory support may be required. The need for oxygen therapy depends on blood gas measurement.

Asthma is the commonest cause of recurrent wheezing. Providing there is no indication of other conditions on history or physical examination, it is justifiable to give a trial of a bronchodilator to confirm the diagnosis. Clinical improvement in wheezing indicates that the bronchospasm is reversible and a diagnosis of asthma can be made. In the older, cooperative child, peak flow measurements before and after the trial are useful.

Some babies wheeze very persistently. If the wheeze is not affecting eating, temperament and growth, this need not arouse too much concern. Such children have been called 'happy wheezers' and the symptoms subside as they grow. Milk allergy is often implicated, but withdrawal of cow's milk protein is only rarely effective. A more important intervention is to stop exposure to cigarette smoke.

Causes of wheeze

Acute asthma

The definition of asthma is episodic, reversible, intrathoracic airway obstruction. Reversibility may occur spontaneously or as a result of therapy. On the basis of this definition it is impossible to diagnose asthma at the time of first presentation of wheeze, but a presumptive diagnosis can be made on the basis of precipitating factors and family history. Chronic asthma is considered on p. 318.

Pathophysiology
Acute asthma is caused by a combination of the following:
- bronchial smooth muscle constriction;
- airway secretion;
- mucosal swelling.

These may be precipitated by allergens, air pollutants, infection, exercise, cold air temperature and emotion. Many children with acute asthma have only a single or few precipitating factors. There is a strong familial element to asthma which appears to be polygenic in nature.

Clinical features Wheeze may be preceded by cough (particularly at night) and episodes of breathlessness where wheeze may not have been heard. Precipitating features such as allergens (dust, pet hairs, mould), recent infection and exercise provocation may be elicited on direct questioning.

On examination growth and chest shape should be recorded. The presence of widespread rhonchi with a generally hyperresonant chest on percussion is typically found during an acute attack. Signs of severe respiratory distress should be noted (see p. 121).

Chest X-ray may show an overinflated chest with no other abnormalities. Signs of infection as the trigger of the wheezing may be seen. Assessment of peak flow will show some reduction from the predicted values and this should be improved after pharmacological treatment thus indicating the reversible nature of the airway obstruction.

ACUTE WHEEZE AT A GLANCE

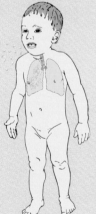

Epidemiology

20% of all children <6 years

Physical examination

Expiratory rhonchi on auscultation
Associated acute clinical features
include cough and respiratory distress

Management

Assess severity of wheeze for evidence of respiratory failure
Assess need for additional oxygen therapy
Investigate causes
Treatment specific to cause

Prognosis

Good for acute wheeze
Long-term outlook dependent on underlying cause

Management There are a variety of highly effective drugs in the management of acute asthmatic attacks. The management of status asthmaticus is discussed in Chapter 10.

- *Betamimetics.* Salbutamol and terbutaline are selective beta-2 adrenoceptor stimulants which cause reversal of broncho-constriction. In acute asthma these may be given in a number of ways (see p. 319).

 Metered inhalation. This requires the child to coordinate inhalation with pressing the metered aerosol and is only possible in children of 5 years and above. Some training is required in this technique.

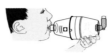 *Spacer device.* The betamimetic is sprayed into a plastic reservoir which is attached to a mask and is held over the child's mouth and nose so that he or she rebreathes the aerosol.

 Nebulizer. This requires an electrically driven nebulizer pump supplied from a clinic. The betamimetic is administered as a very fine aerosol while a mask is held to the patient's face. This requires no coordination and is very useful in small children.

ACUTE ASTHMA AT A GLANCE

Aetiology

Reversible airways obstruction precipitated by a variety of factors:
- Emotional upsets
- Infections
- Irritants (smoke)
- Allergies (house-dust mite, animals, pollens)
- Exercise

History

Persistent cough, particularly nocturnal
Difficulty breathing
Associated with exercise
Symptoms of URTI*
Family history of asthma

Physical examination

Expiratory wheeze (maybe inspiratory too in babies)
Tachypnoea
Subcostal/intercostal retractions
Alar flaring
Hyperresonant chest

NB *Signs and symptoms are variable

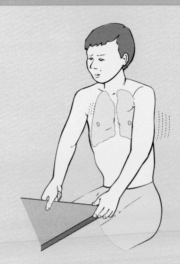

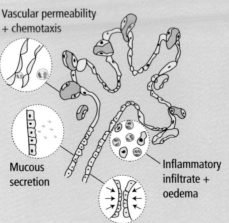

Vascular permeability + chemotaxis

Mucous secretion

Inflammatory infiltrate + oedema

Bronchiolar constriction

Confirmatory investigations

In older child peak flow improved by medication
Chest X-ray non-contributory

Differential diagnosis

URTI
Acute bronchitis
Bronchiolitis in infant
Pneumonia

Management

see Principles of Therapeutics Box, p. 124

Prognosis/complications

Usually good
Rarely life-threatening
May proceed to chronic asthma

Parenteral route. This is best used in children with severe acute asthma (status asthmaticus) and may be combined with other drugs such as intravenous steroids (see p. 321).

• *Xanthine derivatives.* Aminophylline and theophylline may be given in conjunction with betamimetic agents in cases of severe acute asthma. In acute asthma they are used intravenously.

• *Steroids.* These are very valuable in the management of severe asthma, and are of considerable benefit intravenously in status asthmaticus.

Prognosis Acute asthma may be life-threatening and patients still die of this condition. The reason for death is usually that the severity of the acute episode has not been recognized. Children with acute asthma usually respond rapidly to therapy and the management of chronic asthma (p. 319) should prevent frequent recurrences of acute attacks.

Bronchiolitis

Viral infection commonly causes wheezing in infants. The

> ### Principles of therapeutics
> ### Acute asthma
>
> • Assess clinical severity of acute episode
>
> • If severe, measure arterial blood gases and oxygen saturation
>
> • Give inhalational betamimetics
>
> • If status asthmaticus, give intravenous steroids and xanthines
>
> • Closely monitor improvement/deterioration
>
> • Mechanical ventilation if respiratory failure
>
> • Long-term follow-up care (p. 322)

most important viral agent is respiratory syncytial virus (RSV), but others such as parainfluenza virus and adenovirus may also cause wheezing. Pertussis infection may cause acute wheeze.

Bronchiolitis is caused by RSV or, rarely, other viral infections and occurs in epidemics in the winter months. Although RSV infects people of all ages, bronchiolitis is only

BRONCHIOLITIS AT A GLANCE

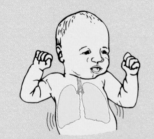

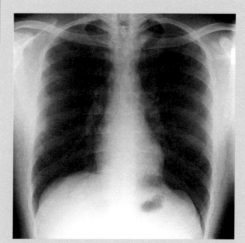

Aetiology

Respiratory syncytial virus, occasionally other viruses
Infants and babies only affected

History

Coryza
Difficulty breathing
Feeding difficulty
Fever*

Physical examination

Widespread wheezing and crepitations
Tachypnoea
Subcostal/intercostal retractions
Nasal flaring
Overinflated chest

NB *Signs and symptoms are variable

Confirmatory investigations

RSV confirmed by immunofluorescence of nasopharyngeal secretions
Chest X-ray shows overinflation of lungs and patchy areas of collapse

Differential diagnosis

Asthma (see text)
Pneumonia

Management

Supportive

Prognosis/complications

Usually good but mortality 1–2%
High proportion go on to have recurrent wheeze through infancy

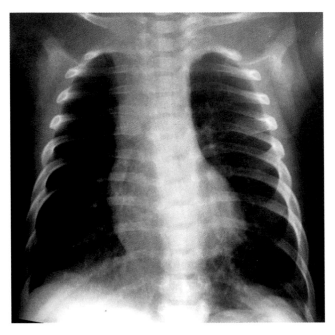

Fig. 4.9 Chest X-ray of an 8-week-old baby with bronchiolitis. The X-ray shows gross over inflation of the lungs clearly seen by the level of the diaphragm and the intercostal spaces. There is also some bronchial wall thickening.

Distinguishing features
Wheezy conditions

Condition	Age	Features
Asthma	Any age, but diagnosed with caution in a child <3 years old	Recurrent wheezing often triggered by a URTI or allergens. Responsive to bronchodilators. Family history of atopy
Wheezy bronchitis	Toddlers	Wheezing with URTI. Often not recurrent but some progress to asthma. May respond to bronchodilators
Bronchiolitis	Babies	Often RSV+. May recur. Often unresponsive to bronchodilators Asthma may develop later in a proportion of babies
Foreign body	Usually toddlers	Unilateral wheezing. May be preceded by choking episode

seen in children below 18 months of age. Infants with congenital heart disease or underlying chronic lung disease may be very severely affected by bronchiolitis.

Clinical features The illness starts with coryza, followed by signs of respiratory distress, including wheeze and cough

as prominent features. Some children develop more severe symptoms including apnoea, and feeding may be affected. Examination reveals an overinflated chest, rhonchi and crepitations on auscultation.

Chest X-ray shows overinflated lungs (Fig. 4.9). Collapse and/or consolidation may be seen in a few cases.

Management Most children are not ill and provided they take feeds well they can be managed at home. Indications for admission to hospital include cyanosis, increasing respiratory distress, apnoea or poor feeding.

Treatment is largely supportive although the antiviral agent ribavirin may be of benefit in severe cases. Respiratory support may be necessary in those babies with underlying lung disease.

Prognosis Most babies recover uneventfully from this condition. Immunity is short-lived and recurrent bronchiolitis is not uncommon. Many babies who suffer from bronchiolitis show a predisposition to recurrence of wheeze through infancy. Death is rare, but occurs in babies who have severe underlying chronic lung disease.

Aspirated foreign body (see also p. 176)

This usually occurs in toddlers who are mobile and put small objects into their mouths. Small plastic or wooden beads and peanuts are the most likely foreign bodies to be aspirated. Peanuts are particularly dangerous as they swell in the airway, becoming firmly lodged and difficult to remove because they tend to fragment.

Clinical features Although acute choking may be noticed by the parent, aspiration of a foreign body may not be immediately recognized. Delay between aspiration and the child presenting is common. The main symptoms are respiratory distress and wheeze. Cough is a prominent feature. There may be asymmetry in chest shape and chest signs with localized rhonchi and crepitations. A localized dull percussion note is detected if collapse has occurred distal to the obstruction. Compensatory emphysema occurs around a collapsed lobe and this will produce a percussion note of increased resonance.

Diagnosis may be made on chest X-ray. This may show segmental collapse or hyperinflation.

Management If aspiration of a foreign body is strongly suspected then bronchoscopy should be performed. Removal of the foreign body is curative.

Complete airway obstruction is a medical emergency and should be treated by the Heimlich manoeuvre (p. 302).

Prognosis If there is delay in diagnosis then bronchiectasis

ASPIRATED FOREIGN BODY AT A GLANCE

Epidemiology

Toddlers most at risk

Aetiology

Peanuts are a particular problem
Foreign body commonly sited in right
main bronchus

History

History of choking*
Cough

Physical examination

Wheeze (may be unilateral)
Asymmetric chest signs

NB *Signs and symptoms are variable

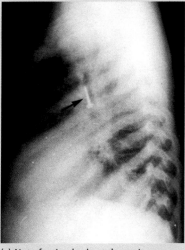

(a) Note foreign body at the carina

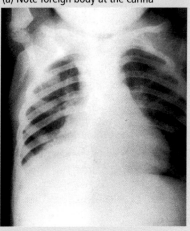

(b) Note collapse of right lower lobe

Confirmatory investigations

Chest X-ray in inspiration and
expiration may show segmental
collapse
Bronchoscopy

Differential diagnosis

URTI
Pneumonia
Asthma
Acute bronchitis

Management

Heimlich manoeuvre if complete
airway obstruction
Bronchoscopy to remove foreign body

Prognosis

Usually good but risk of bronchiectasis
if diagnosis is delayed

---

may occur in the lung distal to the obstruction. In bronchiectasis there is destruction of bronchial architecture. This leaves dilated air sacs which become chronically infected and will eventually require surgical removal.

STRIDOR

Stridor is a noise heard on inspiration and is caused by narrowing of the extrathoracic upper airway. Stridor, as an acute symptom, is very common in young children. The challenge of the condition is to recognize those children with an acute but non-severe self-limiting illness who can be observed at home and those who, if untreated, may develop life-threatening upper airway obstruction. Stridor occurs much more commonly in winter months.

Table 4.16 Causes of stridor

Acute causes
Croup
Acute epiglottitis
Foreign body
Chronic causes
Laryngomalacia
Subglottic stenosis

Pathophysiology

Stridor is most likely to arise from the larynx. The causes of stridor may be either acute or chronic and the commoner causes are listed in Table 4.16. Obstruction of the intrathoracic airway caused by a foreign body is discussed on pp. 125, 176.

The approach to the child with stridor

History

The particular points to enquire about in the history are:
- *Coryza and fever.* The commonest cause of stridor is croup (acute laryngotracheobronchitis) and the stridor is usually preceded by coryzal symptoms and fever. The development of stridor coincides with a barking cough in croup.
- *Nature of the stridor.* The degree of stridor depends on the effort of the inspiratory breath. The stridulous noise is usually louder when the child cries and is softer during sleep.
- *Prodromal symptoms.* Prior to the introduction of *Haemophilus influenza* B (HIb) immunization, the main differential diagnosis of croup was acute epiglottitis. In this condition the prodrome is significantly different from croup, with the child appearing to be much more ill.
- *Aspiration.* Aspiration of a foreign body should always be considered in acute stridor. If a foreign body is a cause of upper airway obstruction the stridor is usually very severe and the child is dramatically ill.

Physical examination

- *Chest signs.* Signs in the chest including crepitations and rhonchi are strongly suggestive of croup and are very uncommon with acute epiglottitis or upper airway foreign body obstruction.
- *Airway obstruction.* Stridor is an important sign because it may proceed to acute airway obstruction, a potentially fatal condition. Do not examine the throat of a child with severe stridor as acute airway obstruction may occur. Examination of the throat should only be undertaken in the presence of an anaesthetist who can intubate the child if necessary. Signs of increasing airway obstruction include:
- cyanosis;
- confusion;
- reduction in stridor with exhaustion;
- drooling with increasing dysphagia.

Investigations

If the child is suspected of having acute epiglottitis or impending respiratory failure, blood should be drawn for a number of investigations (Table 4.17).

Focal points
Evaluation of stridor

- Assess severity of airway obstruction
- Evaluate for systemic features of acute epiglottitis
- Assess likelihood of foreign body aspiration
- If epiglottitis suspected avoid distress to child by not examining throat

---

Table 4.17 Appropriate investigations in children with stridor and their significance

Investigation	Significance
Full blood count	Neutrophilia with excess granulocytes suggests bacterial infection
Blood cultures	To identify *Haemophilus influenzae*
Blood gases	Low Pa_{O_2}, high Pa_{CO_2}, or respiratory acidosis indicates respiratory failure

Management

Stridor caused by croup is usually a self-limiting condition, but in a few cases progressive airway obstruction occurs.

Mild stridor is best managed at home with no specific treatment. Steam is often used to relieve acute stridor. The parents must be instructed to watch for signs of worsening of the condition and to report them immediately. If the child has more severe stridor, hospital admission is necessary for observation, and intubation by an experienced doctor if there are signs of impending airway obstruction.

If acute epiglottitis is suspected urgent transfer to hospital for assessment, antibiotic treatment and intubation is essential as airway obstruction is very likely to develop (see below).

The aim of management is to monitor the child for signs of impending airway obstruction and to intervene prior to this occurring. In hospital, treatment with nebulized steroids or adrenaline may be useful in obtaining symptomatic relief, but severe airway obstruction is most safely relieved by passing a tube via the nose or mouth into the trachea to bypass the obstruction (naso- or endotracheal intubation). This may be very difficult and requires the skills of either an experienced anaesthetist or an ENT surgeon.

Complete upper airway obstruction caused by a foreign body is a medical emergency and if untreated death will rapidly occur. The Heimlich manoeuvre is used as emergency treatment to relieve the obstruction (p. 302).

Principles of management
Stridor

- Initially assess severity of stridor

- Observe for progression in symptoms or signs

- If acute epiglottitis or foreign body is suspected arrange immediate transfer to hospital

- Assess child for incipient airway obstruction

- Intubate if necessary

Distinguishing features
Acute and chronic stridor

	Age	Clinical features
Croup	6–24 months	Coryzal prodrome Barking cough
Acute epiglottitis	2–4 year	Toxicity and high fever Drooling
Foreign body	12–18 months	History and sudden onset
Laryngomalacia	Newborn	Presents at birth and persists Worse on crying Improves with age
Subglottic stenosis	0–6 months	Previous history of intubation Exacerbations with upper respiratory tract infection

Causes of stridor

Croup (acute laryngotracheobronchitis)

This common condition is caused by a parainfluenza virus. It most commonly affects children of 6 months to 2 years of age and causes symptoms initially in the larynx (stridor), and then in the trachea and bronchi (cough and wheeze) hence the term laryngotracheobronchitis. It occurs in winter months and children may have repeated episodes.

Clinical features Croup starts with coryzal symptoms and fever and proceeds to stridor and barking cough. Hoarseness, particularly on crying, is a common feature. The stridor may appear to become acutely worse as a result of associated laryngeal spasm. Further progression down the respiratory tract may cause wheezing and tachypnoea. Although usually mild it may progress rapidly in young children to become very severe. Signs of deterioration include

increased work of breathing, cyanosis and restlessness. Severe deterioration is often accompanied by a reduction in the stridulous noise.

Management Most cases resolve spontaneously. Inhaled steroids are effective in reducing upper airway oedema, but there is no evidence that humidity shortens the duration or severity of the stridor. However, adequate fluids are essential to prevent dehydration. The child must be carefully observed and if obstruction is anticipated intubation should be performed electively.

Acute epiglottitis

This is becoming a rare condition with universal *Haemophilus influenza* B (HIb) immunization of infants. It is caused by infection with the bacterium *Haemophilus influenza* and affects older children (2–4 years).

Clinical features The child presents with signs of toxicity and appears ill. He or she is feverish and often begins to drool as they are unable to swallow. The child with acute epiglottitis adopts a characteristic posture sitting upright with the chin thrust forward. He or she is not hoarse and rarely coughs.

If this condition is suspected, examination of the mouth must not be attempted as acute and total airway obstruction may occur. The child should only be examined with an experienced anaesthetist or throat surgeon standing by. On examination, the epiglottis looks like a bright red cherry arising out of the throat.

Management If epiglottitis is suspected, protection of the airway is the first aim. Investigations may provoke crying which causes airway obstruction and are best done after intubation. Blood cultures will reveal *Haemophilus* and intravenous chloramphenicol or ampicillin is required as soon as the airway is secured. Extubation is usually possible within 48 hours of antibiotic treatment.

Prognosis With airway protection and appropriate antibiotics the prognosis is excellent. Death or severe brain injury may occur if acute airway obstruction occurs.

JAUNDICE

Jaundice is the commonest sign of liver disease, but may also occur as the result of non-liver pathology, notably haemolysis. Neonatal jaundice is discussed in Chapter 6. Jaundice is always a significant sign and the child must be investigated rapidly and fully so that a definite diagnosis can be made.

CROUP AT A GLANCE

Epidemiology

Commonly affects children aged
6 months to 2 years

Aetiology

Parainfluenza virus

History

Stridor and barking cough
Coryza
Fever
Hoarseness*

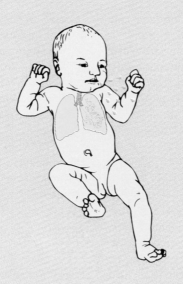

NB *Signs and symptoms are variable

Physical examination

Stridor
Wheezing*
Tachypnoea*
Cyanosis if severe

Confirmatory investigations

Nil

Differential diagnosis

Acute epiglottitis
Foreign body

Management

Humidity and oral fluids
Intubation if exhaustion or imminent
obstruction

Prognosis

Good

ACUTE EPIGLOTTITIS AT A GLANCE

Epidemiology

2 to 4-year-olds

Aetiology

Haemophilus influenzae

History

Ill
Fever
Cough rare

Physical examination

*Don't examine throat if epiglottitis is
suspected*
Ill and distressed
Marked difficulty breathing
Unable to talk or swallow
Drooling
Characteristic sitting posture

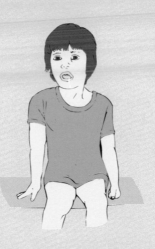

Confirmatory investigations

Epiglottis like a red cherry at
intubation
Blood culture (take only after
intubation)

Management

Intubation
IV chloramphenicol or ampicillin

Prognosis/complications

Prognosis good with prompt diagnosis/
management
Risk of death or severe brain injury if
obstruction occurs

Pathophysiology

Jaundice is caused by accumulation of the yellow pigment, bilirubin, in the skin. Bilirubin metabolism is summarized in Fig. 4.10. Bilirubin is produced as a result of the breakdown of haem from haemoglobin. This is insoluble and referred to as unconjugated. Unconjugated bilirubin is metabolized by the liver cells to a soluble conjugated form and is excreted via the hepatic and bile ducts into the duodenum. Bilirubin and bile salts in the bowel aid the absorption of fats and fat-soluble vitamins. Approximately one half of the conjugated bilirubin is reabsorbed from the bowel as urobilinogen in the enterohepatic circulation. Urobilinogen may be excreted in the urine or remetabolized through the liver. In jaundice, excessive conjugated (soluble) bilirubin may be excreted in the urine which causes the urine to be a dark 'tea' colour.

The causes of jaundice can be divided into those that cause either predominantly unconjugated or conjugated hyperbilirubinaemia. Outside of the neonatal period unconjugated hyperbilirubinaemia is usually caused by haemolysis. Conjugated hyperbilirubinaemia can be divided into either hepatic or obstructive causes (Table 4.18).

The approach to the child with jaundice

History

• *Features of jaundice.* The development of jaundice may occur rapidly as a result of haemolysis. The first sign of more insidious onset of jaundice is a yellow appearance to the sclerae of the eyes. The duration of jaundice should be recorded.
• *Malaise.* Enquire about duration of malaise, abdominal pain and presence of anorexia.
• *Symptoms of anaemia.* Anaemia occurs as the result of haemolysis. Symptoms such as breathlessness may be present and its duration as well as the duration of pallor should be enquired about.
• *Pruritus.* Pruritus refers to intense skin irritation as a result of deposition of bile salts in the skin.
• *Urine.* Colour of the urine should be asked about and later observed. Very dark-coloured urine strongly suggests a conjugated cause of the jaundice.
• *Steatorrhoea.* This refers to frothy, foul-smelling stool which floats in the toilet pan and is commonly described in the majority of children with long-standing cirrhotic liver disease.

Physical examination

• *Growth.* Failure to thrive may occur as the result of any long-standing cause of liver disease.
• *Skin signs.* Scratch marks may be seen on the skin. Signs of long-standing liver disease include spider naevi, clubbing and ascites.
• *Hepatosplenomegaly.* Careful palpation of the liver for enlargement and firmness is important. A hard liver suggests

Table 4.18 Commoner causes of jaundice in childhood. The causes of neonatal jaundice are shown in Table 6.11

Predominantly unconjugated	Predominantly conjugated
Haemolysis	*Hepatic*
Haemolytic disease of the newborn (p. 253)	Hepatitis
Sickle cell disease (p. 92)	Cystic fibrosis
Spherocytosis	Cirrhosis
Hepatic	*Obstructive*
Rare	Hepatitis
	Biliary atresia

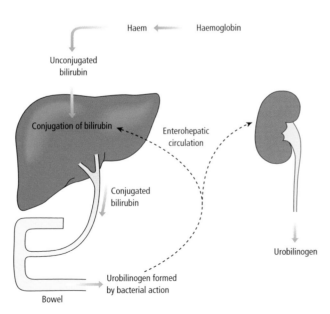

Fig. 4.10 Bilirubin metabolism.

Haemoglobin → Haem

Unconjugated bilirubin

Conjugation of bilirubin

Enterohepatic circulation

Conjugated bilirubin

Urobilinogen

Urobilinogen formed by bacterial action

Bowel

Focal points
Evaluation of jaundice

• Jaundice is first seen in the sclerae

• Dark urine and pale faeces indicate conjugated jaundice

• Presence of anaemia and splenomegaly suggestive of haemolysis

• As part of initial assessment of jaundice measure both conjugated and unconjugated components of serum bilirubin

cirrhosis. Splenomegaly if large may suggest haemolysis, but splenomegaly may also occur as a result of cirrhosis.

The significance of these symptoms and signs in the diagnosis of liver disease is shown in Table 4.19.

Investigations

Basic investigations and their significance are shown in Table 4.20.

Management

Treatment depends on the underlying cause of the jaundice.

Prognosis

The prognosis is dependent on the underlying condition. Jaundice in children is most commonly caused by a self-limiting viral agent which completely resolves. Rarely, chronic liver failure develops following viral infection, and hepatitis B infection is the most likely cause of this.

Where liver disease occurs as the result of an extrahepatic disorder such as cystic fibrosis, the prognosis is most dependent on the underlying condition rather than the liver disease.

Chronic liver failure with cirrhosis carries a poor prognosis, with liver transplantation being the only feasible long-term option.

Causes of jaundice

Viral hepatitis

Hepatitis is caused mainly by viral infections. The causal agents are listed in Table 4.21. The commonest infection is hepatitis A which is spread by faecal contamination of food and water. It is associated with poor hygiene and limited sanitation. The highest incidence for hepatitis A infection in children is 5–15 years of age and the incubation of the virus is approximately 2–6 weeks.

Hepatitis B infection is rare in children and acquired by contamination with blood products. The incubation period of hepatitis B is 2–6 months. The infection is most commonly acquired by vertical transmission from the mother to the baby. Immunization of the newborn infant is possible if the infected mother is recognized antenatally (p. 253). The mother who is hepatitis B antigen positive is highly infectious, but if she has hepatitis B antibodies her baby is protected from vertically transmitted infection.

Clinical features The onset of hepatitis A infection is usually insidious. The child is unwell, with anorexia and nausea, and jaundice appears 5 days later. The liver is tender on palpation, but not enlarged. The urine is dark and the stools may be pale.

Investigations show high liver enzymes (transaminases) with conjugated hyperbilirubinaemia. The virus can be identified serologically and, in the case of hepatitis B, the presence of surface and core antigens must be identified.

Management There is no specific treatment for viral hepatitis. Hepatitis A infection is highly infectious during the prodromal phase, but by the time jaundice is apparent the patient is no longer excreting the virus. Hospital treatment is only required for complications of the condition. Control of cross-infection is essential as a public health measure.

Hepatitis B infection is highly infectious and great care must be taken with handling blood products of infected

Table 4.19 Clinical features of the main causes of jaundice

	Haemolysis	Infectious hepatitis	Cirrhosis
Onset of jaundice	Acute	Acute	Insidious
Dark urine	–	+	+++
Anorexia	–	+++	+
Pruritus	–	–	+++
Anaemia	+++	–	+
Hepatosplenomegaly	+++	–	++
Liver tenderness	+	++	–

Table 4.20 Basic investigations in the jaundiced child with the significance of abnormalities

Investigation	Significance
Haemoglobin (Hb)	Low Hb with increased reticulocytes indicates haemolysis
Bilirubin	Unconjugated excess suggests haemolysis Conjugated excess suggests hepatic or post-hepatic disease
Liver enzymes	Elevated in hepatitis
Alkaline phosphatase	Elevated in cirrhosis or in cases of long-standing jaundice
Serology	Identification of hepatitis virus

Table 4.21 Viral causes of hepatitis

Hepatitis A
Hepatitis B
Hepatitis C (rare)
Epstein–Barr virus
Cytomegalovirus

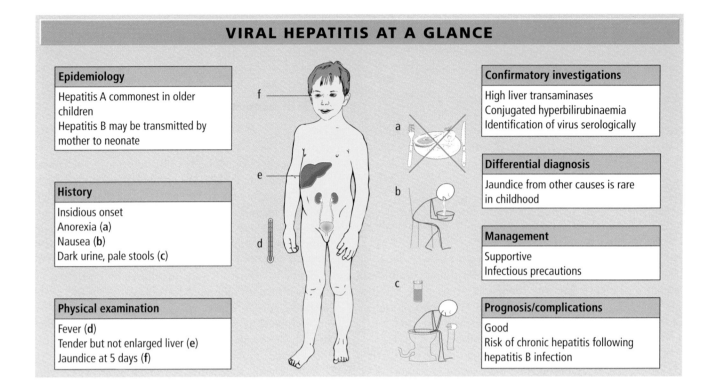

VIRAL HEPATITIS AT A GLANCE

Epidemiology

Hepatitis A commonest in older children
Hepatitis B may be transmitted by mother to neonate

History

Insidious onset
Anorexia (**a**)
Nausea (**b**)
Dark urine, pale stools (**c**)

Physical examination

Fever (**d**)
Tender but not enlarged liver (**e**)
Jaundice at 5 days (**f**)

Confirmatory investigations

High liver transaminases
Conjugated hyperbilirubinaemia
Identification of virus serologically

Differential diagnosis

Jaundice from other causes is rare in childhood

Management

Supportive
Infectious precautions

Prognosis/complications

Good
Risk of chronic hepatitis following hepatitis B infection

---

mothers or children. Immunization of at-risk babies is essential (p. 253) and immunoglobulin infusion is also given to these babies at birth.

Prognosis This is very good following hepatitis A infection. Chronic hepatitis is very rare following infection with the A form and more common following hepatitis B infection. Children who are chronic hepatitis B carriers have an increased risk of subsequent hepatocellular carcinoma in adult life.

Hepatic cirrhosis

This represents the end stage of a number of chronic liver disorders both infectious and metabolic. Cirrhosis in children most commonly follows biliary atresia (p. 253).

Clinical features Jaundice may not be a prominent feature. Failure to thrive as a result of steatorrhoea and vitamin deficiency disorders may be the presenting features (e.g. spontaneous haemorrhages caused by vitamin K deficiency).

Clinical examination reveals an enlarged firm liver which may feel knobbly. Other features of chronic liver disease include spider naevi, ascites, palmar erythema and clubbing.

Investigations must be pursued to identify the underlying cause.

Management This is highly specialized and needs to be undertaken in a recognized centre regularly dealing with chronic liver disease in children. Particular attention must be paid to appropriate nutrition, and correction of fat-soluble vitamin deficiency disorders.
- *Malabsorption.* Lack of bile salts causes steatorrhoea and malabsorption. Diet should be supplemented with medium chain fatty acids which do not require bile salts for their absorption.
- *Vitamin deficiency.* Fat-soluble vitamin deficiency is common in long-standing conjugated jaundice. Vitamins A, D, E and K should be routinely supplemented to avoid deficiency states.
- *Pruritus.* Itching may be very severe. Cholestyramine reduces irritation.
- *Liver transplantation.* This is increasingly becoming a therapeutic resort in end-stage liver diseases. Surgery is limited to a few national centres.

ACUTE ABDOMINAL PAIN

Abdominal pain in children is a very common symptom. Acute and chronic abdominal pain are discussed separately as the presentation and causes are quite different. The problem of recurrent abdominal pain is described in Chapter 5.

When a child presents with acute and severe abdominal pain, the differential diagnosis includes a number of important conditions which require surgical intervention. In practice, many children with acute abdominal pain are referred directly to general surgeons who may have little paediatric experience. It is very important that all children are cared for by medical and nursing staff who have had paediatric training and experience. This includes being looked after in hospital on children's wards where the environment can be made much less frightening.

Pathophysiology

Acute abdominal pain is a common symptom and must be carefully investigated. Acute intra-abdominal pathology may occur in very small babies when a clear history of pain cannot be given by the patient. It is therefore important to consider these causes in all children irrespective of age.

Table 4.22 lists the important and relatively common causes of acute abdominal pain. In some children pain presents acutely and settles spontaneously, only to recur some time later. There may be a gradual merging of episodes of acute abdominal pain with more chronic pain and this can make the categorization of acute and chronic abdominal pain difficult. Table 4.22 therefore overlaps with some conditions described elsewhere.

The approach to the child with acute abdominal pain

History

The description of pain depends on the child's age and verbal skills in describing its intensity, duration and position. In younger children there is very often no clear history of pain.

1 *Pain*. The features of pain in young children include intermittent spasms of screaming for no obvious cause. Pallor during a bout of screaming is an important feature. In older children, the child may be able to point to the area of pain or rub the affected part of the abdomen. Children are not good at localizing the point of maximum pain and often refer to pain all over the abdomen. Ask specifically whether the pain wakes the child at night and whether it is related to eating particular foods. In older children, a description of the pain migrating from the periumbilical area to the right iliac fossa is very suggestive of acute appendicitis.

2 *Blood in stool*. A history of blood in the stool should always be treated seriously. In children with intussusception the classical description is 'redcurrent jelly' stools consisting of blood and mucus.

3 *Associated features*. The history should specifically enquire about the following symptoms and signs. The significance of these in the differential diagnosis is shown in Table 4.23.

- Anorexia (this is a particular feature of acute appendicitis).
- Vomiting and diarrhoea.
- Whether there has been any joint pain or swelling.

Physical examination

Table 4.24 summarizes the important physical signs to look for in a child with acute abdominal pain.

- *General observation*. If the pain is a result of a condition causing peritoneal irritation (peritonism) the child lies very still and movement causes severe pain. Spontaneous move-

Table 4.22 Commoner causes of acute abdominal pain in children

Bowel	Renal	Other
Acute appendicitis	Urinary tract infection	Lower lobe pneumonia
Intussusception	Hydronephrosis	
Mesenteric adenitis	Renal calculus	
Henoch–Schönlein purpura		
Peptic ulceration		
Inflammatory bowel disease		
Intestinal obstruction		
Constipation		
Gastroenteritis		

Table 4.23 Clinical features that distinguish causes of acute abdominal pain

Diagnosis	Clinical features
Acute appendicitis	Tachycardia
	Anorexia
	Peritonism
Intussusception	Intermittent screaming
	Pallor
	'Redcurrent jelly' stool
Mesenteric adenitis	Recent viral infection
	No peritonism
Henoch–Schönlein purpura	Joint pain
	Blood in stool
	Purpura
Urinary tract infection	Dysuria
	Frequency
	Enuresis
Peptic ulceration	Night pain
	Relief by food

ment of the child is an important feature in elucidating the severity of the pain.

• *General examination.* Conditions remote from the abdomen may cause abdominal pain including tonsillitis and mesenteric adenitis or basal pneumonia causing pain referred to the abdomen. The child may have tachycardia and increase in blood pressure in association with pain.

• *Abdomen.* Examination of the acute abdomen may cause extreme agitation in a child who anticipates that the examining doctor will make the pain worse. It is extremely important to reassure the child first, but not to say that 'it will not hurt' as this will be untrue. It is best to precede the examination by an explanation of what will be done and a promise to be as gentle as possible.

The physical examination must be undertaken very carefully and with great sensitivity as the child may anticipate additional pain when the examiner's hand is placed on the abdomen. It may be most appropriate to examine the young child while he or she is lying on his or her mother's lap and sometimes the child's confidence can be gained by placing the examiner's hand on the child's and lightly palpating the abdomen in that manner. This makes the child feel more in control. It is most important to watch the child's face during palpation of the abdomen because this will give a very useful clue as to whether palpation elicits pain. It is obvious that as little additional pain should be inflicted on the child as possible.

The signs of peritonism include great reluctance to move spontaneously, rebound tenderness, guarding and rigidity.

• *Rectal examination.* Although rectal examination may be a considerable intrusion on the child's person, it is an important part of the physical examination in the child who may have an acute appendicitis. It should not, however, be a routine part of all abdominal examinations.

Investigations

If the child has been vomiting, assessment of serum electrolytes and urea is essential to assess the state of hydration. Important investigations in the child with acute abdominal pain are shown in Table 4.25.

Table 4.24 A summary of the systematic approach to examination of the abdomen

---

Observation
General
Does the child look ill?
Is the child moving freely?
Is the child pyrexial?
Is the child tachycardic?
Petechial or purpuric lesions?

Abdomen
Distension?
Is the child holding the abdomen rigid?
Visible peristalsis?
Ask the child to blow out and suck in the stomach. Does this cause pain?

Palpation
Light palpation
Abdominal tenderness?
Rigidity?

Deep palpation
Localized tender area?
Masses?
Guarding?
Rebound tenderness?

Percussion
Ascites? (shifting dullness)

Auscultation
Bowel sounds (increased/absent)

Rectal examination
Tenderness?

Focal points
Evaluation of abdominal pain

• The child with peritonitis lies very still and is reluctant to move

• Signs of peritonism include rebound tenderness, guarding and rigidity

• Pallor and intermittent bouts of screaming suggest intussusception

Table 4.25 Basic investigations in children with acute abdominal pain and their significance

Investigation	Significance
Full blood count	Leucocytosis found in acute appendicitis and urinary tract infection
Urine microscopy and culture	Pyuria and organisms indicate infection
Plain abdominal X-ray	Intussusception (Fig. 4.10) Obstruction
Ultrasound scan	May be particularly helpful in intussusception to exclude renal pathology
Barium enema	For diagnosis and treatment of intussusception (see p. 137)

Management

The most important question to ask oneself when assessing a child with an acute abdomen is whether the child requires a laparotomy. If the child has signs of peritonism (guarding or rigidity, rebound tenderness or severe tenderness on rectal examination) the answer is likely to be yes and a surgical opinion is urgently required. Bowel rupture will rapidly progress to peritonitis and shock. Although acute appendicitis is by far the most likely cause of peritonism there are other rare conditions that can cause this condition. The precise diagnosis is not important because this will be discovered at operation.

Expectant management is appropriate if the child does not have signs of peritonism. Repeated, regular examination of the child's abdomen will determine whether the condition is resolving or getting worse. If there is any doubt as to whether the child has peritonism a surgical opinion may be very valuable.

For non-operative causes of abdominal pain, treatment depends on the underlying condition. The management of the child with recurrent abdominal pain is discussed on pp. 145, 156.

Causes of acute abdominal pain

Acute appendicitis (see also At A Glance Box, p. 136)

This is the commonest cause of an acute abdomen in childhood and occurs in three to four per 1000 children. It can occur at any age including very young infants, but is most common over 5 years of age. It presents most difficulties in diagnosis when it occurs in very young children.

There is no such condition as the 'grumbling appendix'. The child either has an acute appendicitis or not.

Clinical features In older children the presentation may be classical, with the description of pain initially in the periumbilical area moving after a few hours into the right iliac fossa. In young children a history of pain will not be given although the mother will often report that she thinks her baby is in pain. The features of abdominal pain in babies are described above, but the two most important features of acute appendicitis are anorexia and great reluctance to move. Rectal examination must be performed on all children where acute appendicitis is suspected. If there is doubt as to whether the child has acute appendicitis regular re-examination is very important to determine whether the symptoms and signs are getting better or worse.

Investigations Full blood count, electrolytes and urea are essential. Abdominal X-ray is not usually very helpful.

Management Management is always surgical in acute appendicitis. A surgical opinion should be obtained when the diagnosis is suspected.

Prognosis This is very good with skilled surgery. Peritonitis may cause severe illness requiring many weeks for full recovery. If intraperitoneal adhesions occur as a result of peritonitis, later bowel obstruction may occur.

Intussusception

Intussusception is caused by invagination of one part of the bowel into another (Fig. 4.11). The commonest site is the terminal ileum into the caecum. It occurs most frequently

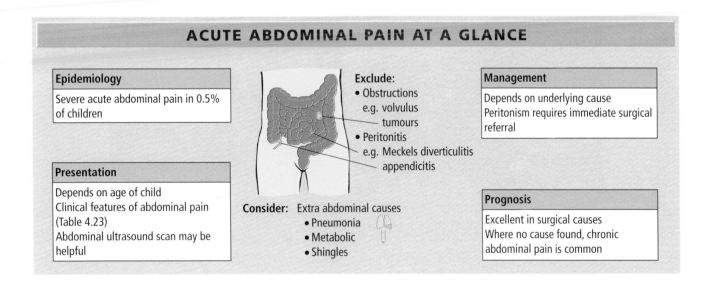

ACUTE ABDOMINAL PAIN AT A GLANCE

Epidemiology

Severe acute abdominal pain in 0.5% of children

Presentation

Depends on age of child
Clinical features of abdominal pain (Table 4.23)
Abdominal ultrasound scan may be helpful

Exclude:
• Obstructions
  e.g. volvulus
  tumours
• Peritonitis
  e.g. Meckels diverticulitis
  appendicitis

Consider: Extra abdominal causes
  • Pneumonia
  • Metabolic
  • Shingles

Management

Depends on underlying cause
Peritonism requires immediate surgical referral

Prognosis

Excellent in surgical causes
Where no cause found, chronic abdominal pain is common

ACUTE APPENDICITIS AT A GLANCE

Epidemiology

Commonest cause of acute abdomen in children over 5 years

History

Classic pain starts periumbilically moving to the right iliac fossa (unobtainable in young children) (**a**)
Anorexia (**b**)
Vomiting in young child (**c**)*
Low grade fever (**d**)*

Physical examination

Rebound tenderness and guarding in the right iliac fossa
Reluctance to move
Rectal exam — marked tenderness against anterior rectal wall

NB *Signs and symptoms are variable

Retro-ileal and pre-ileal 5%
Retrocolic and retrocaecal 75%
Subcaecal and pelvic 20%

Confirmatory investigations

None

Differential diagnosis

Non-specific abdominal pain
Intussusception in infants
Mesenteric adenitis (diagnosis only to be made at laparotomy)

Management

Surgery

Prognosis/complications

Generally good
Risk of peritonitis and adhesions

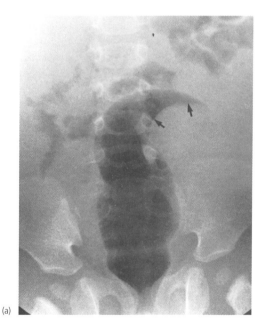
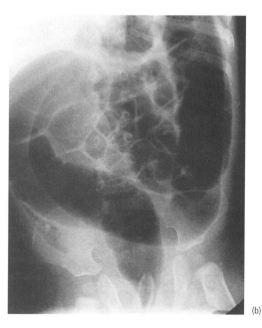
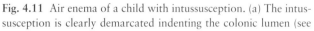

Fig. 4.11 Air enema of a child with intussusception. (a) The intussusception is clearly demarcated indenting the colonic lumen (see arrows). (b) Following reduction, air is now seen in the small bowel.

INTUSSUSCEPTION AT A GLANCE

Epidemiology

Most common from 3 months to 2 years

Aetiology

Most commonly invagination of terminal ileum into caecum

History

Episodic screaming but comfortable between attacks (**a**)
In some children history non-specific passage of 'redcurrant jelly' stool (**c**)*

Physical examination

Pallor at time of screaming
Sausage-shaped mass on right side of abdomen (**b**)*
Blood on rectal exam*

NB *Signs and symptoms are variable

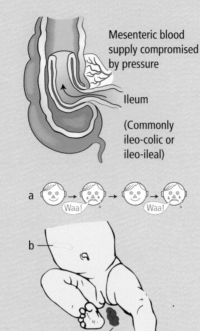

Mesenteric blood supply compromised by pressure

Ileum

(Commonly ileo-colic or ileo-ileal)

Confirmatory investigations

Barium enema

Differential diagnosis

Onset of any acute illness
Otitis media
Appendicitis

Management

Reduction by barium enema
Surgery if barium enema contra-indicated or unsuccessful

Prognosis/complications

Good with prompt diagnosis
Risk of death if diagnosis missed

---

between 3 months and 2 years of age. An enlarged Peyer's patch may form the leading edge of the intussusception and this may occur following a recent viral URTI or gastroenteritis.

Clinical features Classically, the child presents with episodes of severe screaming associated with pallor. The pain is episodic and the child may appear well between colicky episodes. Passage of a 'redcurrent jelly' stool occurs in about 75% of cases and this is an important specific finding. In a proportion of children with intussusception the symptoms and signs may be very non-specific.

Abdominal examination often reveals a sausage-shaped mass in the right side of the abdomen. A plain abdominal X-ray may show signs of bowel obstruction with the typical rounded edge of the intussusception contrasted against the radiolucent lumen of the normal bowel. Ultrasound examination may also be useful in making the diagnosis.

Management In most children the intussusception can be relieved by barium enema examination. This is both diagnostic and curative as the pressure when the barium is inserted can be gradually increased to force back the intussuscepting bowel which can be seen on fluoroscopy. Care must be taken not to use too high a pressure for fear of bowel perforation. Reduction by barium enema should only be used if the history is less than 24 hours and there is no evidence of peritonism or severe dehydration. Surgical reduction is used if barium reduction fails or if the child is unsuitable for barium treatment.

Prognosis Intussusception may be very non-specific in its presentation and is a condition that must always be considered in a child who is acutely but intermittently unwell. Unfortunately, children still die of this condition because the diagnosis is not considered.

Recurrence of the intussusception is uncommon but if this occurs the presence of a polyp should be considered as the cause of the repeated bowel invagination.

Mesenteric adenitis

This condition is often diagnosed where no other cause for acute abdominal pain can be found. It is caused by acute enlargement of intra-abdominal lymph nodes as the result of infection in either the upper respiratory tract, chest or abdomen (gastroenteritis). The acutely enlarged lymph nodes cause pain which may be severe.

Clinical features Children with mesenteric adenitis usually have a recent history of infection and signs may still be

Distinguishing features Acute abdominal pain			
	Age	Clinical features	Management
Acute appendicitis	>5 years	Migration of pain from umbilicus to right iliac fossa	Laparotomy
Intussusception	3–24 months	Pallor and intermittent bouts of screaming	Barium enema reduction
Mesenteric adenitis	Any age	Recent history of infection	Expectant

present in throat or chest. Peritonism and guarding never occur in this condition. It is a diagnosis of exclusion.

Management After other conditions have been excluded the management is expectant.

Prognosis The prognosis is excellent.

THE GENERALIZED CONVULSION

Convulsions are a very common symptom and occur in approximately 20% of children in the first 5 years of life. They are often solitary and do not indicate either that the child will have further convulsions or that he or she will develop epilepsy. The terms fit and seizure are often used synonymously with convulsion. In this section convulsion will be used consistently.

This section deals with the acute investigation and management of the generalized convulsion. The management of epilepsy is discussed in Chapter 10. Neonatal convulsions are dealt with in Chapter 6.

Pathophysiology

Convulsions are caused by synchronous discharge of electrical activity from a group of neurones. Neurones have an excitatory or inhibitory function and cerebral activity is the result of a fine reciprocal balance between these two types of control. Factors that either stimulate a group of excitatory neurones or depress inhibitory ones may throw the system out of balance and precipitate rhythmical firing which in turn causes a clinically observed convulsion.

A convulsion is the clinically apparent manifestation of the discharge through the central and peripheral nervous system. A generalized convulsion is associated with loss of consciousness and involves the face and all four limbs. The immature brain is particularly liable to be subject to

imbalance as a variety of insults may disturb the equilibrium and precipitate convulsions. The commonest trigger factor in children is fever and these are referred to as febrile convulsions (see below).

Convulsions can also be triggered in sensitive children by lack of sleep, a flickering television screen or fast-moving computer games. This is sometimes referred to as reflex epilepsy.

Clinical features

The generalized convulsion or grand mal classically follows a sterotypic sequence:
- aura;
- cry;
- tonic phase (short period of generalized stiffening);
- clonic phase (intermittent muscle contraction and relaxation);
- sleep or drowsiness.

The aura may be visual, auditory or sensory, but is often indescribable in young children, but the mother can often recognize a typical pattern of behaviour. The aura may be absent in febrile convulsions.

The cry stage is common in adolescents, but is not a common feature of younger children. The tonic phase is brief, the child loses consciousness, falls over and becomes stiff.

During the clonic phase, spasms of rhythmical muscle contraction and relaxation of the limb and facial muscles occur. The usual timing of the jerking movements is 1–2 per second. During the clonic phase the child may be incontinent. Clonic movements usually last an average of 2–3 minutes, but in some cases the clonic stage of the convulsion is prolonged lasting more than 20 minutes. A prolonged continuous convulsion lasting longer than 20 minutes is referred to as status epilepticus (see below).

The clonic phase is followed by a period of deep sleep or drowsiness (postictal phase). The child may appear to be confused or irritable after this.

Approach to a child with convulsions

Particular points to consider when seeing a child who is convulsing or is postictal includes:

History

- *Description of the convulsion.* It is very important to obtain an eye witness account of the convulsion so that a 'video' image of the episode can be determined in the clinician's mind. Particular features to enquire about include:
  (i) Duration of the convulsion.

(ii) Previous history of convulsions and any medication for these.

(iii) Was the child unwell or pyrexial before the convulsion?

(iv) If the child is unknown to the doctor, was he or she neurologically and developmentally normal prior to the convulsion.

Physical examination

- *The convulsion.* When a child is seen during a convulsion, note should be taken as to what time the convulsion started and whether it involves all limbs or is focal (confined to one side or one limb). The child's pulse, respiratory rate and general condition should be assessed. If the child is cyanosed then the patency of the airway should be immediately ascertained.
- *Fever.* On examination, the child's temperature should be recorded. Pyrexia following a convulsion, particularly if prolonged, is very common. Even if the child's temperature was not elevated prior to the episode, a period of vigorous muscle activity will elevate body temperature for up to 30 minutes.
- *Focus of infection.* If the child is pyrexial, a source for the infection must be looked for, including examination of the tympanic membranes, throat and chest.
- *Central nervous system examination.* Neurological examination is particularly important as a convulsion may be the first sign of meningitis or other neurological disorders.

Investigations

Investigations are not necessary in all cases, particularly if the child is having repeated febrile convulsions. If the child is pyrexial then a urine culture is useful. Throat swabs should be performed if the child has exudate or marked pharyngitis.

The possibility of meningitis must be considered in any child with a febrile convulsion. If the child is 18 months old or more and has no focal neurological signs or neck stiffness, then a lumbar puncture can be avoided. In younger children a lumbar puncture should be the rule unless there is a very good reason to avoid this procedure.

An electroencephalogram (EEG) is not indicated in every child with a first convulsion. The following are indications for EEG:

- second febrile convulsion;
- any convulsion lasting more than 20 minutes;
- focal (atypical) convulsions;
- convulsion in a child >5 years old.

A convulsion causes considerable disturbance of the EEG and follow-up EEG should be performed more than 6 weeks after the last convulsive episode.

Computer tomography or magnetic resonance imaging brain scans are not indicated unless the child shows focal convulsive activity.

Management

The acute management of a generalized convulsion is discussed here and the long-term management of epilepsy is discussed in Chapter 10.

The convulsing child

Every parent finds the first convulsion a most frightening condition and many children are either rushed to hospital or the GP is urgently summoned as a result of it. If the child is still convulsing when seen by a doctor then the convulsion should be aborted by diazepam medication (see below).

Management of status epilepticus

This is defined as a prolonged convulsion lasting 20 minutes or more, or a series of shorter convulsions with failure to regain consciousness between them. Rapid treatment of a prolonged convulsion is necessary. In hospital, diazepam can be given intravenously by slow injection until the convulsion stops. At home, rectal diazepam can be given by the doctor or the parents if they have been previously shown how to do this.

Subsequent management of the child

If the child is 5 years of age or below and the convulsion is thought to be febrile then long-term treatment is not indicated after the first febrile convulsion. The management of febrile convulsions is discussed below.

If the child is under 5 years and is afebrile or is over 5 years, then epilepsy should be considered as the cause of the convulsion. Long-term maintenance treatment is not necessarily indicated and this problem is discussed in Chapter 10.

Issues for the family

Almost all parents who see their child convulsing for the first time imagine that the child is going to die. This is a terrifying situation for them and they seek medical help rapidly. It is most important to spend time explaining the cause of the fit, first aid procedures and prognosis to the parents. Reassure them that death is extremely unlikely during a convulsion and by following simple first aid measures this can be avoided. Parents whose child has had a convulsion should be instructed in the first aid management of a convulsion. This includes:

- Check airway.
- Lay the child on the floor in the recovery position (semi-prone with the underlying leg flexed at the knee and hip, Fig. 4.12).

- Do not insert objects into the child's mouth.
- Ensure a responsible person stays with the child if a telephone call to a doctor or ambulance is made.
- The child needs medication to abort the convulsion if it lasts longer than 5–10 minutes.

If a child is having regular convulsions then treatment to prevent or abort further convulsions is necessary. In recurrent febrile convulsions, rectal diazepam is the treatment of choice to abort convulsions. The parents must be given clear instructions in how to administer this medication. The rectal diazepam comes in a dispenser that is easily inserted into the child's rectum. The instructions are as follows.

- Put the child in the knee–chest position, lying on his or her side.
- Remove the cap from the rectal diazepam dispenser.
- Insert the nozzle gently through the anus up to the hilt of its spout.
- Squeeze the contents of the tube slowly (over 2–3 minutes) into the child's rectum.
- Remove the applicator, lie the child in the recovery position and stay with him or her.
- The medication is likely to make the child sleepy for several hours.

Prognosis

Children of 5 years of age and below only have a 50% chance of having further convulsions after the first episode. High risk of further convulsions are seen in children with the following adverse features:
- Atypical convulsions.
- Pre-existing neurological abnormality (cerebral palsy, tuberose sclerosis, structural brain anomaly).
- Strong family history of childhood convulsions.
- Prolonged convulsion.

A prolonged convulsion (>20 minutes) carries an increased risk of the child developing temporal lobe epilepsy in later life. The temporal lobe has a high metabolic rate and prolonged convulsing causes 150% increase in oxygen consumption in that part of the brain. This very high metabolic

demand may outstrip the delivery of oxygen and glucose to the area causing autoinfarction of parts of the temporal lobe. This subsequently scars and forms the focus of temporal lobe epilepsy.

Causes of generalized convulsions

Febrile convulsions

These are seizures which occur in children between the age of 6 months and 5 years and are caused by fever. The immature brain is more susceptible to environmental factors and fever may precipitate a grand mal convulsion. They occur in 10% of all children in this age group and the risk is higher if there is a family history.

Clinical features Fever precedes the convulsion, but there may be a sudden rise in body temperature immediately before the convulsion which may not be recognized by the parent. Fever may occur as a result of convulsive activity and fever with convulsion does not necessarily allow the diagnosis of febrile convulsion to be made. The convulsion is usually short-lived, lasting only a few minutes. Status epilepticus occurs in only about 1% of febrile convulsions. In all children with febrile convulsion a careful examination should be performed in order to identify the site of infection. Investigations are described above.

Management The following features should be considered as part of the management of all children with febrile convulsions.
1 *Advice to parents.* If a child has had a febrile convulsion the parents must be shown how to manage subsequent episodes of fever to prevent recurrence of febrile convulsions. This includes:
  - Undress the child.
  - Sponge with tepid water, particularly in groin and axillae.
  - Give paracetamol for its antipyretic effect.
  - An electric fan may be used, but the parents must be warned that this is dangerous if the child pokes his or her fingers in it.
2 *Initial medical management.* If the child is febrile the GP should be called to identify the source of infection as this may need antibiotic treatment or further investigations.
  - Termination of a convulsion lasting for >5–10 minutes.
  - Physical examination to identify any source of infection.
  - Reassurance for the parents and discussion of prognosis.
  - Instruction to the parents on first aid management of further convulsions.

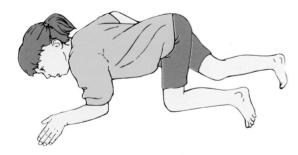

Fig. 4.12 The recovery position.

FEBRILE CONVULSIONS AT A GLANCE

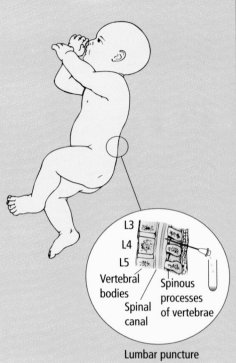

Epidemiology

Occurs between 6 months and 5 years in 10% of children

Aetiology

High fever of any cause particularly at sudden rise

History

Short-lived generalized convulsion
Symptoms of condition causing the fever

Physical examination

High fever
Normal neurological exam following seizure
Signs of infection responsible for fever*

NB *Signs and symptoms are variable

Confirmatory investigations

Lumbar puncture required at first febrile seizure in most cases to exclude meningitis
Investigation for cause of fever if indicated by assessment

Differential diagnosis

Meningitis
Other causes of generalized convulsion

Management

Control of fever
Parental advice regarding management of fever
Treatment of underlying infection if identified
Rectal diazepam for prolonged seizure

Prognosis/complications

Good
Risk of developing epilepsy only 2% in neurologically normal children

L3
L4
L5
Vertebral bodies
Spinal canal
Spinous processes of vertebrae
Lumbar puncture

Principles of management
Febrile convulsions

- Abort convulsion if lasting >10 minutes

- Identify source of infection/fever

- Explain first aid measures if further convulsions

- Teach use of rectal diazepam if convulsions are recurrent

- In children with recurrent febrile convulsions instructions in the use of rectal diazepam.

The parents should be told that the prognosis for brief febrile convulsions is very good and there is no increased risk of epilepsy, provided the child has not had a prolonged or atypical convulsion.

If the child is having repeated convulsions the school should be informed and this is discussed on p. 337.

Continuous anticonvulsant medication for children with febrile convulsions is not frequently given. The indications for this include:
- more than four convulsions per year;
- prolonged seizures (>20 minutes);
- where there is existing underlying neurological abnormality.

Prognosis Children with uncomplicated febrile convulsions are at no greater risk of subsequent epilepsy than children without febrile convulsions. A prolonged convulsion lasting more than 20 minutes may predispose to temporal lobe epilepsy (see above).

5 Common Symptoms and Complaints of Childhood

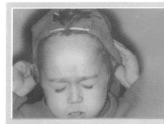

Introduction, 142
The crying baby and colic, 142
Causes of crying in babies, 143
Recurrent abdominal pain, 144
Non-organic causes of recurrent abdominal
    pain, 147
Organic causes of recurrent abdominal pain,
    148
Headache, 149
Causes of headache, 150
Leg pain and limp, 152
Causes of leg pain and limp in childhood, 153
Chest pain, 155
Causes of chest pain, 156
Non-organic pain in childhood, 156
Vomiting, 156
Causes of vomiting in childhood, 158
Acute diarrhoea, 160
Causes of acute diarrhoea, 162
Chronic diarrhoea, 162
Causes of chronic diarrhoea in
    childhood, 165
Constipation, 168
Causes of constipation, 170

Soiling and encopresis, 172
Blood in the stool, 172
Causes of rectal bleeding, 173
Cough, 173
Causes of cough in childhood, 175
Fits, faints and funny turns, 178
Types of fits, faints and funny turns, 179
Urinary symptoms: dysuria, 183
Causes of dysuria, 183
Urinary symptoms: polyuria and
    frequency, 183
Causes of urinary frequency, 184
Causes of polyuria, 184
Urinary symptoms: diurnal enuresis, 185
Causes of diurnal enuresis, 185
Urinary symptoms: nocturnal enuresis, 186
Urinary symptoms: haematuria, 188
Causes of haematuria, 189
Rashes and skin lesions, 190
Rashes of acute onset, 191
Conditions causing acute generalized rashes
    in childhood, 193
Conditions causing acute vesicular
    rashes, 197

Conditions causing purpuric rashes, 198
Conditions causing acute wheals, 200
Chronic skin problems, 201
Common chronic skin conditions in
    childhood, 203
Birthmarks, 206
Common birthmarks, 206
Discrete skin lesions, 207
Common discrete skin lesions, 208
Itching, 211
Conditions causing itching, 211
Nappy rash, 213
Swollen joints, 214
Causes of swollen joints in childhood, 216
Pyrexia of unknown origin, 220
Specific causes of pyrexia of unknown origin
    in childhood, 222
Recurrent infection, 222
Causes of serious recurrent infection, 223
Swellings in the neck, 225
Conditions causing swellings in the
    neck, 226
Oedema, 229

A Doctor came hurrying round, and he said:
'Tut-tut, I am sorry to find you in bed.
Just say "Ninety-nine," while I look at your chest . . .'
. . . And ordered him Nourishment, Tonics and Rest,
'How very effective,' he said as he shook
The thermometer . . .
The Doctor next morning was rubbing his hands,
And saying, 'There's nobody quite understands
These cases as I do . . .'.

The Dormouse and the Doctor
A.A. Milne

Introduction

This chapter deals with those symptoms and complaints that commonly present in general practice or in paediatric outpatients, as opposed to problems that present more acutely (Chapters 4 and 9), or through child health surveillance (Chapter 3). An approach to diagnosing each problem is discussed, with details of the most important causative conditions and their distinguishing features.

In all these conditions the most important aspects of the diagnostic process are clinical and, if a careful history and physical examination are performed, investigations can be kept to a minimum.

THE CRYING BABY AND COLIC

Babies, or rather their parents, often present complaining of excessive crying. The crying is usually periodic and related to discomfort, stress or temperament. However, and particularly if of acute onset, it may indicate a serious problem. Infantile colic is a term used to describe periodic crying that affects young infants usually in the first 3 months of life.

Teething is very often blamed for crying, but there is little evidence that systemic disturbances such as fever, facial rashes and diarrhoea are caused by teething. When a baby seems to have a very irritable temperament, particularly if accompanied by possetting and vomiting, the diagnosis of reflux oesophagitis should be considered.

Babies are generally more irritable than older children when ill from any cause, and may well be off their feeds for a while. A common condition that causes severe distress, particularly at night, in the baby and young child is otitis media (see p. 105), which may occur in the absence of fever or catarrh. A serious cause of acute distress is intussusception (see p. 135) which precipitates severe paroxysmal crying. The common causes of crying are listed in Table 5.1.

Approach to the crying baby

The purpose of the clinical evaluation is to ensure that there is no organic basis to the crying, and to identify psychosocial factors that may be exacerbating the problem.

History

• *What are the characteristics of the cry?* Experienced parents can usually differentiate their baby's cries. If they are concerned that he or she is in pain, this needs to be taken seriously. Colic characteristically occurs late in the day. Acute otitis media may cause a baby to wake at night in pain. Crying associated with feeds may suggest reflux oesophagitis. The sudden onset of severe paroxysmal crying should suggest intussusception.

• *Is the baby ill?* Ill babies are usually more irritable than usual, and often go off their feeds. Enquiry into fever and a complete review of systems is needed.

• *How are the parents coping?* Babies are very sensitive to stress in the home, and existing stress levels increase with an incessantly crying baby. Gaining an idea of stress levels and coping strategies are important in managing the problem.

Table 5.1 Causes of crying in babies

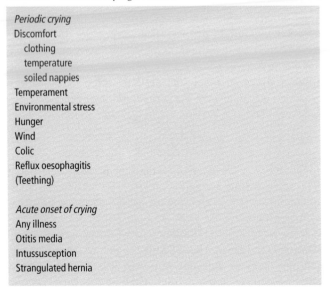

Periodic crying
Discomfort
clothing
temperature
soiled nappies
Temperament
Environmental stress
Hunger
Wind
Colic
Reflux oesophagitis
(Teething)
Acute onset of crying
Any illness
Otitis media
Intussusception
Strangulated hernia

Physical examination

• *Growth.* Poor growth is a worrying sign which suggests the baby is not receiving enough milk.

• *Evidence of illness.* A complete physical examination including inspection of the tympanic membranes must be carried out. In intussusception the baby can be seen to be experiencing paroxysms of severe distress.

Management

All babies cry, and even the most experienced parents at times may have difficulty in understanding what is distressing their baby. New parents have often had little previous experience of babies and need to learn how to handle their infant, and to respond to his or her needs.

Infants who waken and cry consistently at short intervals may not be receiving enough milk. However, it is important to appreciate that infants cry for reasons other than hunger. They may have discomfort from some other cause, such as too much clothing, soiled or wet nappies, swallowed air or illness. It is inadvisable to fall into the pattern of offering frequent feeds, or of holding and feeding to pacify all crying.

Unfortunately, and sadly too often, breast-feeding is thought by mother or health professional to be inadequate and supplements started. If the baby is thriving, and often when he or she is not, artificial feeds are of no benefit, and the mother and baby discover this too late when lactation has ceased.

Stress has a particular role. Babies are very sensitive to stress within the family and usually respond by crying. The crying itself, of course, can induce stress in the calmest of families, and can exacerbate already stressful situations.

Medical management, once a physical problem has been excluded, involves reassurance and support for the parents. Additional on-going support can often be provided at home visits by the local health visitor.

Causes of crying in babies

Colic

The term 'colic' describes a common symptom of paroxysmal crying which occurs in babies principally under 3 months of age, and which is presumed to be of intestinal origin. Certain infants are particularly susceptible to colic. It may be associated with hunger and swallowed air, or discomfort and distension caused by overfeeding.

Clinical features The clinical pattern is characteristic. The attack usually begins suddenly, with crying which often lasts more or less continuously for several hours. The face may be

COLIC AT A GLANCE

Epidemiology

Babies under 3 months old

Aetiology

Presumed to be intestinal in origin

History

Crying for several hours, often late in the day
Face flushed, legs drawn-up*
Abdomen distended*
Relief on passing flatus or faeces*

NB *Signs and symptoms are variable

Physical examination

Normal

Confirmatory investigations

None

Differential diagnosis

Discomfort and stress
Reflux oesophagitis
Acute onset:
• intussusception
• otitis media

Management

Reassurance and support

Prognosis/complications

Usually resolves by 3 months old

---

flushed, the abdomen distended and tense, the legs drawn up and the hands clenched. The attack may end when the infant is completely exhausted, but often there is relief when faeces or flatus are passed. Attacks commonly occur late in the afternoon or evening. Careful physical examination is important to eliminate the possibility of intussusception, strangulated hernia or other disorders.

Management Holding the baby, or carrying him or her in a sling close to the parent can soothe, and secure swaddling occasionally helps. No effective remedies have been found, although recent research suggests that sucrose may be effective. Changes of infant formula, although commonly tried, are rarely helpful. Support and sympathy are important in successful management of the problem, which resolves spontaneously over a few months.

Reflux oesophagitis (p. 158)

If oesophagitis is suspected a trial of antacids, thickeners or H_2 antagonists can be empirically given, although in severe cases further investigation is merited.

RECURRENT ABDOMINAL PAIN

Recurrent abdominal pain is one of the commonest symptoms presenting in children with 10–15% of school-age children at some point experiencing it. Of these, only 1 in 10 are found to have an organic problem, the majority having no identifiable cause for the pain. The commoner causes of recurrent abdominal pain are listed in Table 5.2. The problem of the child with acute abdominal pain is discussed in Chapter 4.

Approach to the child with recurrent abdominal pain

Abdominal pain can accompany almost any chronic childhood disorder, although luckily, it is rarely the only manifestation of serious disease. The purpose of the clinical evaluation is to determine as rapidly as possible whether there is an organic cause for the pain and, if not, to provide appropriate reassurance and support rather than let the anxiety linger that there is a serious problem which has not been identified.

History

A complete history is required, reviewing the child's lifestyle and habits as well as focusing on symptoms appertaining to each organ system.

• *Nature of the pain.* The character of the pain can help in identifying the cause. The child may be able to describe if the pain is colicky or constant, and how it is related to daily activities, bowel habit or diet. Even if the child cannot describe the pain, the site can often be located. Non-organic pain is classically periumbilical, and it has been said that the further the pain is from the umbilicus, the greater the chances that an aetiology can be identified. A diary kept by the family can be quite helpful in clarifying the frequency of episodes and their relation to other events.

• *Symptoms relating to abdominal organs.* Symptoms

Table 5.2 The more common causes of recurrent abdominal pain

Idiopathic

Psychogenic

Gastrointestinal
Irritable bowel syndrome
Oesophagitis
Peptic ulcer
Inflammatory bowel disease
Constipation
Malabsorption
Giardiasis

Urinary tract
Infections

Hepatic
Hepatitis

Pancreas
Pancreatitis

Gynaecological
Dysmenorrhoea
Pelvic inflammatory disease
Haematocolpos
Ovarian cyst

Other
Abdominal migraine
Lead poisoning

Focal points
Evaluating recurrent abdominal pain

• Obtain a full picture of the pattern of episodes of pain

• Identify symptoms related to the various abdominal organs

• Determine whether there are any constitutional symptoms

• Decide if the pain is likely to be organic or functional in origin

• Obtain a picture of the psychosocial circumstances and the effect the pain has on the child's activities

---

related to specific organ systems may give clues to an organic cause. Constipation, diarrhoea or vomiting suggest a gastrointestinal cause, and frequency and dysuria suggest urinary tract aetiology. Enquiry into gynaecological symptoms should not be forgotten in this age group.

• *General constitutional symptoms.* The presence of general constitutional symptoms such as anorexia, weight loss and fever are important indicators that there is a serious underlying cause.

• *Emotional and family problems.* The assessment must always include enquiries into emotional and family problems, as these commonly are associated with abdominal pain. It is important to establish the extent to which symptoms are interfering with the child's life at home and at school.

• *Family history.* The presence of gastrointestinal disease in the family, especially peptic ulcers, may be relevant.

Physical examination

A complete physical examination must be carried out and should not be limited to the region below the diaphragm and above the pelvis.

• *Growth.* Height and weight measurements are particularly important, as weight loss indicates serious pathology. If the problem is long-standing, fall off in growth may also occur.

• *General examination.* Signs of pallor, jaundice and clubbing should be sought.

• *Abdominal examination.* The abdomen needs to be examined for signs of hepatomegaly, splenomegaly, enlarged kidneys or a distended bladder.

• *Anorectal examination.* This is not routine in children, but should be carried out if there are symptoms of constipation, or any suspicion of sexual abuse.

Investigations (Table 5.3)

If the symptoms are significant, a full blood count, sedimentation rate, stools for ova and parasites, and urinalysis and culture can be helpful as inflammatory bowel disease, chronic urinary tract infection (UTI) and gastrointestinal parasites may present with abdominal pain alone. Further investigations should only be carried out in response to findings suggestive of a particular disease process.

On the basis of a thorough clinical evaluation and a minimum of investigations, it is usually possible to distinguish functional pain from organic pain. Table 5.4 summarizes the characteristic features.

Management

The management of abdominal pain depends on the aetiology. Analgesics are usually unhelpful. The strategy described

Investigation	What are you looking for?
Blood tests	
Full blood count	Anaemia, eosinophilia, infection
Sedimentation rate or plasma viscosity	Elevated in inflammatory bowel disease
Liver function tests	Liver dysfunction
Urea and electrolytes	Renal failure
Amylase	Pancreatitis
Urine test	
Urinalysis and culture	Urine infection
Stool	
Ova and parasites (× 3 samples)	Gastrointestinal parasites, e.g. giardiasis
occult blood	Gastrointestinal blood loss, e.g. inflammatory bowel disease or peptic ulcer
Ultrasound	
Abdominal and pelvic	Urinary obstruction at all levels, organomegaly, abscesses, pregnancy, ovarian cyst and torsion
X-ray	
Plain abdominal	Constipation, renal calculi if radiopaque, lead poisoning
Barium swallow and follow-through	Oesophagitis and reflux, peptic ulcer, Crohn's disease, congenital malformations of the gut
Barium enema	Ulcerative colitis
Endoscopy	Oesophagitis and reflux
	Peptic ulceration
	Colitis

Table 5.3 Useful investigations in assessing the child with recurrent abdominal pain

	Organic	Non-organic
Characteristics	Day and night Character depends on underlying cause	Periodic pain with intervening good health Often periumbilical If psychosomatic may be related to school hours
History	Weight loss and/or reduced appetite Lack of energy Recurrent fever Organ specific symptoms, e.g. change in bowel habit, polyuria, menstrual problems, vomiting Occult or frank bleeding from any orifice Family history of gastrointestinal problems	Otherwise healthy child
Physical exam	Ill appearance, growth failure, swollen joint	Normal, thriving child
Preliminary investigations	Anaemia, leucocytosis, raised sedimentation rate or eosinophilia on blood count Abnormal urinalysis and/or culture	Normal

Table 5.4 Features differentiating organic and non-organic causes of abdominal pain

in An approach to the child with non-organic recurrent pain on p. 156 may be helpful.

Non-organic causes of recurrent abdominal pain

Idiopathic recurrent abdominal pain

The majority of children presenting with recurrent abdominal pain have no identifiable organic cause. In this circumstance the expression 'recurrent abdominal pain' is often used as a diagnostic term, in itself implying that the pain is functional rather than organic.

Clinical features Children with recurrent abdominal pain suffer very real pain which can be severe. The periodicity of the complaint and the intervening good health are characteristic of the syndrome. The children are often described as being sensitive, highly strung and high achieving individuals, although this is by no means always true.

Management and prognosis Management must be directed towards reassurance, maximizing a normal lifestyle and minimizing school absence (see An approach to the child with recurrent pain, p. 156). In the majority of children the pain resolves over time.

Psychogenic abdominal pain

In some children the abdominal pain is truly psychosomatic and related to stress at home or at school. Obviously these underlying causes must be addressed. In most cases simply indicating the link and explaining that children tend to experience tummy-aches in a similar way to which adults experience headache is enough to reassure the parents and child.

Some children utilize abdominal pain, whether real or fictitious, to their own ends, so missing school or unpleasant events. In this circumstance confrontation is not usually helpful. An understanding attitude, while maintaining that absence from school is unnecessary, is a good approach.

Irritable bowel syndrome

The term 'irritable bowel syndrome' is sometimes used instead of 'recurrent abdominal pain', particularly if there are minor gastrointestinal symptoms, and no psychological stresses identified. It has been suggested that the discomfort results from a dysfunction of the autonomic system of the gut.

Clinical features The bowel pattern may be described as varying from pellets to unformed stool. Flatus can also be a

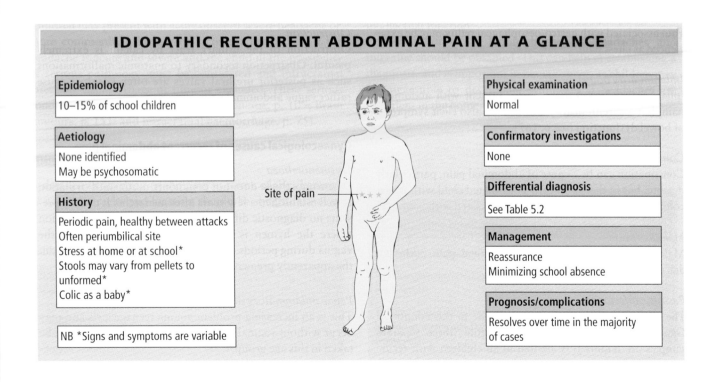

IDIOPATHIC RECURRENT ABDOMINAL PAIN AT A GLANCE

Epidemiology
10–15% of school children

Aetiology
None identified
May be psychosomatic

History
Periodic pain, healthy between attacks
Often periumbilical site
Stress at home or at school*
Stools may vary from pellets to unformed*
Colic as a baby*

NB *Signs and symptoms are variable

Site of pain

Physical examination
Normal

Confirmatory investigations
None

Differential diagnosis
See Table 5.2

Management
Reassurance
Minimizing school absence

Prognosis/complications
Resolves over time in the majority of cases

Physical examination

A careful physical examination is important in order to determine whether there is any evidence of serious pathology. In the severe, acute headache the key clinical features to be assessed are the presence of fever, meningeal signs, level of consciousness, focal neurological signs and signs of raised intracranial pressure. In persistent or recurrent headaches there are usually no signs. However, it is important to exclude the following:

• *Hypertension.*
• *Signs of raised intracranial pressure.* Signs are slow pulse, high blood pressure, papilloedema and enlarging head circumference in the preschool child.
• *Focal neurological signs.* These signs are dependent on the site of the lesion. Cerebellar signs of nystagmus, ataxia and intention tremor, or signs of cranial nerve palsies indicate an infratentorial tumour. Signs of focal spasticity indicate a cerebral lesion, while delayed growth and puberty and visual field defects indicate a pituitary tumour.
• Evidence of dental caries, sinus tenderness and carotid bruits should also be sought.

Investigations

Investigations are rarely indicated unless there is evidence of raised intracranial pressure or neurological signs. In this circumstance a computer tomography (CT) scan or magnetic resonance imaging (MRI) scan is indicated.

Management

Simple analgesia with paracetamol is usually adequate. If the headaches persist the approach described on p. 156 (An approach to non-organic pain) may be helpful.

Causes of headache

Tension headaches

Tension headaches usually develop towards later childhood. They are thought to be caused by persistent contraction of neck and temporal muscles.

Clinical features Headaches which are constricting or band-like in nature tend to occur towards the end of the day, but do not interfere with sleep. There may or may not be evidence that the child is under stress. Often other members of the family suffer from similar headaches.

Management The family needs to be reassured that there is no serious underlying pathology. In terms of treatment, rest

Features of concern in the clinical evaluation
• Acute onset of severe pain
• Headache intensified by lying down
• Associated vomiting
• Fall-off in school performance or regression of developmental skills
• Consistently unilateral pain
• Cranial bruit
• Hypertension
• Papilloedema
• Fall-off in growth

and sympathy is often all that is required. Simple analgesics such as paracetamol may be given, but dependency should be avoided. Any underlying stress and tensions in the child's life need to be addressed. It is important that school absence is kept to a minimum, and the school may have to be approached directly to develop a strategy for when headaches develop in school hours.

If others at home experience headaches it helps to advise minimizing attention to them as children can be quite susceptible to the symptoms of others.

Prognosis The headaches often resolve spontaneously or become less frequent.

Migraine

Migraine is another common cause of headache in the school-age child, and is thought to result from constriction, followed by vasodilatation and pulsation of the intracranial arteries.

Clinical features Onset is usually in late childhood or early adolescence. Classically the attack is preceded by an aura (caused by constriction of the vessels), which is often visual in nature, but may consist of other fleeting neurological sensations. Within a few minutes a throbbing unilateral headache occurs accompanied by nausea and vomiting. Sleep usually ends the attack. In younger children the attack is often bilateral with no aura, nausea or vomiting. Rarely, complicated migraine occurs when focal neurological symptoms and signs are present. The migraine headache always causes some reduction in the child's ability to function normally.

There is often a history of repeated vomiting or travel sickness when the child was younger, and a positive family history is usually present.

TENSION HEADACHES AT A GLANCE

Epidemiology

Common in later childhood

Aetiology

Possibly caused by contraction of neck and temporal muscles

History

Constricting/band-like pain
No interference with sleep
At end of day*
Stress at home or school*
Family history of headaches*

NB *Signs and symptoms are variable

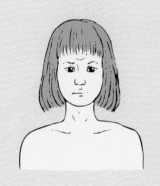

Physical examination

Normal

Confirmatory investigations

None

Differential diagnosis

Migraine
(Causes of raised intracranial pressure)

Management

Reassurance
Simple analgesics

Prognosis/complications

Usually spontaneous resolution

There is no confirmatory test for migraine and diagnosis is made on the presence of some of the following:

- episodic nature;
- aura;
- visual disturbance;
- nausea in 90% of cases;
- unilateral headache;
- family history;
- impairment of normal function during an attack.

Management   First line treatment is rest, with simple analgesia. In some children attacks are precipitated by certain foods such as chocolate, cheese or nuts, and withdrawal of these items from the diet can be helpful. If attacks are frequent prophylaxis with propranolol or pizotifen should be considered. Sumatriptan, a 5-hydroxy-tryptamine agonist, is useful in aborting acute migraine attacks in adolescents. It is not recommended for use in childhood.

Prognosis   Migraine headaches often persist into adulthood, but may undergo remission spontaneously.

Raised intracranial pressure

Brain tumours, abscesses and chronic subdural haematomas are rare causes of headache in childhood.

Clinical features   Headaches which are caused by a rise in intracranial pressure are classically exacerbated by lying down and so it is concerning if a child wakes from sleep with headaches. The headache is often accompanied by vomiting with little associated nausea. Raised intracranial pressure may cause elevated blood pressure, bradycardia, papilloedema and altered neurological function.

The location of the pain is a good localizing sign for the site of the lesion. The commonest tumours are infratentorial in site, causing signs of cerebellar or brain stem dysfunction. Supratentorial tumours may be located in the hypothalamic–pituitary axis causing endocrine or visual problems, or may be located in the cerebrum causing epilepsy or spasticity.

Management   CT and MRI scans are reliable in detecting intracranial space occupying lesion. Treatment depends on the pathology of the lesion.

Hypertension

Hypertension is usually asymptomatic in childhood, but headache can be a symptom, and measurement of blood pressure is of course mandatory in any child presenting with headache.

Other causes of headache

Headaches often accompany minor systemic infections. Dental caries, sinusitis and otitis media are all treatable causes of headache and signs of these problems should be

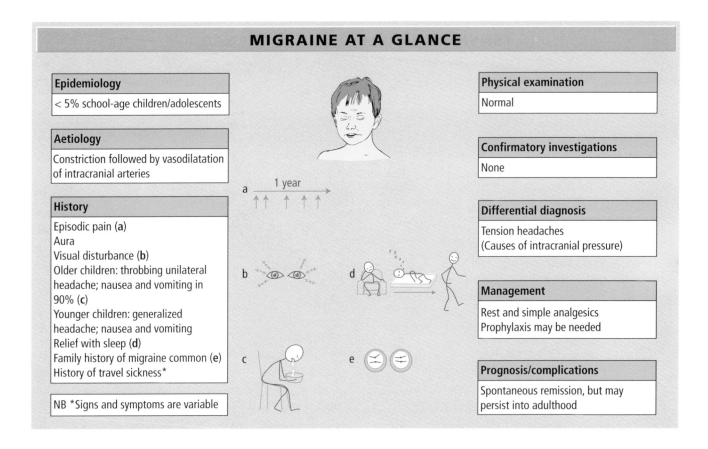

MIGRAINE AT A GLANCE

Epidemiology

< 5% school-age children/adolescents

Aetiology

Constriction followed by vasodilatation of intracranial arteries

History

Episodic pain (**a**)
Aura
Visual disturbance (**b**)
Older children: throbbing unilateral headache; nausea and vomiting in 90% (**c**)
Younger children: generalized headache; nausea and vomiting
Relief with sleep (**d**)
Family history of migraine common (**e**)
History of travel sickness*

NB *Signs and symptoms are variable

Physical examination

Normal

Confirmatory investigations

None

Differential diagnosis

Tension headaches
(Causes of intracranial pressure)

Management

Rest and simple analgesics
Prophylaxis may be needed

Prognosis/complications

Spontaneous remission, but may persist into adulthood

Distinguishing features—Headache in childhood

	Character of the headache	Timing of the headache	Associated features	Physical examination
Tension	Constricting, band-like	Towards the end of the day	Nil	Normal
Migraine	Throbbing, unilateral		Nausea, vomiting, aura, photophobia, family history	Normal
Raised intracranial pressure (RICP)	Worse on lying down, may be localized to site of lesion	Early morning Waking at night	Vomiting without nausea, other features depend on site of lesion	Slow pulse High BP Papilloedema Enlarging HC Focal signs

sought on clinical evaluation. Eye strain is often blamed for headaches, although there is little evidence for this. However, it does no harm to recommend an assessment of visual acuity.

LEG PAIN AND LIMP

The complaint of leg pain alone, unaccompanied by physical signs is usually non-organic in nature. Limp, however, is likely to have an underlying organic explanation. The causes of leg pain and limp are listed in Table 5.6.

Approach to the child with leg pain or limp

In a child presenting with acute or recurrent leg pain, a good history and physical examination should differentiate non-organic from organic causes. Investigations may be required to identify the aetiology where organic disease is suspected.

Table 5.6 Causes of leg pain and limp in childhood

Organic
Transient synovitis
Septic arthritis
Legg–Calvé–Perthes disease
Slipped capital femoral epiphysis
Trauma
Osteomyelitis
Neoplastic disease
Systemic disease
Non-organic
Growing pains

Focal points
Evaluating leg pain and limp

• Organic and non-organic causes can be differentiated on clinical grounds (see Table 5.8)

• Important features suggestive of organic disease are a child's refusal to walk, a limp and any physical signs

• Pain in the hip is referred to the knee, so children presenting with knee pain require a full examination of the leg and groin

History

The history should focus on the characteristics of the pain and any systemic symptoms that the child might have.

• *Character of the pain.* Pain as a result of organic causes tends to be persistent, occurring day and night and interrupts play as well as schooling. Particularly significant is a limp or refusal to walk. Organic pain is often unilateral or located to a joint. By contrast, non-organic pain usually occurs at night and primarily on school days. It does not interfere with normal activities, and the parents report a normal gait. It is often bilateral and located between joints.

• *Systemic symptoms.* Systemic symptoms such as weight loss, fever, night sweats, rash and diarrhoea point to organic causes.

Physical examination

The child should be examined lying down and then walking. It should be remembered that pain in the hip is referred to the knee, so that a child presenting with knee pain requires a full examination of the leg and groin.

• *The limb.* Signs of point tenderness, redness, swelling and

Table 5.7 Laboratory tests helpful in distinguishing organic and non-organic leg pain

Investigation	Significance
Blood count	Leukaemia
	Infections
	Collagen vascular disease
Plasma viscosity	Infections
	Collagen vascular disease
	Inflammatory bowel disease
	Tumours
X-ray	Bone tumours
	Infection
	Trauma
	Avascular necrosis
	Leukaemia
	Slipped capital femoral epiphysis
Bone scan	Osteomyelitis
	Stress fractures
	Malignant tumours
Muscle enzymes	Damage to muscle cells

muscle weakness or atrophy should be sought. The joints need to be examined for limitation of movement. In non-organic pain the examination is normal although minor changes such as coolness or mottling of the leg may be found.

• *General examination.* Evidence of fever, rash, pallor, lymphadenopathy or organomegaly should be sought and are suggestive of infectious or systemic causes.

Investigations

If the leg pain is thought to be pathological the investigations listed in Table 5.7 may be indicated.

Management

In the child where no organic cause is suspected, the approach described on p. 156 may be helpful.

Causes of leg pain and limp in childhood

Transient synovitis

Transient synovitis is the commonest cause of limp in young children, usually affecting boys aged 2–8 years. It is a benign condition, the major significance being the possibility of overlooking septic arthritis of the hip.

	Organic	Non-organic
Characteristics	Day and night	Only at night
	Interrupts play	Primarily school days
	Unilateral	No interference with normal activities
	Located in joint	Located between joints
	Limp or refusal to walk	Bilateral
		Normal gait
History	Weight loss	Otherwise healthy child
	Fever	
	Night sweats	
	Rash	
	Diarrhoea	
Physical examination	Point tenderness	Normal examination or minor changes
	Redness	such as coolness or mottling of leg
	Swelling	
	Limitation of movement	
	Muscle weakness or atrophy	
	Fever, rash, pallor, lymphadenopathy, organomegaly	

Table 5.8 Features differentiating organic and non-organic causes of leg pain

Clinical features There is a sudden onset of limp with hip and/or knee pain. A mild UTI may precede the symptoms. On examination there is limited abduction, extension and internal rotation of the hip. Transient synovitis can be differentiated from septic arthritis by the lack of systemic symptoms and signs, a normal white cell count, normal or only mildly elevated erythrocyte sedimentation rate (ESR), and a normal hip X-ray.

Management and prognosis Transient synovitis lasts for a few days or weeks and treatment consists of rest and simple analgesia.

Septic arthritis of the hip (see also pp. 115, 217)

Septic arthritis of the hip is a serious cause of pain in the infant and toddler. The child, who may appear toxic, holds the leg in a flexed and abducted posture. However, as opposed to septic arthritis in other joints, the hip may not appear swollen or hot to the touch. The management of the child suspected as having septic arthritis is discussed on p. 217.

Growing pains

Growing pains is a term used for the common complaint of leg pain in children where organic disease has been excluded. The complaint tends to occur in the 3–6-year-old age group. The term 'growing pains' is a misnomer as the pain does not appear to be related to growth, but may be caused by oedema in the fascial sheaths.

Clinical features Limp is not a feature. The pain classically occurs at night, often after a day of vigorous activity. These children also not infrequently experience headaches and abdominal pain.

Management Symptoms usually respond to heat and massage and may need simple analgesia. As in all cases of functional pain, psychosomatic factors should be considered. The approach described on p. 156 may be helpful.

Legg–Calvé–Perthes disease

Legg–Calvé–Perthes disease (avascular necrosis of the femoral head) is a relatively common condition affecting children, principally boys, between the ages of 4 and 10 years. It may follow on from an episode of transient synovitis. The aetiology of the avascular necrosis is unknown.

Clinical features The condition is initially painless but, once a crush fracture develops, pain in the hip or knee, and limp are major features. Diagnosis is made by X-ray (Fig. 5.1) or bone scan.

Management and prognosis Treatment involves bracing or traction and recovery may take 2–3 years.

Slipped capital femoral epiphysis

Slipped capital femoral epiphysis is a condition classically occurring in overweight sedentary teenage boys.

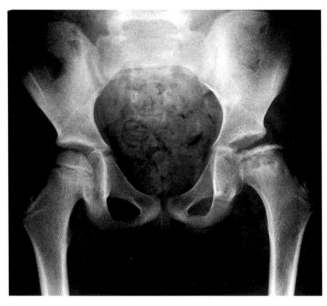

Fig. 5.1 X-ray of the hips of a 5-year-old child with Legg–Calvé–Perthes disease. Note the increased density, flattening and fragmentation of the left capital femoral epiphysis.

Clinical features Pain is experienced in the groin or medial side of the knee, often gradual in onset. On examination the hip is held in abduction and external rotation with limitation of internal rotation. X-ray confirms the diagnosis.

Management Treatment is surgical.

Trauma

Trauma when acute is an obvious cause of leg pain; however, chronic pain may result from stress fractures or prolonged healing of muscle haematomata. It is therefore worth enquiring into a preceding traumatic event when a child presents with persistent or recurrent leg pain.

Osteomyelitis (see p. 222)

Osteomyelitis can present subclinically as well as acutely. There may be associated swelling, erythema, tenderness and decreased movement of the limb. The sedimentation rate is high, the white cell count elevated and diagnosis can be made radiologically or by bone scan.

Neoplastic disease

Neoplastic disease is the most potentially serious of all causes of limb pain. Malignant tumours are usually palpable as a tender mass, which is seen as a destructive bony lesion on X-ray. Benign tumours also occur and may also present as a mass or pain. Leukaemic bone disease is harder to diagnose. The pain is described as deep and throbbing and often wakes the child at night. Diagnosis is often made on the blood count but X-rays are only sometimes helpful.

Systemic disease

Children with haemophilia may have leg pain as a result of bleeding into the tissues. Leg pain caused by sickling crisis is a cardinal sign in sickle cell anaemia. Swelling of the joints (see p. 214) rather than arthralgia is usually seen in the collagen vascular diseases.

CHEST PAIN

Chest pain is a relatively common complaint which is usually benign and self-limited, but generates a lot of anxiety because of the connotations that chest pain has for adults. Table 5.9 shows the causes of chest pain in childhood.

Approach to the child with chest pain

History

The history is important as there are rarely any physical signs. The duration, frequency, quality and location of the pain should be ascertained, and whether there is any exacerbation or relief with position, exertion, eating, coughing or stress.

Physical examination

Physical examination should focus on the presence of fever or weight loss, signs of trauma and altered breathing patterns, as well as inspection of the chest and spine and a good respiratory and cardiac assessment.

Investigations

Investigations in terms of blood counts, sedimentation rate, chest X-ray and electrocardiogram (ECG) are rarely required but may provide extra reassurance.

Table 5.9 Causes of chest pain

Idiopathic
Psychogenic
Stitch
Musculoskeletal
Oesophagitis/gastro-oesophageal reflux
Cardiovascular (very rare)

Management

Management should consist of acknowledging the pain, providing relief for the symptoms in terms of rest and simple analgesics, explaining the phenomenon and reassuring the family of the benign nature of the problem.

Causes of chest pain

Stitch

This familiar pain is thought to be caused by peritoneal ligament stress occurring when exercising in the upright posture.

Musculoskeletal pain

Musculoskeletal pain can occur as a result of muscle strain, cough trauma and stress fracture. Costochondritis as manifested by pain at the costochondral junctions is not uncommon and is often preceded by an upper respiratory tract infection (URTI) or exercise.

Oesophagitis/gastro-oesophageal reflux

See p. 158.

NON-ORGANIC PAIN IN CHILDHOOD

There is nothing that abateth so much the strength as pain
Ambrose Pare, 17th century physician

Children commonly experience recurrent headaches, stomach aches and leg pains, often occurring in combination. Luckily the cause is rarely organic, but none the less the complaint can be serious in terms of discomfort, the anxiety produced in the family and the degree of dysfunction, especially in terms of school absenteeism that may result. The approach taken for all these complaints needs to be a thorough clinical assessment to exclude identifiable pathology, and a minimum of investigations. Reassurance and understanding are essential in the management of these children.

VOMITING

The return of small amounts of food during or shortly after eating is called regurgitation. When this occurs in a baby at or after a milk feed it is known as posseting. More complete

Approach to the child with non-organic recurrent pain

- Assure the parents and child that no major illness appears to be present. In particular, rule out and focus on diagnoses which concern the family

- A diagnosis of psychosomatic pain should not simply be made by exclusion of pathology. Positive emotional and psychological causes must be identified

- In the child where neither an organic nor a psychosomatic cause is found, it can be helpful to label the diagnosis such as tension headache, or growing pains, while qualifying this with an explanation that the aetiology is unknown

- Identify those symptoms and signs which the parents should watch for and which would suggest the need for a re-evaluation

- Do not communicate to the parents that the child is malingering

- Develop a system of return visits to monitor the symptom. Having the family keep a diary of pain episodes and related symptoms can be helpful

- During return visits allow time for both the child and parent to uncover stresses and concerns

- Make every effort to normalize the life of the child, encouraging attendance at school and participation in regular activities

emptying of the stomach is called vomiting. Rumination refers to chronic regurgitation which is often self-induced by the baby. If it occurs with growth failure, psychological factors should be suspected.

Vomiting is one of the commonest symptoms of infancy, if not of childhood. Its causes are listed in Table 5.10. Vomiting may be associated with a variety of disturbances, both trivial and serious. It is most commonly associated with gastroenteritis (p. 162), but may accompany any infection from minor ailments such as otitis media to more serious illnesses such as pyelonephritis. It may be the first symptom of a potentially lethal disease, such as meningitis or pyloric stenosis.

Approach to the vomiting child

In the infant the first step is to differentiate simple regurgitation from vomiting. If vomiting is truly the problem, the underlying diagnosis can usually be suspected by a thorough history and physical examination.

History

- *General well-being.* The general health of the child, and particularly appetite, is a guide to the severity of the complaint. Significant vomiting is likely to be accompanied by

Table 5.10 Common causes of vomiting

Infancy
Gastroenteritis (p. 162)
Gastro-oesophageal reflux
Overfeeding
Anatomic obstruction
   pyloric stenosis
   intussusception (p. 135)
Systemic infection particularly meningitis, pyelonephritis

Childhood
Gastroenteritis (p. 162)
Systemic infection
Toxic ingestion or medications (p. 309)
Whooping cough (p. 51)

Adolescence
Gastroenteritis (p. 162)
Systemic infection
Migraine (p. 150)
Pregnancy
Bulimia (p. 352)

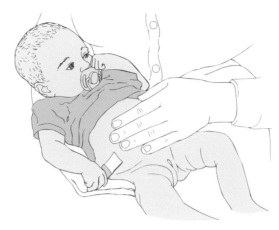

Fig. 5.2 Palpation of the abdomen for pyloric stenosis.

Focal points
In the evaluation of vomiting

• In the infant differentiate posseting from vomiting

• Look for evidence of infection whether gastroenteritis or extragastrointestinal

• Determine whether the child is dehydrated

• In the infant with projectile vomiting palpate the abdomen carefully for pyloric stenosis

• Suspect reflux in the infant or child with physical disability if there is failure to thrive, blood-stained vomitus, irritability, aspiration or apnoea

• Exclude hypertension as a cause

---

poor weight gain, if not weight loss. Fever suggests an infective cause.

• *Characteristics of the vomiting.* The history should be able to differentiate posseting and regurgitation from true vomiting. Vomiting from infectious causes tends to be non-projectile, whereas the vomitus in pyloric stenosis can be dramatically projected over some distance. Paroxysms of coughing such as occur in whooping cough can precipitate vomiting. Blood-stained vomiting indicates inflammation in the upper gastrointestinal tract. Bile-stained vomitus is a

serious sign, suggestive of intestinal obstruction and must be investigated urgently.

• *Associated symptoms.* Gastroenteritis and other infections are usually accompanied by diarrhoea. Constipation suggests intestinal obstruction. Irritability or pain may accompany infection or reflux. Aspiration and apnoea are worrying signs of gastro-oesophageal reflux.

• *Adolescence.* In adolescents the focus of questions is somewhat different and needs to include symptoms of migraine, and consideration of gynaecological causes. Bulimia rarely presents as vomiting as the adolescent is careful to hide the symptom.

Physical examination

• *General examination.* A full examination is required to exclude infection in sites other than the gastrointestinal tract, particularly if there is fever. Severe infection such as meningitis or pyelonephritis can present with vomiting. Poor weight gain is indicative of dehydration in the short term, and malnutrition in the longer term. Hypertension should be excluded.

• *Signs of dehydration.* Persistent vomiting leads to dehydration. The signs of dehydration are described on p. 117.

• *The abdomen.* The abdomen may be tender in gastroenteritis with increased bowel sounds. In the rare event of intestinal obstruction the bowel sounds are tinkling or absent. In the vomiting infant, palpation of an 'olive' (Fig. 5.2) is diagnostic of pyloric stenosis.

Investigations

Investigations are usually only required if significant reflux is suspected, in which case pH monitoring and a barium meal may be indicated.

Worrying features in the vomiting child

- Bile-stained vomitus*

- Blood in the vomitus

- Drowsiness

- Refusal to feed

- Malnutrition

- Dehydration

* This suggests intestinal obstruction and is always a serious sign which must be investigated urgently.

Causes of vomiting in childhood

Gastro-oesophageal reflux

Gastro-oesophageal reflux is a very common occurrence in babies and also in children with developmental disabilities, such as severe cerebral palsy. It results from a chronically lax gastro-oesophageal sphincter, or frequent spontaneous decreases in sphincter tone, which allows reflux of stomach contents back up the oesophagus.

Clinical features The symptoms range from trivial posseting to life-threatening episodes. Common problems are vomiting, oesophagitis, aspiration and, to a lesser extent, apnoea. Vomiting is the commonest complaint and may cause failure to thrive. Oesophagitis causes irritability and anorexia, and should be particularly suspected if there is blood in the vomitus or occult blood in the stools. Opisthotonos (arching of the back) and other head posturing may be associated and is possibly an attempt to reduce the pain associated with acid reflux. Aspiration can manifest itself as episodes of choking and must be suspected in the baby with recurrent episodes of pneumonia. Reflux can also cause reflex apnoea and bradycardia. The relationship to acute life-threatening events (see p. 312) is controversial.

Investigations In mild cases a careful clinical assessment is sufficient, and confirmation of the diagnosis is made by the response to treatment. In more severe or complex cases a barium swallow can be helpful, although results should be interpreted with caution as reflux is an episodic event which may not be demonstrable during the short exposure time of the X-ray, and also because it can be seen in normal asymptomatic children. The severity and frequency of reflux can be documented by continuous pH monitoring (usually 24

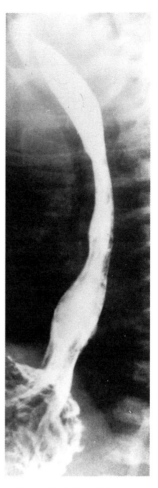

Fig. 5.3 Barium swallow of a baby with gastro-osophageal reflux. The barium can be seen refluxing up the entire oesophagus.

hours) with a probe placed in the lower third of the oesophagus. Oesophagoscopy with biopsy is the best technique for demonstrating oesophagitis, which may also be suspected if a ragged mucosal outline is seen on the barium meal (Fig. 5.3).

Management In mild uncomplicated cases, propping the child, thickening the feeds and attending to burping may resolve the problem. If oesophagitis is present H_2 receptor antagonists such as ranitidine or frequent use of antacids can be helpful. Cisapride, a motility stimulant, reduces the severity of reflux in infants, although response to therapy may take a few weeks. If symptoms do not respond to a good trial of medical agents, or if recurrent aspiration and apnoea are major problems, surgery is indicated, the commonest procedure being Nissen fundoplication.

GASTRO-OESOPHAGEAL REFLUX AT A GLANCE

Epidemiology

Common in babies, and children with Down's syndrome and severe cerebral palsy

Aetiology

Lax gastro-oesophageal sphincter

History

May be asymptomatic
Vomiting*
Irritability and anorexia*
Choking*
Apnoea*
History of pneumonia*

Physical examination

Normal
Chest signs if aspirating*
Failure to thrive*
Opisthotonous*

NB *Signs and symptoms are variable

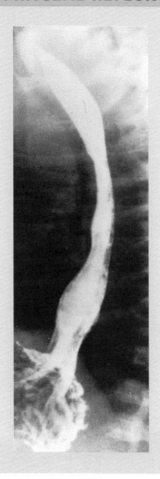

Confirmatory investigations

Response to trial of antireflux medication
Barium swallow: reflux visualized
pH monitoring: increased acidity in oesophagus
Oesophagoscopy: oesophagitis

Differential diagnosis

Normal posseting
Colic in young babies
Other causes of vomiting (p. 157)
Other causes of recurrent pneumonia
Other causes of apnoea (p. 313)

Management

Thickened feeds and propping
Medication: H_2 receptor antagonist and motility stimulant
Surgery: Nissen fundoplication required if aspirating, apnoea or poor response to medication (rare)

Prognosis/complications

Reflux resolves in most normal children by the time they are eating solids/ walking

Pyloric stenosis

Pyloric stenosis is caused by hypertrophy and hyperplasia of the pylorus muscle. It usually develops in the first 4–6 weeks of life, and is commonest in first-born male children.

Clinical features The vomiting is characteristically projectile and generally occurs during or immediately after feeding (although not necessarily every feed). The vomitus is not bile-stained, but may be blood-tinged. The infant is hungry and is prepared to take another feed immediately. Physical examination reveals weight loss and varying degrees of dehydration. In advanced cases the infant may be moribund. Visible peristalsis from the left upper quadrant to the right is most prominent immediately after a feed or just prior to vomiting. Careful palpation (Fig. 5.2) should reveal a hard mobile tumour (the pylorus) which feels like an acorn or an olive just to the right of the epigastrium. Once the tumour has been palpated there is no need for barium studies or ultrasound. However, if the diagnosis is suspected, but the tumour not palpable, the diagnosis can be confirmed by ultrasound (Fig. 5.4). If vomiting is protracted the loss of acidity from the stomach results in hypochloraemic alkalosis and reduced sodium and potassium levels in the serum (see p. 361).

Management Treatment is surgical. The Ramstedt procedure consists of splitting the pylorus muscle, without penetrating the mucosa. If the infant is dehydrated, rehydration must take place prior to surgery with replacement of sodium, chloride and potassium (see p. 118). Oral feeds can be gradually given within hours postoperatively.

Regurgitation and posseting

Within limits, regurgitation is a natural occurrence, especially during the first 6 months or so of life. It can be reduced by winding the baby during and after a feed, by gentle handling, by preventing the baby from becoming upset and swallowing air before feeding and by propping the baby after a feed.

PYLORIC STENOSIS AT A GLANCE

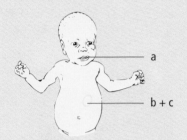

Epidemiology

Age 4–6 weeks
Mainly boys
7 boys : 1 girl
Age 1–10 weeks

Aetiology

Hypertrophy and hyperplasia of the pylorus muscle

History

Projectile vomiting during or just after feed (**a**)
Infant hungry immediately after vomit
Constipated

Physical examination

Weight loss +/– dehydration
Visible peristalsis from left upper quadrant to right upper quadrant (**b**)
Mobile olive-sized tumour palpable to right of epigastrium during feed (**c**)

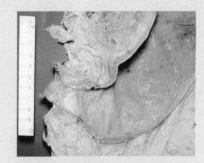

Confirmatory investigations

Abdominal ultrasound (not needed if 'olive' felt)
Hypochloraemic alkalosis (see p. 361)
Low serum sodium and potassium

Differential diagnosis

Posseting
Gastro-oesophageal reflux
Gastritis
Systemic infection

Management

Rehydration
Surgical correction: Ramstedt procedure

Prognosis/complications

Excellent following surgery

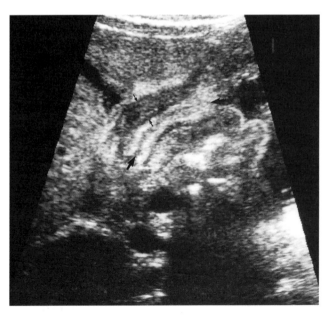

Fig. 5.4 Ultrasound of a baby with pyloric stenosis. Arrows indicate the elongated pyloric canal (thick arrow) and thickened pyloric muscle (thinner arrow).

Providing the child is gaining weight and generally contented, the family can be reassured that it is simply a laundry problem, and that the baby will grow out of it by the time a more upright posture is achieved by the age of 1 year. If very troublesome, and the baby is not breast-fed, food thickeners can be added to the milk.

ACUTE DIARRHOEA

Diarrhoea is defined as an increase in the frequency, fluidity and volume of faeces. Children are likely to experience as many as three acute severe episodes in the first 3 years of life. These episodes are almost invariably infectious in aetiology, although the infection may be extrinsic to the gastrointestinal tract. The causes of acute diarrhoea are shown in Table 5.11.

Approach to the child with acute diarrhoea

In the evaluation of diarrhoea the clinical assessment needs to focus on whether the child needs treatment for associated problems, namely dehydration or non-gastrointestinal infection, rather than the underlying cause of the gastroenteritis.

History

- *A description of the illness.* A good description of the illness, and whether there has been an increase in number, volume or fluidity of the stools provides a guide as to whether the child is likely to be dehydrated. The presence of blood, mucus, abdominal pain and fever suggest a bacterial cause, which is important to recognize for public health reasons.
- *Is there evidence of dehydration?* Apart from frequency of liquid stools there are other clues as to whether the child is likely to be dehydrated. If the child is urinating infrequently (less than three times in 24 hours is a guide) a degree of dehydration is likely to be present. A history of weight loss is also important.
- *Other symptoms.* Symptoms such as earache, dysuria or coryza might suggest an infection outside of the gastrointestinal tract.
- *Other affected individuals.* Identifying other individuals with diarrhoea within the family or child care setting might suggest a cause such as food contamination or provide useful epidemiological information.

Physical examination

- *Assessment of hydration.* This is covered in detail in Chapter 4 (see p. 116). The state of alertness, moistness of mucous membranes, presence of tears, skin turgor, sunken fontanelle and eyes, and pulse rate should be assessed.
- *Signs of any extragastrointestinal infection.* Otitis media, tonsillitis and chest infections commonly cause diarrhoea.
- *Weight.* The child should always be weighed. If a recent weight is available weight loss would provide important evidence of dehydration. In any event the weight is a valuable baseline if the child deteriorates.

Investigations (Table 5.12)

If the child is not dehydrated, nor the stools bloody, investigations are not generally necessary unless the child is hospitalized or has been exposed to others with proven bacterial gastroenteritis. Stool microscopy and culture is indicated if there is blood and mucus in the diarrhoea. Rotavirus can be detected by stool immunoassay. If extragastrointestinal infection is suspected, confirmation may be required from blood and urine cultures or X-ray.

Management

Fluids

The management of dehydration is covered in Chapter 4. If signs of dehydration are mild or absent the child can be managed at home. Cow's milk is usually stopped and it is traditional to give clear fluids for the first day. In the toddler and older child dilute apple juice or a flat cola drink may be offered, but babies should be given oral rehydration fluids which provide electrolytes and calories in the appropriate balance. If the child is breast-fed, this should be continued.

Solids are gradually introduced and bananas, rice, apple

Table 5.11 Causes of acute diarrhoea

Viral gastroenteritis
Bacterial gastroenteritis
Shigella
Escherichia coli
Salmonella
Campylobacter
Infections outside the gastrointestinal tract
Antibiotic induced

Focal points
Evaluating diarrhoea

- Assess the degree of hydration (Table 4.10, p. 117)
- Look for evidence of infection outside of the gastrointestinal tract
- Identify features suggestive of bacterial gastroenteritis

Table 5.12 Investigations to be considered in acute diarrhoea

Investigation	Indication	Condition identified
Stool microscopy and culture	Blood and mucus in the stool	Bacterial gastroenteritis
Stool immunoassay	Hospitalized child	Rotavirus
Blood count	High fever	Possible bacterial infection
Blood and urine culture, chest X-ray	Suggestion of extra gastrointestinal infection in clinical evaluation	Bacterial infection

sauce and toast (the BRAT diet) are foods that are generally recommended. Milk is sometimes reintroduced in diluted form, but there is no evidence that this gradual introduction is beneficial, and may result in the child receiving inadequate calories. If diarrhoea is persistent the child's state of hydration must be rechecked to determine whether more aggressive management is required.

Use of antiemetics and antidiarrhoeal agents
These agents have no place in the management of diarrhoea in young children. They are ineffective and have a high incidence of side-effects.

Causes of acute diarrhoea

Viral gastroenteritis

Viral infection is the commonest cause of gastroenteritis in young children and rotavirus is the main agent responsible for winter epidemics.

Clinical features Diarrhoea usually begins after 1–2 days of low-grade fever, vomiting and anorexia, although in the younger child the onset is often more rapid.

Management and prognosis Management is discussed on p. 118. Antibiotics should not be given as they encourage gut superinfection with other organisms. The diarrhoea usually resolves within a week.

Bacterial gastroenteritis

Bacterial gastroenteritis presents a similar picture to viral gastroenteritis. The commonest pathogens are *Escherichia coli*, shigella, salmonella, and campylobacter.

Clinical features The clinical features are described in the Distingushing features of the common causes of gastroenteritis box (below). Particularly noteworthy is the fact that meningismus and febrile fits occur with shigella infection, and that bloody stools are characteristic of shigella or campylobacter.

Management and prognosis Antibiotics should not be used in uncomplicated gastroenteritis caused by salmonella, shigella or *E. coli* as they tend to prolong the carrier state. Campylobacter infections should be treated with oral erythromycin. If there is a clinical suspicion of septicaemia in association with gastroenteritis, the child should be admitted to hospital and treated with appropriate antibiotics intravenously. The general management of diarrhoea is covered on p. 118.

Other causes of acute diarrhoea

Other causes of acute diarrhoea include any form of infection, particularly in the young child. These commonly include URTIs, chest infections, otitis media and UTI. If infections such as otitis media, UTI or pneumonia are detected, the appropriate antibiotic should be given. Of the non-infective causes of diarrhoea, intussusception is a serious condition that may present with bloody (characteristically 'redcurrant jelly') stools (see p. 135). Antibiotic therapy in itself commonly causes diarrhoea.

CHRONIC DIARRHOEA

Chronic diarrhoea is a common complaint particularly in infants and young children. However, there is a large variation in normal bowel patterns (Table 5.13) at this age and before launching into any form of assessment, a good

Distinguishing features — Common causes of gastroenteritis

	Rotavirus	Shigella	Escherichia coli	Salmonella	Campylobacter
Age	<2 years	1–5 years	<2 years	Any	Any
Season	Winter	Usually late summer	Usually late summer	Usually late summer	Usually late summer
Vomiting	Common	Common	Common	Common	
High fever	Common	Common			
Fits		10%			
Pain		Common			Marked
Stool	Watery	Watery, blood, mucus, pus	Loose	Loose and slimy	Watery, blood, mucus

ACUTE GASTROENTERITIS AT A GLANCE

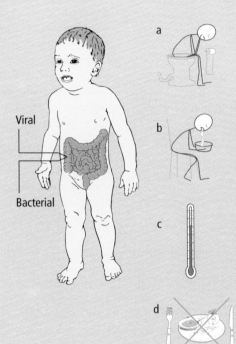

| **Epidemiology** |
| Common in all ages |

| **Aetiology** |
| Viral, particularly rotavirus |
| Shigella |
| *E.coli* |
| Salmonella |
| Campylobacter |

| **History** |
| Diarrhoea (**a**) |
| Abdominal pain* |
| Malaise* |
| Vomiting* (**b**) |
| Fever* (**c**) |
| Anorexia* (**d**) |
| Febrile fits in shigella* |
| Bloody stools in shigella, Campylobacter |

| **Physical examination** |
| Tender abdomen |
| Sore anus |
| Dehydration* |

| NB *Signs and symptoms are variable |

Viral

Bacterial

N.B. Prevent and treat dehydration

| **Confirmatory investigations** |
| Usually none in primary care setting |
| Stool culture if prolonged course, bloody stools or hospitalized |

| **Differential diagnosis** |
| Infections outside the gastrointestinal tract |
| Antibiotic-induced diarrhoea |

| **Management** |
| Fluid management of dehydration |
| Antibiotics not usually indicated, even for bacterial causes |
| Antidiarrhoeal agents should not be prescribed |

| **Course/complications** |
| Usually resolves spontaneously, although may take days to weeks |
| Carrier state may follow salmonella and shigella |
| Temporary lactose intolerance may develop |

description of the stool pattern should be obtained in order to be sure that diarrhoea is really a problem.

Causes of chronic or recurrent diarrhoea are shown in Table 5.14. Broadly speaking the diarrhoeal illnesses of childhood can be divided into malabsorption, inflammation and infections. However, for the purpose of classification it is useful to divide them according to the characteristics of the stool.

Approach to the child with chronic diarrhoea

Clinical evaluation should differentiate the healthy child with loose frequent stools from the child with a medical problem. It should identify any worrying features suggestive of a pathological process and should lead one to request appropriate investigations so that a definitive diagnosis can be made.

History

• *Bowel pattern.* The history should include details of the bowel pattern in terms of increase in number, volume and

fluidity of the stools, so that an idea as to whether the pattern is abnormal or not can be obtained. A description of the stools' appearance, consistency and presence of blood or mucus is helpful in terms of differentiating the diagnosis, but odour and 'flushability' are usually not.

• *Precipitating events.* The problem may have been precipitated by an episode of acute infective diarrhoea, or troublesome foods may be identified. Identifying other

Table 5.13 Normal stool patterns

0–4 months	
Breast-fed	2–4 per day (range 1–7) yellow to golden, porridgy consistency, pH 5. Infrequency of stools is also normal (up to once per week)
Bottlefed	2–3 per day, pale yellow to light brown, firm, pH 7
4 months–1 year	1–3 per day, darker yellow, firmer
After 1 year	Formed, like adult stool in odour and colour

Table 5.14 Common causes of chronic or recurrent diarrhoea

Watery
Non-specific diarrhoea
Toddler diarrhoea
Lactose intolerance
Parasites—*Giardia lamblia*
Cow's milk protein allergy
Overflow diarrhoea in constipation

Fatty
Cystic fibrosis
Coeliac disease

Bloody
Ulcerative colitis
Crohn's disease

Focal points
Evaluating chronic or recurrent diarrhoea

- Check that the stool pattern is really abnormal for age

- Attempt to classify the character of the stool—watery, fatty or bloody

- Identify any features suggestive of significant pathology, e.g. weight loss or poor weight gain, abdominal pain

---

affected individuals in the family or in child care may be helpful.
• *Associated symptoms.* It is important to determine whether the diarrhoea is an isolated problem in an otherwise healthy child or whether there are concomitant symptoms. Weight loss or abdominal pain are particularly significant.
• *Review of symptoms.* As many diseases can cause failure to thrive with rather non-specific bowel symptoms, a complete review of symptoms is required.
• *A symptom diary.* As in most recurrent and chronic problems, requesting the family to keep a diary is helpful in assessing the severity and pattern of the symptom.

Physical examination

• *Growth measures.* Height, weight and head circumference must be recorded and compared with earlier measurements if available. Poor weight gain is suggestive of a process requiring further evaluation. These measures also serve as a critical baseline if the diarrhoea persists for any length of time.
• *Other features.* Examination should include an evalua-

tion of hydration, pallor, abdominal distension, tenderness and finger clubbing.
• *General examination.* As diseases of many different organ systems can cause failure to thrive a complete examination is required.
• *Anorectal examination.* Any significant degree of diarrhoea will cause perianal irritation, particularly if the child is still in nappies. Rectal examination is not routinely indicated but should be considered to rule out impaction (if soiling is considered as the diagnosis) and to obtain a sample of the stool.

Laboratory investigations (Table 5.15)

If a child is thriving and there are no accompanying symptoms or signs, laboratory investigations are rarely necessary. However, if there is concern that a pathological process is present, investigations are required and should differentiate the malabsorptive, inflammatory and infective causes of chronic and persistent diarrhoea.

Malabsorption
The commonest causes of malabsorption in childhood result from pancreatic insufficiency, protein intolerance and lactose intolerance.
• *Pancreatic insufficiency.* In pancreatic insufficiency (as occurs in cystic fibrosis), low chymotrypsin levels are found in the stool, and on microscopic inspection fat globules are visualized.
• *Protein intolerance.* The commonest form of protein intolerance is coeliac disease. Coeliac antibodies are useful as a screening test. If positive, or there are other concerns that malabsorption is present, jejunal biopsy is required to confirm the diagnosis.
• *Sugar malabsorption.* Sugar malabsorption, of which secondary lactose intolerance is the commonest, is suggested by the presence of reducing substances in the stool and a low pH. The low pH results from bacterial production of organic acids from the unabsorbed sugar. The breath hydrogen test is another indirect measure of carbohydrate malabsorption; an oral dose of the sugar being tested is given, and if it is not absorbed the enteric bacteria act on it to produce hydrogen gas, which is measured in the expired air.

Inflammation
Faecal blood loss would suggest inflammatory bowel disease or food sensitivity. A very high plasma viscosity or ESR level is supportive of inflammatory bowel disease. The diagnosis is made by barium studies and endoscopy.

Infection
Repeated examination of at least three stool specimens should identify parasitic infection of which *Giardia lamblia*

Table 5.15 Laboratory investigations in the assessment of chronic diarrhoea

Investigation	Finding	Significance
Blood		
Full blood count	Anaemia	Blood loss, malabsorption or poor diet
	Eosinophilia	Parasites or atopy
Plasma viscosity or sedimentation rate	High	Non-specific finding, but if very high suggestive of inflammatory bowel disease
Coeliac antibodies	Present	Screening test for coeliac disease
Stool		
Occult blood	Positive	Cow's milk intolerance, inflammatory bowel disease
Ova and parasites	Positive	Parasite identified
Reducing substances and pH*	Positive and low pH	Sugar intolerance (usually lactose)
Chymotrypsin	Low	Pancreatic insufficiency
Microscopy for fat globules	Globules seen	Fat malabsorption (usually pancreatic insufficiency)
Other		
Urine culture and sensitivity	Positive	Urinary tract infection
Sweat test	Elevated Na+ concentration	Cystic fibrosis
Breath hydrogen test	High H_2	Sugar intolerance
Jejunal biopsy	Flattened villi	Coeliac disease
Barium meal and enema	Characteristic lesions	Inflammatory bowel disease
Endoscopy	Characteristic lesions	Inflammatory bowel disease

* This is performed by mixing stool with water and testing it with Clinitest tablets (as for urinary glucose).

is the commonest. Urine culture excludes chronic UTI as a cause for diarrhoea.

Causes of chronic diarrhoea in childhood

Non-specific diarrhoea

Many children have episodes of loose, frequent stools for which no cause is found. These may follow on from an acute episode of gastroenteritis. If the child is well and thriving, reassurance is all that is required, with monitoring of growth for the duration of symptoms. Treatment is unnecessary and the use of antidiarrhoeal agents in children is contraindicated.

Toddler diarrhoea

Non-specific diarrhoea is very common in the toddler age group. It is likely to be caused by a rapid gastrocolic reflex.

Clinical features Parents commonly describe the appearance of particles of food, particularly meat fibres, peas and beans in the stool. The child may have a large fluid intake, particularly of fruit juices. The diagnosis should only be made if the child is thriving.

Management and prognosis In some instances a reduction in fluid intake can be helpful, but usually, if the toddler is thriving, reassurance is all that is required. In some cases of frequent stooling with severe parental anxiety, loperamide may be used to slow bowel transit time. As the child matures the symptoms resolve.

Lactose intolerance

Secondary lactose intolerance is common in the baby and young child. During an acute episode of gastroenteritis the superficial mucosal cells containing lactase are stripped off, resulting in high levels of lactose in the bowel which prolongs the diarrhoea. Congenital lactose intolerance is extremely rare.

Clinical features The diarrhoea, which is watery in nature, follows an acute episode of gastroenteritis. The diagnosis is suspected if the gastroenteritis persists for several days particularly if the temperature has resolved. Laboratory evidence is found in a low stool pH (<6.0) and the presence of reducing substances (lactose) in the stool (>0.5%). It is rarely necessary to perform lactose challenge or breath hydrogen tests.

Management and prognosis In the bottle-fed baby an empirical change of infant formula to soy milk formula (which contains non-lactose sugar) can be tried. The baby should revert to cow's milk once symptoms are resolved. The breast-fed baby needs no change of milk, and symptoms should eventually resolve.

Coeliac disease (Fig. 5.5)

Coeliac disease results from a permanent inability to tolerate gluten, a substance found in wheat and rye.

Clinical features Most children present before the age of 2 years with failure to thrive, irritability, anorexia, vomiting and diarrhoea, although some have few symptoms. Examination classically shows abdominal distension, wasted buttocks, irritability and pallor. The stools are pale and foul. Additional physical signs may include mouth sores, a smooth tongue, excessive bruising, finger clubbing and peripheral oedema.

The range of clinical features is very wide and some have mild symptoms such that the diagnosis is sometimes only made in adulthood. The most constant features are decrease in weight gain and linear growth.

Investigations Anaemia is common, usually with an iron deficient picture, but folate too may be low. Most children

eating significant amounts of fat will have steatorrhoea and the faecal smear will demonstrate fat globules. Detection of coeliac antibodies can be used as a screening test, but a definitive diagnosis must be made by jejunal biopsy. The characteristic finding is subtotal villous atrophy (Fig. 5.6).

Management Response to a gluten-free diet, which consists of eliminating all wheat and rye products, is usually prompt, with an improvement in mood, resolution of diarrhoea and good growth. The diet is quite constricting, but special gluten-free products are now widely available. As the disorder is caused by a permanent intolerance to gluten, the diet must be continued indefinitely. Before consigning the child to this life-long dietary restriction it is recommended that he or she is rechallenged with gluten after a minimum period of 2 years (to allow for full villi regeneration) and the biopsy is repeated.

Prognosis The prognosis is excellent provided the child adheres to the diet.

Cystic fibrosis (see also p. 176)

One of the manifestations of cystic fibrosis is pancreatic insufficiency, and infants more often present with diarrhoea and failure to thrive rather than with respiratory symptoms seen in older children.

Clinical features Symptoms include frequent, bulky, greasy stools and failure to gain weight even when food intake appears large. A history of frequent chest infections and cough may, but not always, be elicited. A protuberant abdomen, decreased muscle mass, poor growth and delayed maturation are typical signs.

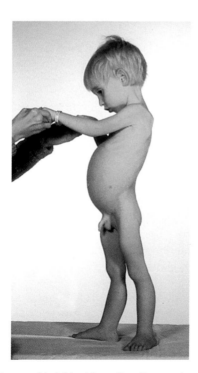

Fig. 5.5 A 2-year-old child with coeliac disease, showing marked abdominal distension and wasted buttocks.

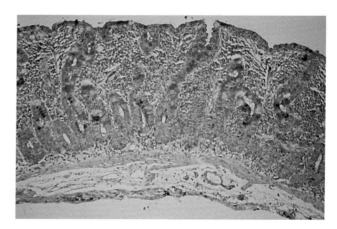

Fig. 5.6 Histology of a jejunal biopsy taken from a child with coeliac disease, showing atrophy of the villi.

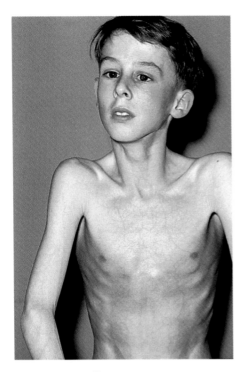

Fig. 5.7 A boy with cystic fibrosis.

Investigations Examination of the stool demonstrates fat globules and a low chymotrypsin level. A sweat test is required to make the diagnosis (see p. 365). A chest X-ray is usually normal in the early stages.

Management Children require dietary adjustment, pancreatic enzyme replacement and supplementary vitamins to correct their loss of pancreatic function and inadequate digestion of fat and protein. Pancreatic enzyme supplements have to be taken with all meals and snacks. The diet should be high in energy and protein, and there is no need to restrict fat. Dietary supplements are often needed at times of illness or if there is anorexia. All patients require supplements of vitamins A, D and E. Extra salt is needed in hot weather or if the child is febrile to replace losses in sweat.

The other aspects of management are covered on p. 176.

Prognosis The outlook for cystic fibrosis used to be very poor, with death occurring in the early years. Current average life expectancy is about 30 years.

Inflammatory bowel disease

Inflammatory bowel disease is a cause of chronic diarrhoea in late childhood and adolescence. Both Crohn's disease and

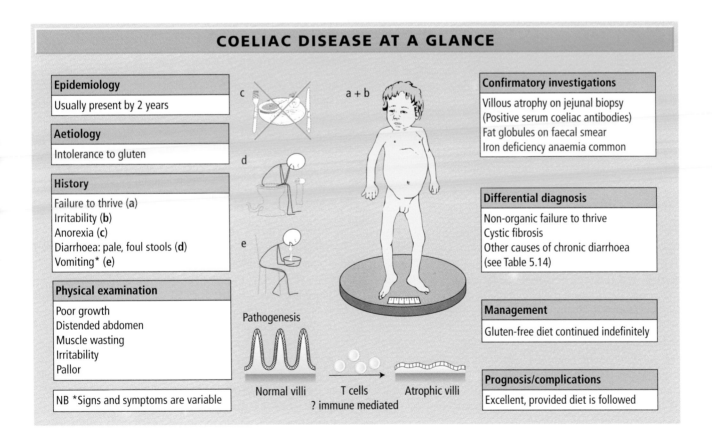

COELIAC DISEASE AT A GLANCE

Epidemiology

Usually present by 2 years

Aetiology

Intolerance to gluten

History

Failure to thrive (a)
Irritability (b)
Anorexia (c)
Diarrhoea: pale, foul stools (d)
Vomiting* (e)

Physical examination

Poor growth
Distended abdomen
Muscle wasting
Irritability
Pallor

NB *Signs and symptoms are variable

c

a + b

d

e

Pathogenesis

Normal villi   T cells   Atrophic villi
? immune mediated

Confirmatory investigations

Villous atrophy on jejunal biopsy
(Positive serum coeliac antibodies)
Fat globules on faecal smear
Iron deficiency anaemia common

Differential diagnosis

Non-organic failure to thrive
Cystic fibrosis
Other causes of chronic diarrhoea
(see Table 5.14)

Management

Gluten-free diet continued indefinitely

Prognosis/complications

Excellent, provided diet is followed

ulcerative colitis are characterized by unpredictable exacerbations and remissions. The underlying cause for these conditions is unknown. The diagnosis is suspected from the history and a persistently elevated sedimentation rate is supportive. The diagnosis is confirmed by barium studies and endoscopy.

Crohn's disease

Clinical features Crohn's disease presents with recurrent abdominal pain, anorexia, growth failure, fever, diarrhoea, oral and perianal ulcers and arthritis.

Management Remission can be induced by nutritional programmes based on elemental diets. This approach is as effective as steroids and avoids the hazard of growth impairment. Surgical resection may be indicated in localized disease.

Prognosis The inflammatory activity continues to remit and exacerbate throughout life.

Ulcerative colitis

Clinical features Ulcerative colitis presents with diarrhoea containing blood and mucus. Early on these episodes may be short-lived and thought to be simply infective in nature. Systemic upset in terms of pain, weight loss, arthritis and liver disturbance may occur.

Management Treatment is by corticosteroid enemas or suppositories. Sulphasalazine may be given orally, and steroids, immunosuppressive therapy and even colectomy may be required in severe cases.

Prognosis Most cases starting in childhood are severe in terms of activity and extent of involvement. There is a high risk of colonic cancer developing later in life.

Parasites

The commonest parasite causing diarrhoea in Britain is *Giardia lamblia*, which commonly causes outbreaks in day-care nurseries. It is endemic in some overseas holiday destinations and infection may be related to travel abroad.

Clinical features The infected child may either be asymptomatic or have a combination of diarrhoea, weight loss and abdominal pain. The diagnosis is made on microscopic examination of the stool. Three separate specimens are required as excretion of the cysts can be irregular. The blood count may show eosinophilia and the parasite can be detected in duodenal aspirate (obtained when jejunal biopsy is undertaken for coeliac disease).

Management Treatment is with metronidazole and, in an outbreak, asymptomatic carriers should be treated.

Prognosis Treatment failure is common.

Cow's milk protein intolerance

Allergy to cow's milk protein is rare and often over-diagnosed.

Clinical features Cow's milk protein intolerance is a cause of chronic diarrhoea and vomiting. Classically the diarrhoea is bloody, and urticaria, stridor and bronchospasm may occur. Very rarely, the sensitivity can be life-threatening. The condition is less common in babies who have been breast-fed.

The diagnosis is clinical. Symptoms should subside within 1 week of withdrawing cow's milk from the diet. The child should be rechallenged after a period of time (in hospital if the original symptoms were severe), and observed for recurrence of symptoms.

Management and prognosis Treatment consists of removing cow's milk from the diet. Soy milk infant formulas provide adequate nutrition for the young baby and child. In most cases the intolerance is transitory, usually resolving in 1–2 years. Prolonged breast-feeding reduces the likelihood of cow's milk intolerance.

Overflow diarrhoea in constipation

The soiling that results from constipation is sometimes interpreted as being diarrhoea. A careful bowel history is required along with evidence of constipation on abdominal and rectal examination. Treatment is obviously directed towards resolving the constipation.

CONSTIPATION

In normal children there is a wide range in frequency of bowel movements. In the past, children were trained to open their bowels each morning and this regularity is still seen in elderly patients. With less rigid ideas of child-rearing, most children have no set pattern to their toilet habits. Some will have more than two movements per day and others go several days with none. The diagnosis of constipation should therefore be based on hardness of stools and painful defaecation rather than infrequency of bowel movements alone. This rule of thumb is particularly relevant in the exclusively breast-fed infant where it can be normal for the baby to pass only one stool in 10 days.

Constipation is common, and is nearly always functional

Distinguishing features — Conditions causing chronic diarrhoea

	Characteristics of diarrhoea	Associated features	Age of child
Non-specific diarrhoea	Loose watery stools	Thriving child, may follow episode of acute gastroenteritis	Any age
Toddler's diarrhoea	Loose with undigested food in stool	Thriving child, may have large fluid intake	Toddler
Lactose intolerance	Watery, low pH, reducing substances in stool	Follows acute gastroenteritis	Baby and toddler
Giardiasis	Watery	Weight loss and abdominal pain variable	Any age, common in nurseries
Cow's milk protein allergy	Watery, may be bloody	May have urticaria, stridor or bronchospasm	Babies
Functional constipation	Soiling rather than diarrhoea	Constipated stool palpable per abdomen or per rectum	Any age
Cystic fibrosis	Fatty	Failure to thrive, respiratory symptoms	Usually infancy
Coeliac disease	Fatty	Failure to thrive, irritability, muscle wasting, abdominal distension	Usually late infancy, but can be any age
Inflammatory bowel disease	Bloody in ulcerative colitis	Weight loss, exacerbations and remissions, abdominal pain and anorexia in Crohn's disease	Late childhood and adolescence

in nature. The causes are listed in Table 5.16. Organic causes are rare, the most important being Hirschsprung's disease.

Approach to the child with constipation

The purpose of the evaluation is principally to assess the severity of the complaint in order to evaluate the need for treatment. Rare organic causes can be ruled out on the basis of the history and physical examination.

History

• *Description of symptoms.* Is the child truly constipated or are the stools infrequent but normal? The hardness of the stool, painful defaecation, crampy abdominal pain and the presence of blood on the stool or toilet paper indicate the former, although long-standing constipation can be painless.
• *Constipation history.* Constipation is often precipitated by a period of fluid depletion, as in hot weather, or during a febrile illness or one where vomiting has occurred. When constipation is chronic it is often not possible to recall the onset. Mismanagement of toilet training can be a factor. Constipation starting during infancy is suggestive of Hirschsprung's disease, whereas functional constipation usually has a later onset. Previous history of an anal fissure is significant.
• *Associated symptoms.* Bowel obstruction results in constipation, but rarely presents as constipation alone. Vomiting and abdominal pain are accompanying symptoms.

Focal points
Evaluating constipation

• Assess the severity of the constipation

• Attempt to identify a precipitating cause

• Constipation from infancy, in conjunction with failure to thrive suggests Hirschsprung's disease

Table 5.16 Causes of constipation

Acute
Fluid depletion
Bowel obstruction

Chronic
Functional constipation
Hirschsprung's disease
(Breast-fed babies)

• *Diet.* A dietary history is important in order to base subsequent advice on dietary management of constipation.

Physical examination

• *Growth.* Review of the growth chart is needed as Hirschsprung's disease is accompanied by failure to thrive.

- *General examination.* Hard indentable faeces are often palpable in the left lower quadrant of the abdomen and above.
- *Anorectal examination.* Rectal examination is by no means always indicated but will reveal hard stools. Inspection of the anus is important as fissures may be found and, in addition, signs of sexual abuse could indicate a less benign reason for pain on defaecation.

Investigations

A plain X-ray of the abdomen may show enormous quantities of faeces in the colon (Fig. 5.8). However, this investigation is not usually required. The diagnostic test for Hirschsprung's disease is rectal biopsy, and is indicated if the history goes back to infancy and the child has shown poor growth.

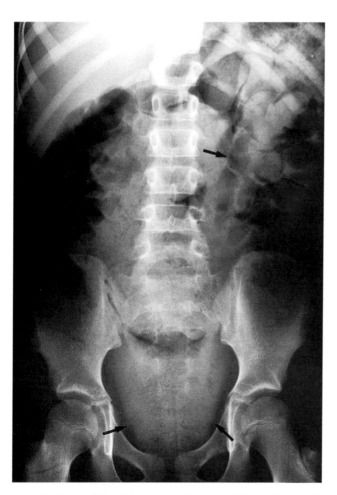

Fig. 5.8 X-ray of the abdomen of a 12-year-old boy with chronic constipation. The rectum and sigmoid colon are grossly distended by faeces, as indicated by the arrows.

Causes of constipation

Fluid depletion

A child may become fluid depleted during hot weather or following a febrile illness, particularly if vomiting has occurred. The problem can usually be resolved by increasing the fluid intake. Occasionally laxatives may be required, particularly if a fissure has developed. A simple episode of constipation can be responsible for the development of more chronic constipation (see below).

Bowel obstruction

Bowel obstruction is rare in childhood and results from congenital malformations of the gut. The presentation is usually an acute abdomen (see p. 132) rather than constipation.

Functional constipation

Chronic constipation often stems from an episode when passage of a large hard stool is painful or causes an anal fissure. The child responds by withholding further stools in order to avoid pain. The stools remain in the colorectum where water is reabsorbed, and the stools become harder and even more painful to pass. Eventually the cycle becomes self-perpetuating and the rectum so stretched that dilatation of the colon may occur resulting in megacolon (Fig. 5.8).

Constipation is a particular problem in immobile children with physical disabilities.

Clinical features It is often not possible to recall the start of the cycle of constipation, and the parent and doctor are simply faced with the chronically constipated child, who may also be soiling (see below).

Management Management can be divided into three stages (Table 5.17):
1 evacuation of the constipated stools and retraining of the bowel;
2 maintenance to prevent relapse;
3 vigilance that the cycle does not recommence.

Prognosis Constipation often recurs. However, provided active management is started early, the problem is usually controllable.

Hirschsprung's disease (see also p. 241)

Hirschsprung's disease should be considered if the constipation goes back to infancy and particularly if the child is failing to thrive, with marked abdominal distension. Rectal examination classically shows an empty rather than an impacted rectum.

Breast-fed babies

Beyond the first few weeks of life the fully breast-fed infant normally develops infrequent bowel movements. One movement every 4 or 5 days is common, and one in 10 days is not abnormal. The stools are soft and semiliquid. These babies are not constipated, but inexperienced mothers often become alarmed at the infrequency of their baby's motions. No treatment is required.

Table 5.17 Practical management of constipation

Stage 1: Evacuation of the bowel	*Diet:* in simple cases this alone is effective (see adjacent box)
	Laxatives: stool softeners such as lactulose can be prescribed. The dose can safely be increased on a daily basis until the stools become liquid, when it should be reduced. The aim should be to attain soft stools almost to the point of diarrhoea and to sustain this for at least 2 weeks. Bowel stimulants such as Senokot may also be prescribed
	Enemas: rarely required
Stage 2: Maintenance	Stools should be kept soft either by diet or laxatives for 3–6 months
	Children should be encouraged to have daily bowel movements by sitting on the toilet at a fixed time once or twice each day for 5–10 minutes
Stage 3: Vigilance	Treatment should be started at the first indication of recurrence of hard stools

Foods that can promote good bowel habits

High fibre foods
Wholewheat bread and flour
Bran
High fibre breakfast cereals
Fruit (particularly the peel)
Vegetables
Beans
Nuts

Stool softeners
Fluids of any sort
Orange juice
Prune juice
Fruit

CONSTIPATION AT A GLANCE

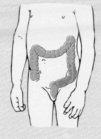

Epidemiology
Any age, but particularly problematic in immobile disabled children

Aetiology
Cycle of painful defaecation and withholding

History
Infrequent hard stools
Painful defaecation
Abdominal pain*
Soiling*

NB *Signs and symptoms are variable

Physical examination
Indentable mass in left lower quadrant
Hard stool on rectal examination (PR not often indicated)
Anal fissure*

Confirmatory investigations
Faecal loading +/– megacolon on plain abdominal X-ray (investigation not usually indicated)

Differential diagnosis
Hirschsprung's disease

Management
Dietary advice
Laxatives

Prognosis/complications
Problem may recur periodically

SOILING AND ENCOPRESIS

Soiling

The term soiling is used in two contexts. The first is when a child is not toilet trained by the usual age of about 2 years, and it is certainly seen to be a problem if this has not been achieved by the age of 4 years. Immaturity in acquiring bowel continence may result from inappropriate toilet training. A programme of regular toilet training needs to be instituted, with much positive reinforcement for successes.

The second situation where the term is used is when faecal staining of underwear results from leakage of liquid stool around impacted faeces when a child is constipated. In this circumstance it is sometimes mistaken for diarrhoea. The problem must be approached by addressing the underlying constipation (see above). Resolution of the soiling will occur as a result.

Soiling in both circumstances is a problem causing social inconvenience and embarrassment for both the child and the family.

Encopresis

Encopresis refers to the voluntary passage of formed stool in inappropriate places (including underwear) by a child who is mature enough to have acquired bowel continence. The term is also sometimes confusingly and inappropriately used in reference to soiling.

Encopresis is indicative of behavioural difficulties, often of a severe nature. Simple behavioural management in terms of understanding and encouragement, and the use of positive reinforcement may be attempted, but more intense psychiatric or psychological help is usually necessary.

BLOOD IN THE STOOL

The appearance of blood in the stool is usually alarming. The commonest cause is constipation, whether an anal fissure is visualized or not. Apart from dysentery, the other causes (Table 5.18) are not common, but demand evaluation.

Approach to the child with blood in the stool

History

- *The stool.* Constipation and dysentery are easily differentiated on history. A description of the stool is helpful, and the parent or child should be able to describe whether the blood is outside the stool, indicating the lower bowel as the site of bleeding (usually constipation), or whether it is

Table 5.18 Causes of blood in the stool

Infancy
Anal fissure
Dysentery and salmonella
Milk allergy
Intussusception

Older children
Anal fissure
Dysentery and salmonella
Inflammatory bowel disease
Intussusception
Henoch–Schönlein purpura
Intestinal polyp

mixed in with the stool, which indicates pathology higher up. In intussusception the blood is characteristically described as being like 'redcurrant jelly'. Blood from the upper intestinal tract is usually digested and appears as melaena, and has a black, tarry consistency, and a characteristic odour.

- *Pain.* Pain is a useful symptom. Constipation severe enough to cause bleeding is usually associated with significant pain on defaecation. In intussusception (p. 135) the baby has rhythmical attacks of screaming from abdominal pain. A description of pain in the older child may suggest peptic ulcer or inflammatory bowel disease.
- *Other sites of bleeding.* Bleeding from other sites would indicate a more generalized bleeding disorder.

Physical examination

- *General examination.* High fever occurs with dysentery. If significant blood has been lost the child may appear anaemic. The rash of Henoch–Schönlein purpura is usually characteristic (purpura on the extensor surfaces, see Fig. 5.18).
- *The abdomen.* In any of the conditions resulting in rectal bleeding the abdomen may be tender. In constipation, faecal loading may be palpable in the left lower quadrant and above.
- *Anal and rectal examination.* The anus must be inspected. The commonest finding is an anal fissure (see Fig. 5.9) which results from a large hard stool being extruded. Signs of more gross trauma would indicate abuse. In the absence of a fissure, a rectal examination may be indicated to confirm constipation or to obtain a stool sample for culture or occult blood.

Investigations

Investigations are not required if a diagnosis of constipation is made. Bloody diarrhoea requires stool culture to confirm dysentery. If intussusception is suspected an urgent barium enema is required for diagnosis and treatment (see p. 136). Inflammatory bowel disease requires confirmation, radiologically and endoscopically.

Causes of rectal bleeding

Anal fissure (Fig. 5.9)

The underlying cause of an anal fissure is the passage of a large hard stool which tears the delicate rectal mucosa. Constipation is exacerbated further as the child withholds stool to prevent the severe pain that is experienced on defaecation. Treatment consists of aggressively treating the underlying constipation (see p. 171), to the point of very soft stools, so that the anal fissure is not reopened at each bowel movement. Application of anaesthetic jelly may allow some relief of pain at defaecation.

Milk allergy

Bloody diarrhoea is a rare manifestaion of cow's milk allergy in babies. Microscopic gastrointestinal blood loss is common in infants fed whole cow's milk early.

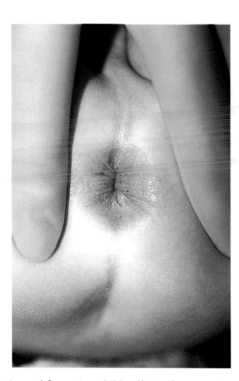

Fig. 5.9 An anal fissure in a child suffering from constipation with rectal bleeding.

COUGH

The purpose of this section is to discuss the child presenting with troublesome and persistent cough, but who is not acutely ill. The problem of the child presenting with respiratory distress (of which cough is usually a feature) is covered on p. 119, and the febrile child with cough on p. 101.

Illnesses causing cough (Table 5.19) vary with age, although the commonest cause of cough for all ages is infection affecting the upper or lower respiratory tract. A cough may persist and perpetuate itself after any illness, as coughing can injure the tracheal mucosa making it more susceptible to irritation. Passive exposure to smoking exacerbates coughing and respiratory disease.

In infancy, URTIs can be particularly troublesome as the infant's ability to feed can be affected (see below). Bronchiolitis, which affects the small airways (see p. 124) is a disease which is specific to this age. If cough is chronic in infancy, serious causes must be considered as congenital anomalies of the airways and aspiration of stomach contents can present in this way.

In the preschool years exposure to respiratory illnesses increases, and cough is very common. Bronchitis is a rather

Table 5.19 Causes of cough by age

Infancy
Infections
upper respiratory tract
bronchiolitis
pneumonia
Congenital malformations of the airway
Gastro-oesophageal reflux
Cystic fibrosis
Preschool
Infections
upper respiratory tract
croup
acute bronchitis
pneumonia
Foreign body
Asthma
Cystic fibrosis
Passive smoking
School-age to adolescence
Asthma
Infections
upper respiratory tract
Cigarette smoking
Postnasal drip
Psychogenic

non-specific term used either in relation to a productive cough (acute bronchitis) or bronchospasm. It is important to appreciate, however, that chronic bronchitis is not a paediatric disease. Asthma (see Chapter 4, p. 122, and Chapter 10, p. 318) often presents for the first time in the preschool years, and may be manifested by cough rather than wheeze. Foreign bodies are also common, and the cough may occur some time after the episode of choking has been forgotten.

In older children asthma and minor infections are the commonest causes of cough. Smoking must be considered as a cause of cough in adolescence.

Approach to the child with a cough

History

• *What does the cough sound like?* The sound of the cough can give a clue to the aetiology (Table 5.20). The rattling sound of mucus in the tracheobronchial tree is quite distinctive from either a dry laryngeal cough or the wheezy cough of asthma.

Focal points
Evaluating cough

• Transmitted sounds from the upper airways are commonly heard and should not be confused with crepitations

• Observation of tachypnoea, intercostal or subcostal retractions and alar flaring are often more important signs than findings on auscultation

• Asthma commonly presents with cough in young children rather than wheezing

• High fever in itself does not indicate lower respiratory tract infection

• In a child with chronic or persistent cough, look for evidence of chronic lung disease

---

Table 5.20 Characteristics of coughs

Loose, productive	Bronchitis, wheezy bronchitis, cystic fibrosis, bronchiectasis
Wheezy	Asthma, wheezy bronchitis
Barking	Croup
Paroxysmal (with or without vomiting)	Cystic fibrosis, pertussis, foreign body
Nocturnal	Asthma, sinusitis
Most severe on waking	Cystic fibrosis, bronchiectasis
With vigorous exercise	Exercise-induced asthma, cystic fibrosis, bronchiectasis
Disappears with sleep	Habit cough

• *Sputum.* Asking for a description of sputum is of limited value as young children swallow sputum, rather than expectorate. The older child, however, may be able to cooperate. Persistent purulent sputum suggests suppurative lung disease such as cystic fibrosis or bronchiectasis. In asthma sputum is clear and tenacious. Bloody sputum, if not from nasopharyngeal irritation, is suggestive of a foreign body.

• *Timing of the cough.* The timing of the cough can be helpful. A non-productive nocturnal cough suggests bronchospasm or postnasal secretions. A productive cough on rising suggests bronchiectasis or cystic fibrosis. Paroxysms of coughing suggest either a foreign body or pertussis, and coughing related to eating points to aspiration.

• *Is the cough acute, persistent or recurrent?* Cough may persist for weeks even after a mild respiratory infection. However, persistent cough in conjunction with other signs may indicate a chronic lung condition. Recurrent coughing, particularly at night, is suggestive of asthma. Diaries kept by parents are valuable if the cough is persistent or chronic.

• *Is the child ill?* Fever indicates infection, but does not differentiate between upper and lower respiratory tract infection. If the child is ill, lower respiratory tract infection must be considered (see Pneumonia, p. 106).

• *Associated symptoms and precipitating factors.* Coughing associated with wheezing strongly points to asthma, and the presence of other atopic manifestations in the child or the family helps in diagnosis. Exacerbations during the spring and summer suggest an allergic aetiology. An episode of choking might be recalled suggesting inhalation of a foreign body. Chronic symptoms of diarrhoea suggest cystic fibrosis.

• *Does anyone smoke in the family?* Passive smoking has an irritant effect on the young airway and can cause cough in itself. It also predisposes to asthma and infections. Adolescents may not confess to smoking, particularly if accompanied by a parent.

• *Past medical history.* A history of previous chest infections, particularly if confirmed radiologically, should suggest chronic lung disease.

Physical examination

• *Growth.* Weight and height should be assessed in all children as poor growth occurs in chronic conditions such as cystic fibrosis, bronchiectasis, immunodeficiency or severe asthma.

• *Signs of respiratory distress.* The presence of tachypnoea, subcostal and intercostal retractions and alar flaring indicate significant respiratory distress and are often more significant than auscultation findings in childhood. Tachypnoea may be the only sign of serious respiratory pathology.

• *Examination of the chest.* Examination of the chest is

obviously important. However, findings on auscultation must be interpreted cautiously by the newcomer to paediatrics. Transmitted sounds from the upper airways are commonly heard in the child with a cold, and must be differentiated from crepitations. Focal chest signs are less reliable in indicating the site of infection. Expiratory wheezing suggests the diagnosis of asthma, but may not be present between attacks unless the asthma is severe. Decreased air entry indicates bronchial obstruction from any cause.

• *Other signs*. The association of cough with clubbing suggests the possibility of suppurative lung disease or associated cardiac pathology. Signs of atopy such as eczema or allergic appearing eyes point towards a diagnosis of asthma.

Investigations (Table 5.21)

Investigations are required if a child has evidence of pneumonia or chronic lung disease. Too often chest X-rays are repeatedly obtained in children with asthma.

If a foreign body is suspected, chest fluoroscopy is required to look for mediastinal shift on inspiration.

Evidence of serious chronic lower respiratory tract disease in children

• Persistent fever

• Restriction of activity

• Failure to grow or gain weight

• Clubbing

• Persistent tachypnoea

Table 5.21 Investigations and their relevance in a child with cough

Investigation	Relevance
Full blood count	Raised white count and shift to the left with bacterial infection
	Possible eosinophilia in asthma
Blood culture	Lower respiratory tract infection
Pernasal swab	To identify pertussis
Chest X-ray	Lower respiratory tract infection
Chest X-ray and barium swallow	Congenital anomalies of the airway, gastrointestinal reflux
Sweat test	Cystic fibrosis
Videofluoroscopy and bronchoscopy	Aspirated foreign body
Trial of bronchodilators +/– peak flow measurements	Asthma

Bronchoscopy is needed to confirm the diagnosis and remove the foreign body.

A sweat test for cystic fibrosis is indicated if the cough symptoms are accompanied by poor growth or abnormal stools. As asthma is the commonest cause of recurrent cough, diagnosis using tests of peak flow are desirable when the child is old enough to cooperate.

Management

Antibiotics are too often prescribed for cough in the primary care setting. They have no place for URTIs, and should only be given if there is good evidence of infection of the lower tract. A good trial of bronchodilators, delivered by a technique appropriate for age, is required when asthma is suspected or diagnosed (see p. 123).

Cough is unusual in that treatment is often directed at the symptom rather than the cause. In general, little is to be gained by treating a cough *per se* unless it disrupts sleep or school.

There are two categories of medication: expectorants and cough suppressants. Expectorants are commonly prescribed but have never been shown to be effective, although they may have a good placebo effect. As regards cough suppression, codeine is the most effective medication, although the non-narcotic dextromethorphan provides an alternative. These medications should only be prescribed for a limited period. Constipation is a problematic side-effect of codeine.

Other therapeutic considerations include humidification of air if the cough seems to be triggered by drying of the mucous membranes. Lozenges in older children can help soothe coughs arising from irritation of the pharynx.

Smoking is an important cause and exacerbator of cough. Every effort must be made to discourage exposure, whether passive or active.

Causes of cough in childhood

Upper respiratory tract infection

In infancy, URTIs can be particularly troublesome for two reasons. First, infants are obligatory nose breathers, so nasal congestion can cause dyspnoea which is particularly problematic during feeding. Secondly, vomiting may be triggered by the cough or result from swallowing quantities of mucus.

Respiratory infections occur particularly frequently when babies and children first start nursery or school and are exposed to a wide variety of minor respiratory infections. The less robust will contract cold after cold to their parents' great anxiety.

Post-nasal drip secondary to catarrh is disputed to be a possible cause of cough. It is possible that the cough in this circumstance is more related to mouth breathing with drying and inflammation of the pharynx.

Chest infection

Chest infection is a generic term which includes bronchitis, bronchopneumonia and pneumonia. Viral infection is the commonest cause, but may be difficult to distinguish from bacterial infection. The pattern of infecting organism varies with age. *Chlamydia pneumonia*, bronchiolitis (see p. 124) and pertussis (despite immunization) (p. 51) are infections of particular importance in infancy. *Mycoplasma pneumonia* is a common respiratory infection between the ages of 10 and 15 years and tends to have an insidious onset and subacute course. Pneumonia is discussed in detail in Chapter 4.

Cystic fibrosis must be excluded if recurrent chest infections occur. Bronchiectasis and tuberculosis are rare but serious causes of chronic cough.

Asthma

Asthma is a very important cause of cough in childhood and must be considered in any child with a persistent or recurrent cough. It is covered in detail in Chapter 10 (p. 318).

Aspiration of foreign body (see also p. 125)

Children, particularly toddlers, may aspirate a foreign body without the parent realizing that this has occurred.

Clinical features Usually there is an immediate episode of coughing or choking, or a history of such an episode days or weeks earlier. However, the child may present with cough alone. As the commonest place for the foreign body to lodge is the right main bronchus (Fig. 5.10), there may be signs of right lung collapse and unilateral wheezing.

Management If an inhaled foreign body is suspected, videofluoroscopy or flexible bronchoscopy should be performed. Mediastinal shift is observed on inhalation. Bronchoscopy is required to remove the foreign body.

Cystic fibrosis

Cystic fibrosis is the commonest cause of suppurative lung disease in children in the UK. It is inherited as an autosomal recessive condition, one in 25 of the population being carriers. In northern Europe the commonest mutant gene is delta *F508*.

This gene codes for a protein which controls sodium and chloride transport across the apical membrane of secretory

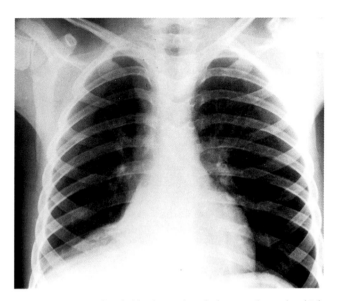

Fig. 5.10 X-ray of a child admitted with fever and cough which failed to respond to treatment. At bronchoscopy a Dinky car steering wheel was found in the right intermediate bronchus. The chest X-ray shows collapse of the right middle and lower lobe with loss of definition of the right hemidiaphragm and right heart border.

epithelial cells. The mutation leads to a high salt content of sweat, and thick secretions produced by the epithelial cells of some organs. Clinically, in the lungs, the thick mucus obstructs the small airways and predisposes to infection. In the pancreas, the ducts become obstructed and fibrosis develops. Similarly, biliary cirrhosis and obstruction of the vas deferens with male infertility may occur.

Most patients present with meconium ileus (Obstruction of the bowel by thick meconium, p. 240) at birth, or with diarrhoea and failure to thrive in infancy, often with respiratory problems. Others present beyond infancy with chronic and persistent respiratory symptoms. Some centres screen for cystic fibrosis at birth (see p. 49).

Clinical features
• *Respiratory tract.* The lungs are normal at birth, but the child later develops a tendency to frequent and prolonged infections. As the disease progresses, sputum is produced and the cough becomes chronic. Clubbing develops early, and in severe cases there may be chest deformity and growth retardation. The rate of progression of lung disease is very variable.
• *Intestinal tract* (see p. 166). Most children show evidence of malabsorption caused by exocrine pancreatic insufficiency. Symptoms include frequent, bulky, greasy stools and failure to thrive. A protuberant abdomen, decreased muscle mass and poor growth are typical signs.

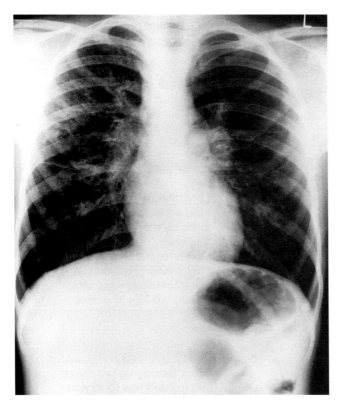

Fig. 5.11 Chest X-ray of a boy with cystic fibrosis. There is gross overinflation of the lungs with hilar enlargement and ring shadows caused by bronchial wall thickening and bronchiectatic change.

Investigations (see p. 365)

The diagnosis of cystic fibrosis is made by sweat test (see Fig. 12.6). Sweat is collected by pilocarpine iontophoresis. A low voltage electric current is used to carry pilocarpine into the skin of the forearm and to locally stimulate the sweat glands. Sweat is collected by filter paper and then analysed for sodium and chloride concentrations. Elevated levels (>60 mmol/L Na in a minimum sample of 100 mg sweat) are diagnostic of cystic fibrosis.

The chest X-ray in advanced cystic fibrosis shows patchy collapse, consolidation, cystic and linear shadows and overinflation (Fig. 5.11).

Sputum typically cultures *Haemophilus* species, *Staphylococcal aureus* or *Pseudomonas aeruginosa*.

Management
• *Respiratory tract.* The aim of treatment is to drain secretions, prevent infections and treat them promptly and effectively when they occur. Parents are taught how to carry out regular postural drainage. Antibiotic therapy is often required, intravenously or orally, at high dosage for prolonged periods.
• *Malabsorption and diet.* Pancreatic enzyme supplements (e.g. pancreatin) have to be taken with all meals and snacks, but may not control the malabsorption entirely. Children need to eat a high protein, high calorie diet, supplemented with fat soluble vitamins. Extra dietary supplements may be required at times of illness and for older children with anorexia. Extra salt is needed during hot weather and if the child is febrile.

Prognosis

Cystic fibrosis remains a life-limiting condition although the outlook has improved greatly in recent years so that average life expectancy is now 30–40 years. Infants with severe lung disease may die early, but in general, with good treatment, most individuals can lead relatively normal lives in the childhood years. Growth may slow down in later childhood and puberty may be delayed. In adulthood, the slow progression of lung disease eventually becomes disabling.

Cystic fibrosis may affect other systems. Diabetes develops in some children during adolescence. Most males are azospermic, but have unimpaired sexual function.

Distinguishing features — Causes of cough

	Fever	Features of cough	Respiratory signs
Upper respiratory tract infection (URTI)	+/–	Non-productive	None, other than transmitted sounds
Pneumonia	+	Productive	Alar flaring, intercostal, subcostal retractions, +/– dullness to percussion, diminished breath sounds
Asthma	– or +/– if URTI present	Wheezy, often nocturnal or on exercise	Alar flaring, intercostal, subcostal retractions, expiratory wheeze (but may be absent at time of examination)
Foreign body	– (until infection develops)	Often preceded by choking episode	Wheeze, diminished breath sounds on right

BREATH-HOLDING SPELLS AT A GLANCE

Epidemiology
Occur in babies and toddlers

Aetiology
Breath-holding or reflex anoxia

History
Cyanotic type (a):
• breath-holding precipitated by crying
• cyanosis
• extension of limbs
• loss of consciousness*
Pallid type (b):
• triggered by trauma, cry may be absent
• pallor and collapse
Rapid recovery from spell
No postictal phase

NB *Signs and symptoms are variable

(a) Cyanotic type

(b) Pallid type

Physical examination
Normal after event

Confirmatory investigations
None
Normal EEG

Differential diagnosis
Apnoeic spells
Infantile spasms
Febrile convulsions
Hypoglycaemia

Management
Reassurance

Prognosis/complications
Resolve by school age

or other minor injury, which triggers vagal reflex overactivity, causing transient bradycardia and circulatory impairment.

Clinical features The child may or may not start to cry but then turns pale and collapses. There is transient apnoea and limpness, followed by rapid recovery. The typical history, and absence of postictal drowsiness can help to distinguish these attacks from epilepsy.

Management The electroencephalogram (EEG) is normal, and this can help to establish the diagnosis. Reassurance is all that is required.

Prognosis The attacks disappear spontaneously prior to school age.

Night terrors

Night terrors usually have their onset in the preschool years.

Clinical features The child wakes from sleep confused and disorientated, does not recognize his or her parents and appears very frightened. Signs of autonomic activity in terms of dilated pupils, sweating, tachypnoea and tachycardia may be observed. Some minutes may pass before the child becomes orientated again and he or she does not usually recall the event. Night terrors are sometimes mistaken for epilepsy.

Management and prognosis Night terrors require simple reassurance. They are benign and usually self-limited.

Benign paroxysmal vertigo

These episodes are characterized by acute attacks of vertigo in young children aged 1–4 years old, and are thought to be caused by a disturbance of vestibular function.

Clinical features During a typical attack the child suddenly becomes unsteady on the feet, appears frightened and may clutch at the parent. There is no alteration of consciousness and the child reverts to normal within a few minutes. The condition is often mistaken for epilepsy, the distinguishing feature being the preservation of normal alertness during an attack.

Management and prognosis Reassurance alone is required. The episodes usually resolve within 1–2 years.

Epilepsy: partial, myoclonic and absence seizures (p. 333)

The diagnosis and management of absence, myoclonic and partial seizures are covered in detail in Chapter 10, but a description is given here to help in differentiating these fits from the other conditions described in this section.

Simple absence seizures (petit mal)

Simple absence seizures (petit mal) are fleeting episodes of impaired consciousness, which are unassociated with falling or involuntary movements.

Myoclonic seizures

Myoclonic seizures take the form of shock-like jerks often resulting in sudden falls. They most commonly occur in children with neurological conditions.

Simple partial seizures

Simple partial seizures usually consist of twitching or jerking of one side of the face, an arm or a leg. Consciousness is usually retained or is only slightly impaired.

Complex partial seizures (temporal lobe seizures)

Complex partial seizures (temporal lobe seizures) are attacks with altered or impaired consciousness associated with strange sensations, hallucinations or semipurposeful movements, such as chewing, sucking or swallowing motions which usually lasts a few minutes.

Infantile spasms

Infantile spasms are a form of myoclonic epilepsy with a particularly poor prognosis. The characteristic flexion spasms ('jack-knife' or 'salaam spasms') last a few seconds and occur in clusters.

Syncope

Syncope, or fainting, occurs when there is hypotension and decreased cerebral perfusion. Syncope is not uncommon, particularly in teenage girls reacting to painful or emotional stimuli. It also occurs in the teenage years in individuals with poor vasomotor reflexes who faint on standing up rapidly or during prolonged standing.

Clinical features Blurring of vision, light-headedness, sweating and nausea precede the loss of consciousness which is rapidly regained on lying flat. There may be a history of an unpleasant stimulus or prolonged standing.

Management and prognosis Syncope is rarely a symptom of cardiac arrhythmias or poor cardiac output in childhood. The evaluation should therefore include a clinical cardiac examination, standing and lying blood pressure and an ECG if there is any doubt as to the cause of the faint. Simple syncope usually becomes less of a problem in adulthood.

Hysterical seizures

Hysterical, psychogenic or pseudoseizures are problems which may mimic epilepsy and not infrequently occur in children with a genuine epileptic condition.

Clinical features Features suggestive of these seizures are:
- episodes provoked by emotional stimuli;
- gradual rather than abrupt onset;
- unusual aura;
- asynchronous flailing movements;
- an abrupt change of the episode in response to a stimulus.

Incontinence, bodily injury and postictal drowsiness are conspicuously absent.

Management EEG recording can be helpful in making the diagnosis, and a full psychological assessment is required if the diagnosis is suspected.

Hyperventilation

Excitement in some children, particularly teenage girls, may precipitate hyperventilaton to the point of losing consciousness.

Clinical features The diagnosis is usually evident in that breathing is excessive and deep, and tetany may also occur. A history of tingling lips and pins and needles may be reported.

Management Rebreathing into a paper bag restores the child back to normality. If episodes occur frequently, psychological therapy may be required.

Tics

Tics are rapid, repetitive, brief, involuntary movements such as blinking, jerking or facial grimacing. They are common particularly in school-age children and are intensified by anxiety, fatigue or excitement. They may resemble simple or complex partial seizures, but can be differentiated by the fact that they can be controlled voluntarily and are not associated with an alteration in consciousness.

Hypoglycaemia and other metabolic conditions

Metabolic disturbance, including hypoglycaemia, may cause loss of consciousness with seizures or a less dramatic alteration in consciousness. An underlying metabolic problem

Distinguishing features — Various fits, faints and funny turns in infants and preschool children

	Characteristic features	Precipitating event	EEG
Apnoea and ALTE	Usually found limp or twitching	None apparent	
Breath-holding spells (cyanotic)	Stops breathing, becomes cyanotic and extends, may lose consciousness. Then becomes limp and breathes normally. No postictal state	Always precipitated by crying from pain or anger	Normal*
Reflex anoxic spells (pallid)	Turns pale and collapses. Rapid recovery	Bump on head or other minor injury	Normal*
Night terrors	Wakes from sleep disorientated and frightened. May be autonomic signs		Normal*
Benign paroxysmal vertigo	Sudden unsteadiness. Frightened and clings to parent. No postictal state	None	Normal*
Infantile spasms	Jack-knife spasms occurring in clusters. Developmental regression	Often occur on waking	Hypsarrythmia
Epilepsy	As for the school-age child		

* EEG not required to make the diagnosis.

Distinguishing features — Various fits, faints and funny turns in the school-age child

	Characteristic features	Precipitating event	EEG
Syncopal attacks	Blurred vision, light-headedness, sweating and nausea, resolves on lying down	Painful or emotional stimulus, prolonged standing	Normal*
Hyperventilation	Excessive deep breathing, sometimes tetany. Resolves on breathing into a paper bag	Excitement	Normal*
Hysterical seizures	Gradual onset, asynchronous flailing movements, no incontinence or postictal state	Often an emotional stimulus	Normal unless the child has in addition genuine epilepsy
Tics	Rapid, repetitive, brief, involuntary movements which can be voluntarily controlled	Anxiety and fatigue	Normal*
Simple absence epilepsy	Fleeting vacant look	None	Characteristic three per second spike and wave activity
Myoclonic epilepsy	Shock-like jerks causing sudden falls. Most common in children with known neurological condition	None	Abnormal
Partial epilepsy	Twitching or jerking of face, arm or leg	None	Abnormal
Complex partial epilepsy	Altered or impaired consciousness with strange sensations or semipurposeful movements such as chewing or sucking. May be a postictal phase	None	Discharges arising from the temporal lobe

* EEG not required to make the diagnosis.

should be suspected in a child if there are features such as significant vomiting, developmental delay, dysmorphism, hepatosplenomegaly or micro- or macrocephaly. Hypoglycaemia may be suspected if there is a temporal relationship of the episode to food.

URINARY SYMPTOMS: DYSURIA

Dysuria, or pain on micturition, is commonly experienced by little girls secondary to vulval irritation and inflammation. Urinary tract infection is less frequently a cause but needs to be considered, particularly if fever is also present. The principal causes of dysuria are listed in Table 5.23.

Approach to the child with dysuria

History

A history of UTIs or symptoms such as frequency, fever and abdominal pain suggest urine infection. Anal itching indicates irritation resulting from threadworms.

Physical examination

The perineal area should be inspected for signs of inflammation and poor hygiene, and evidence of a discharge may be found in underwear.

Investigations

Urinary tract infection should be ruled out by urine culture. If itching is a problem, the child needs to be investigated for threadworms (see p. 212) or empirically treated with mebendazole.

Management

The management, providing there is no urinary infection, lies in improving hygiene and reducing factors which lead to inflammation of the area.

Causes of dysuria

Urinary tract infection (see p. 111)

Urinary tract infection often causes dysuria. It is discussed in Chapter 4.

Other causes

Poor hygiene, bubble bath sensitivity and threadworms all irritate the delicate skin and mucous membranes and cause soreness. Poor hygiene may be a particular problem in young girls who have just achieved independent toileting but may not wipe themselves well or wash carefully. Paradoxically, bubble baths and soaps also cause dysuria by irritating the sensitive skin in this area.

Another cause is enterobiasis. In a child infested with threadworms, the worms may emerge from the anus and enter the perineal area causing both itching and soreness. Candida infection is often overdiagnosed as a cause of dysuria in children who are out of nappies.

URINARY SYMPTOMS: POLYURIA AND FREQUENCY

Polyuria and frequency may be difficult to differentiate on clinical grounds unless urine volume measurements are made, so these two problems are considered together. Both may result from organic disease (Table 5.24) but may also, and more commonly, arise from psychogenic causes.

Approach to the child with polyuria and frequency

The importance of the clinical evaluation is to differentiate the psychogenic causes of frequent or excessive urination from organic disease which must then be identified.

History

- *Pattern of urination*. It may be possible to differentiate

---

Advice for girls with dysuria

- Daily baths or washing with simple, non-perfumed soap or, if not too dirty, water alone

- Bubble baths and talcum powder should be avoided

- Girls should only wear pure cotton knickers and preferably skirts. Constricting clothing such as nylon tights or tight trousers trap moisture and exacerbate irritation

- A barrier cream or nappy cream may help

- An empirical trial of mebendazole against threadworms can be given

---

Table 5.23 Causes of dysuria

Urinary tract infections (see p. 111)
Irritation secondary to poor hygiene
Sensitivity to bubble baths or washing powder
Irritation secondary to threadworm infestation (p. 212)

Table 5.24 Causes of frequent and excessive urination

Urinary tract infection
Psychogenic causes
Diabetes mellitus
Diabetes insipidus
(Chronic renal failure)

frequency and polyuria by taking a good history. In general, parents are more aware of the child who frequently urinates rather than the child who passes large quantities of urine at normal intervals. In the child with recently attained bladder control, any condition causing polyuria or frequency is likely to cause enuresis. If symptoms are absent through the night a psychogenic cause is likely, although the reverse cannot be stated. Urinary tract infections may be associated with dysuria, abdominal pain and fever, although they may be asymptomatic.

• *Thirst and pattern of drinking.* The key question to determine whether polyuria, rather than frequency alone, is present, is to establish whether the child is experiencing thirst. Thirst and polydipsia always accompany polyuria, whether of organic or psychogenic aetiology. Organic causes of polyuria precipitate thirst secondary to decreased hydration and, conversely, excessive drinking for any reason will result in increased urine output. However, thirst does not accompany problems causing frequency without polyuria.

• *Behaviour.* As the commonest causes of both frequency and polyuria are psychogenic, enquiring into behavioural and emotional issues is important.

• *Past medical history.* A history of poor growth, weight loss and head injury are significant in identifying the child with a chronic illness.

Physical examination

The physical examination rarely contributes to the diagnosis of the child presenting with these urinary symptoms. Height and weight measurements are important if only to provide a baseline for the future. Signs of dehydration and weight loss are clearly concerning. It is good practice to examine the abdomen for bladder distension, kidney size and abdominal masses.

Investigations

The most important bedside action is to obtain a sample of urine and carry out urinalysis prior to culture. Sugar in the urine is indicative of diabetes mellitus. Blood and protein would suggest a UTI, and a low specific gravity would suggest polyuria, whether caused by diabetes insipidus or psychogenic polydipsia.

Causes of urinary frequency

Urinary tract infection

The treatment of UTI is covered in Chapter 4, and the management of recurrent infections later in this chapter.

Psychogenic causes

Young children around the time of acquiring bladder control often test and try their parents by frequent demands for the potty or toilet. This may cause irritation on the part of the parents, but is rarely a major diagnostic problem. At a later age children often experience frequency and sometimes urgency when excited or frightened and this too can usually be handled sensibly. More rarely, urinary frequency can be an indicator of more serious emotional problems and stress.

Causes of polyuria

Psychogenic or habitual polydipsia

The commonest cause of polyuria is polydipsia. Obviously a child who drinks excessively will pass very large quantities of dilute urine. Usually the problem is simply one of habit, particularly in the toddler who is attached to a bottle. Very rarely, polydipsia can be a sign of significant psychopathology.

Psychogenic polydipsia can usually be differentiated from true diabetes insipidus by withdrawing fluids. In the former, urinary output is reduced. In long-standing cases the kidneys may become 'washed out' by chronic polyuria and may take a period to recover normal concentrating capacity. If there is serious concern that diabetes insipidus is present, the trial of fluid withdrawal must be carried out in hospital as the child in this case can become seriously dehydrated.

Diabetes mellitus (see also p. 325)

Unlike adults, children with diabetes mellitus rarely present with chronic polyuria. They are usually diagnosed within a few weeks of the onset of symptoms of polyuria and weight loss, often before diabetic acidosis has developed. The diagnosis can be made on the presence of large quantities of sugar in the urine on dipstick, and is then confirmed by random blood glucose levels. The management of diabetes mellitus is covered in Chapter 10.

Diabetes insipidus

Diabetes insipidus is a rare condition where there is an inability to concentrate urine.

Chronic renal failure

Polyuria occurs in chronic renal failure caused by the loss of the kidney's ability to concentrate urine. It is unlikely to be the presenting symptom.

URINARY SYMPTOMS: DIURNAL ENURESIS

Diurnal enuresis can be defined as a lack of bladder control during the day in a child old enough to maintain bladder continence. In our culture this usually occurs by the age of $2^{1}/_{2}$ years, but can be delayed beyond this. Most children experiencing daytime enuresis also have nocturnal enuresis. In contrast to nocturnal enuresis alone, which is nearly always non-organic in nature, diurnal enuresis requires exclusion of organic disease (Table 5.25).

Approach to the child with diurnal enuresis

Organic conditions can usually be excluded on clinical grounds, provided a thorough evaluation takes place. A neurological problem must be suspected if a child has an abnormal gait and coexisting bowel disturbance. A neurogenic bladder may result from either an upper or lower motor neurone lesion, and features which suggest this problem are a distended bladder, abnormal perianal sensation and anal tone, and abnormal neurological findings in the legs.

History

- *Is the enuresis primary or secondary?* It is important to ascertain the age at which toilet training was achieved. The enuresis is primary if bladder control was never attained and secondary if a relapse in control has occurred.
- *Is the child ever dry?* Most enuresis is intermittent through the day, but if continuous dampness or leakage of urine occurs, an organic problem such as ectopic ureter must be suspected.

Table 5.25 Causes of diurnal enuresis

Organic
Urinary tract infection
Neurogenic bladder
Congenital anomalies
Constipation (or rarely other pelvic masses)
Physiological
Urgency incontinence
Psychogenic

Focal points
Evaluating diurnal enuresis

- Establish if the enuresis is primary or secondary
- The commonest organic cause is urinary tract infection
- Continuous leakage of urine indicates an anatomic cause
- Features of a neurogenic bladder include a distended bladder, abnormal perianal sensation and anal tone, and abnormal neurological findings in the legs

- *Are there other symptoms?* Accompanying symptoms of dysuria, frequency and haematuria or prior UTI suggest a UTI. Neurogenic bladder is suspected in a child with coexisting bowel and gait difficulties.

Physical examination

The genitalia, abdomen, anus and legs need to be examined, and if possible the urinary stream observed (in girls it is easier to listen than observe).
- *The abdomen.* A distended bladder suggests bladder outlet obstruction. This can be caused by abdominal masses—hard faeces or otherwise.
- *The genitalia.* If the history suggests continuous wetting the vulval area must be inspected for seepage of urine.
- *The back and legs.* The back and legs must be examined as a midline lipoma, hairy patch, spinal deformity or abnormal neurological evaluation of the legs suggest the presence of spina bifida occulta (see p. 237) with neurogenic bladder.
- *The anus.* Abnormal perianal sensation and anal tone are suggestive of a neurogenic bladder. Pelvic masses which may be obstructing the urinary outlet can be assessed on rectal examination.

Laboratory investigations

The only baseline tests required are a urinalysis and urine culture, and even the latter is probably unnecessary in boys.

If organic causes are suspected imaging of the urinary tract by ultrasound, renal scan, intravenous pyelogram and uroscopy may be indicated, along with spinal X-rays

Causes of diurnal enuresis

Urinary tract infection

Although UTI usually presents with symptoms of dysuria, frequency, abdominal pain and/or fever, it is important to exclude infection by urine culture in all enuretic children. The management of UTI is dealt with elsewhere (see p. 112).

Neurogenic bladder

Enuresis can result from neurological dysfunction of the bladder. Usually it is evident that the child already has a neurological problem such as cerebral palsy or spina bifida, and gait disturbance or inadequate bowel control generally accompany the complaint. The neurological dysfunction can range from the spastic small bladder which empties suddenly without warning, to the large hypotonic bladder which fills to capacity and overflows.

The finding of hairy patches or lipoma overlying the lower spine suggests a spinal anomaly responsible for the problem. Neurogenic bladder dysfunction is serious, not only because of the difficulties of incontinence, but also because such children are at risk for damage to the kidneys.

Congenital anomalies

The commonest congenital urinary tract anomalies causing enuresis are ectopic ureters in girls and posterior urethral valves in boys. The ectopic ureter commonly ends in the vagina, causing continuous dampness and dribbling. Posterior urethral valves cause lower urinary tract obstruction and bladder distension with overflow incontinence. Both conditions are treated surgically.

Pelvic masses

Pelvic masses, the commonest being faecal impaction, may lead to stress incontinence which is particularly troublesome when running, coughing or lifting.

Urgency incontinence

In this condition, which is common in women too, bladder spasms lead to abrupt voiding. There is usually a life-long history of urgency, but it is sometimes triggered by a UTI. Children may become very distressed by the problem and are usually well motivated to tackle it. Treatment involves voiding at frequent intervals and training the child to increase control by practicing stream interruption exercises, such as those recommended in antenatal classes.

Psychogenic enuresis

When stressed, young children are likely to wet themselves. Common triggers are the birth of a sibling or school entry. In the latter circumstance the child may be too shy or embarrassed to ask permission to go to the toilet. These children are helped by sympathy and support both at home and at school.

Enuresis may be part of a wider behavioural problem, where the child becomes resistant and negative about using the toilet. Bowel continence may also be affected. Usually the toilet training has been highly pressurized, either in terms of endless lecturing or physical punishment. Management should be directed towards reducing pressure on the child and giving positive encouragement.

URINARY SYMPTOMS: NOCTURNAL ENURESIS

Nocturnal enuresis or bedwetting can be defined as being a problem when it occurs during more than one night a month. It is very common, occurring in 30% of children at

Distinguishing features—The causes of diurnal enuresis

Pathology	Enuresis	Suggested by
Urinary tract infection (UTI)	Secondary	Frequency, dysuria
Neurogenic bladder	Primary or secondary, depending on problem	Distended bladder, abnormal perianal sensation and anal tone, abnormal neurological findings in the legs Spinal deformity, lipoma and hairy patch
Congenital anomalies	Primary (or secondary if triggered by UTI)	Continuous leakage of urine Distended bladder Urinary tract infection in the preschool years
Constipation	Secondary	Infrequent stools Faecal mass palpable in abdomen and per rectum
Physiological	Primary or secondary	Life-long history of urgency
Psychogenic	Primary or secondary	Stress such as sibling birth or starting school Behaviour problems

4 years old, 10% at 6 years old, 3% at 12 years old and 1% at 18 years old. Enuresis may be primary (dryness never achieved) or secondary (a relapse of bladder control). Unlike diurnal enuresis, an organic problem is rarely implicated (Table 5.26), although it is usual to exclude infection, particularly if the problem is secondary rather than primary.

In nocturnal enuresis, various mechanisms have been implicated such as immaturity of the pathways for voluntary bladder control, inadequate nocturnal antidiuretic hormone secretion, small bladder capacity, and deep sleeping. Boys are affected more than girls and the problem frequently runs in families.

Approach to the child with nocturnal enuresis

History

The history may reveal stresses which have triggered the enuresis, and the birth of a sibling, moving to a new house or family dissention are common triggers. As enuresis frequently runs in families, particularly among the males, it is important to enquire into a family history. It is interesting how often fathers seem to conceal this information from their suffering sons.

Although organic causes are less likely, it is important to enquire into symptoms of UTI and polydipsia which may give clues to more serious causes of the enuresis.

Physical examination

The physical examination usually contributes little to the management of nocturnal enuresis. Relevant signs would be as described in the section on diurnal enuresis.

Investigations

Urinary tract infection should be excluded by urinalysis and culture.

Management

Intervention is usually delayed until a child is 7 years old and at a stage of maturity when he or she can take some responsibility for tackling the problem. Needless to say, even before

Table 5.26 Causes of nocturnal enuresis

| *Common* |
| Delayed maturation (often familial) |
| Emotional difficulties |
| |
| *Rare* |
| Urinary tract infection |
| Causes of polyuria (see Table 5.24) |

NOCTURNAL ENURESIS AT A GLANCE

Epidemiology

10% of children at 6 years, decreasing to 3% at 12 years
More common in boys

Aetiology

Various physiological mechanisms suggested

History

May be primary or secondary enuresis
Stresses at home*
Family history of enuresis* (a)

Physical examination

Normal

NB *Signs and symptoms are variable

Confirmatory investigations

None

Differential diagnosis

Rarely can be UTI
Causes of diurnal enuresis
(see Table 5.25)

Management

Intervention usually only indicated for children aged 7+ years
Behavioural incentives
Enuresis alarm
Vasopressin

Complications

Good with appropriate management, although 1% still enuretic at 18 years

a

this age wet beds can cause a lot of tension within the family and embarrassment for the child.

Preliminary tactics

Parents usually try tactics such as fluid restriction in the evening and lifting a child from bed to urinate at night with varying degrees of success. Understanding how prevalent bedwetting is in childhood, and how counter-productive it can be to address the problem at too early an age, can help relieve the frustration and exasperation of some parents.

Behavioural management

Many children respond to good behavioural management in the form of star charts and rewards for dry nights provided they are mature and motivated enough to try. A more intensive behavioural approach is the use of the enuresis alarm which is triggered by urine touching a sensor attached to the pyjama bottoms or sheet. The child is woken in time to complete voiding in the toilet. This alarm is very successful in training the motivated child and is often not required beyond a period of 2–3 weeks. It is best to reserve this method until the child is responsible enough to connect the alarm system him or herself and to change clothes and bedding too, if necessary.

Medication

Medication is an alternative to the alarm system. In the past the antidepressant imipramine was used, and was generally effective for the duration of administration, but children frequently relapsed when it was discontinued. More recently, vasopressin has become available by nasal spray or orally. Some children respond to a course of treatment by remaining dry, but others relapse on withdrawing the medication. Vasopressin can also be effectively used to ensure a dry night on an occasional basis when required, such as at cub camp or staying with a friend.

URINARY SYMPTOMS: HAEMATURIA

Haematuria may be gross, and evident to the eye, or micro-scopic and identified on dipstick or microscopy of the urinary sediment. It may occur as an isolated symptom or accompanied by signs of a systemic disorder.

The commoner causes of haematuria are shown in Table 5.27. The commonest cause is UTI, whether bacterial or viral. Another important cause in childhood is acute glomerulonephritis, in which glomerular damage is inflicted by the formation of immune complexes, most commonly following a streptococcal infection.

Table 5.27 Causes of haematuria

Urinary tract infection
Trauma
Acute glomerulonephritis
Stones and hypercalciuria
Congenital anomalies
Tumour
Bleeding disorder
Exercise
Drugs

Focal points
Evaluating haematuria

- Identify the site of the urinary tract damage by the colour of the urine and microscopy of the sediment

- Measure blood pressure

- Palpate carefully for renal masses

Blunt or penetrating injury to the abdomen may injure the kidney and cause haematuria, and if there is a urinary tract malformation, even minor trauma to the flank can result in bleeding. Renal stones are rare and can result from chronic infection or excessive secretion of calcium and other metabolites. The commonest tumour is Wilms' tumour which may present with haematuria, but more commonly presents with a loin mass.

Approach to the child with haematuria

History

- *What colour is the urine?* The colour of the urine indicates the site of the damage. Haematuria originating from the kidney is brown or Coca-cola coloured, that from the bladder or urethra has a red to pink colour and may contain clots. Not all red urine is caused by blood. Urine may turn red on consumption of certain foods, notably beetroot and blackberries.
- *Are there other urinary symptoms?* The presence of frequency and dysuria suggest a UTI.
- *Is there pain?* Abdominal pain or renal colic suggest a clot, calculus or obstructive malformation.
- *Was there a precipitating factor?* Trauma to the loin or abdomen can cause kidney damage. Upper respiratory tract or skin infections often precede acute glomerulonephritis. Intense exercise may precipitate haematuria.

Table 5.28 Investigations and their relevance in haematuria

Investigation	Relevance
Urinalysis	Red cell casts and proteinuria indicate a glomerular lesion. Pyuria and bacteriuria point to infection
Urine culture	Urinary tract infection
Full blood count	Anaemia
ASO titre and throat culture	Recent streptococcal infection often precedes acute glomerulonephritis
Serum creatinine, urea and electrolytes	Elevated creatinine and urea indicate impaired renal function
24 hour urine for creatinine, protein and calcium	Creatinine clearance quantifies the degree of renal impairmant
Serum C3 level	Low C3 is specific for certain types of glomerulonephritis
ANF/autoantibodies	Positive in systemic lupus erythematosus
Abdominal/pelvic ultrasound and IVP	Structural abnormalities of the kidney
Renal biopsy	Required if haematuria is persistent with proteinuria, hypertension or impaired renal function

• *Family history.* A family history of a bleeding disorder, hypertension or kidney disease may be relevant.

Physical examination

• *Blood pressure.* Measurement of blood pressure is mandatory in any child presenting with haematuria. Hypertension suggests renal malfunction and the child should be admitted to hospital.
• *Oedema.* Oedema is found periorbitally and at the ankles. It can be a feature of glomerulonephritis.
• *Renal mass.* The abdomen needs to be palpated carefully for tenderness, and for renal masses. If a mass is found the most likely diagnosis is hydronephrosis, polycystic kidneys or tumour.

Investigations (Table 5.28)

A dipstick test of urine is not a precise diagnostic test. If haematuria is suspected or identified, urinalysis is required on the sediment of a centrifuged sample of urine. The presence of red cell casts and proteinuria indicate the glomeruli to be the source of the damage.

Urinalysis and culture is required in any child with haematuria, but beyond this investigations are guided by clinical evaluation. If acute glomerulonephritis is suspected, confirmation of streptococcal infection is required by throat

culture, antistreptolysin (ASO) titre and complement (C3) levels, and serum creatinine concentration to assess renal function. Further investigations are only required in this condition if renal failure ensues or the course is atypical for poststreptococcal disease.

Causes of haematuria

Acute glomerulonephritis

Acute glomerulonephritis results from immunological damage to the glomerulus. The commonest form in childhood occurs as a result of the formation of immune complexes following infection by a nephritogenic form of streptococcus. Haematuria characteristically occurs 1–2 weeks after a throat or skin infection. Other forms of glomerulonephritis are much rarer and only need to be considered if the course of the illness is atypical.

Clinical features The presenting complaint is the appearance of smoky or Coca-cola coloured urine. The child may otherwise be asymptomatic, although malaise, headache and vague loin discomfort may occur. Oedema may be seen around the eyes, and the backs of the hands and feet. Urine microscopy shows gross haematuria with granular and red cell casts. Proteinuria is also evident. In most children mild oliguria only occurs, but the course may be complicated by renal failure, hypertension, seizures and heart failure.

Management Evidence that the condition is the poststreptococcal form is sought by taking a throat swab and

Distinguishing features
Haematuria

Condition	Urine	Symptoms	Possible signs
Urinary tract infection	Bloody	Dysuria, frequency, urgency	
Glomerulonephritis	Smoky, Coca-cola coloured, granular and red cell casts	Malaise, oliguria	Hypertension, oedema
Renal stone	Bloody	Renal colic	
Tumour	Bloody	Abdominal pain	Renal mass
Congenital anomalies	Bloody	Painless	Renal mass

ACUTE GLOMERULONEPHRITIS AT A GLANCE

Prevalence

Age 3+ years

Aetiology

Immunological damage to the glomerulus, usually caused by immune complexes resulting from streptococcal infection

History

Smoky/Coca-cola coloured urine (a)
Malaise/headache* (b)
Loin discomfort* (c)
Throat or skin infection 1–2 weeks previously* (d)

Physical examination

Oedema*: periorbital and backs of hands/feet (1)
Hypertension* (2)

Confirmatory investigations

Gross haematuria
Urinalysis: haematuria, proteinuria
Urine microscopy: granular and red cell casts
Throat swab/ASO titre for streptococcal infection
Low C3 (as opposed to normal in nephrotic syndrome)

NB *Signs and symptoms are variable

Differential diagnosis

UTI
Other causes of haematuria (see Table 5.27)

Management

Monitor fluid balance and creatinine clearance
Salt and water restriction if oliguric
Diuretics and hypotensive agents for hypertension
Rarely dialysis
Penicillin to eradicate streptococcus in child and family
Renal biopsy if course is atypical

Prognosis/complications

Good prognosis for post-streptococcal glomerulonephritis
Usually resolved by 10–14 days
Complications include:
• renal failure
• hypertension
• seizures
• heart failure

Pathophysiology

Epithelial cell
Foot processes
Glomerular basement membrane
Urine space
Endothelial cell cytoplasm
Blood space
Endothelial cell
Circulating immune complexes
IgG
Subepithelial 'hump' granular deposits of IgG immune complexes
Triggers local inflammatory response

ASO titre. Low complement (C3) levels provide further evidence. There is no specific therapy for glomerulonephritis and the management is similar to that of acute renal failure. Creatinine clearance and fluid balance need to be monitored, and if oliguria develops, salt and water restriction is imposed. Diuretics and hypotensive drugs are needed if there is hypertension, and rarely, peritoneal dialysis is required.

Eradication of streptococcal infection with penicillin is recommended to limit the spread of nephritogenic organisms, but there is no evidence that it affects the course of the disease. Members of the family should also be cultured, and if the organism is found, treated with penicillin.

Prognosis The long-term prognosis for poststreptococcal glomerulonephritis is excellent. Other forms have a poorer prognosis. The illness usually resolves in 10–14 days, but if renal impairment persists a renal biopsy is justified to define the nature of the glomerular pathology.

Exercise haematuria

Gross or microscopic haematuria may follow vigorous exercise. The source of bleeding is probably in the lower urinary tract. It resolves within 48 hours of cessation of exercise.

RASHES AND SKIN LESIONS

Parents commonly bring their child to the doctor for diagnosis of rashes and skin lesions. In most situations a diagnosis

Table 5.29 Types of skin lesion

Type of lesion	Description	Example
Macules	Discrete flat lesions of any size or shape that are pink or red in colour. Characteristically they fade on pressure	Rubella Roseola
Papules	Solid palpable projections above the surface of the skin	Insect bite
Maculopapular	Mixture of macules and papules which tend to be confluent	Measles Drug rash
Purpura and petechiae	Purple lesions caused by small haemorrhages in the superficial layers of the skin. In general they indicate a serious condition. Characteristically they *do not fade on pressure*. Petechiae are tiny purpuric lesions	Meningococcaemia Idiopathic thrombocytopenic purpura Henoch–Schönlein purpura Leukaemia
Vesicles	Raised fluid filled lesions <0.5 cm in diameter. If large they are called bullae	Chicken pox
Wheals	Raised lesions with a flat top and pale centre of variable size	Urticaria
Desquamation	A loss of epidermal cells producing a 'scaly' eruption	Post-scarlet fever Kawasaki's disease

can be made clinically, and treatment, if required, given without further investigation. Experience is required to identify these skin manifestations and the process of identification can be likened to the identification of wild flowers or bird-spotting—if you have encountered it before you are likely to recognize it again. It is important, however, to learn to describe the features, just as in bird-spotting, this increases one's powers of observation and enhances the learning process.

The various types of skin lesion are described and illustrated in Table 5.29.

Approach to the child with a rash or skin lesion

Unlike almost any other condition in medicine, it is reasonable to examine the child presenting with a rash or skin lesion before embarking on a detailed history, so that the approach can be modified to suit the likely diagnosis.

Description of the rash or lesion

If one is unsure of the correct dermatological term the lesions should be carefully described according to their characteristics. The following terms or features are important to include:
- raised or flat;
- crusty or scaly;
- colour;
- blanching on pressure;
- size of the lesions;
- distribution (discrete, generalized or limited to certain sites in the body).

Other features

The age of onset, changes in the rash over time, current health and any accompanying features contribute to the diagnosis.

On the basis of this brief evaluation, the problem can be classified according to the following criteria:
- acute onset of rash;
- chronic rashes;
- nappy rash;
- individual skin lesions;
- birth marks;
- itchy conditions.

Each of these types of skin manifestation is discussed in the following sections.

RASHES OF ACUTE ONSET

Most children presenting with acute onset of a rash have one of the common infectious diseases of childhood, and are unwell with a temperature. Most of these exanthematous conditions require only supportive treatment and so specific diagnosis is often not critical. However, the exceptions are the purpuric conditions which may be life-threatening and must be identified promptly. The other reason for accurately diagnosing exanthematous conditions is for public health purposes so that epidemics can be recognized. The common rashes of acute onset are listed in Table 5.30.

Approach to the child with a generalized rash of acute onset

History

• *Is the child ill or febrile?* Most of the exanthematous diseases are accompanied by fever and malaise. In measles and meningococcaemia the child is often very ill. Measles is suspected if the three 'C's (coryza, cough and conjunctivitis) are present. In roseola the rash appears once the fever falls after 3–5 days. In rubella, fifth disease and non-specific viral exanthems the child often appears remarkably well. In

Henoch–Schönlein purpura (HSP) and idiopathic thrombocytopenic purpura (ITP) fever is usually absent. Scarlet fever is preceded by tonsillitis.
• *Is the rash itchy?* Itchiness suggests chicken pox if the rash is vesicular, or an allergic response. In the latter it is worth enquiring into possible allergens such as food, washing powder, soaps and lotions. However, the allergen is rarely identified.
• *Are there associated symptoms?* These are particularly important in the purpuric conditions. In ITP bleeding may occur from the gums and nose and bruising may be evident. In HSP, arthritis and abdominal pain, melaena and haematuria commonly occur. In hives, wheezing or stridor are rarely present.
• *Past medical history.* A previous attack of an infectious disease makes a further attack unlikely, but there is a high incidence of inaccurate diagnoses, particularly of the maculopapular rashes. An immunization history is obviously relevant. An atypical rash commonly follows some 10 days after measles, mumps and rubella (MMR) vaccination.
• *Contact with anyone ill.* It is important to enquire whether anyone else in the family, or at school or nursery has been diagnosed as having an infectious disease.

Physical examination

The rash
A good description of the rash is required focusing on the following.
• *Characteristics.* Is the rash macular, papular, maculopapular, purpuric or petechial, vesicular or wheals? An important part of the examination is to test the rash for blanching as purpuric and petechial rashes do not blanch on pressure, whereas maculopapular rashes do.
• *Distribution.* Measles and rubella both start on the face and work their way down the body. Roseola and chicken pox are mostly on the trunk. Both HSP and fifth disease have characteristic distributions.
• *The presence of an enanthem.* An enanthem should be sought in the mouth. In chicken pox the vesicles rapidly break down so that shallow ulcers are seen. In measles Koplick spots (appearing like grains of salt on a red background) are seen during the prodromal period only.

General examination
A complete physical examination is required, although other than the findings of fever and possibly lymphadenopathy rarely contributes to the diagnostic process.

Investigations

In general, the viral exanthems do not need confirmation of the diagnosis serologically, unless for public health reasons.

Table 5.30 Common rashes of acute onset in childhood

Macular and maculopapular	Measles
	Rubella
	Roseola
	Scarlet fever
	Fifth disease
	Non-specific viral illnesses
Vesicular	Chicken pox
	Hand, foot and mouth disease
Purpuric	Meningococcaemia
	Henoch–Schönlein purpura (see p. 199)
	Idiopathic thrombocytopenic purpura (see p. 199)
Wheals	Urticaria

Focal points
Evaluating generalized rash of acute onset

• Decide if the rash is macular, maculopapular, vesicular, purpuric or wheals

• Determine if the child is febrile or ill

• If the rash is petechial or purpuric and the child is unwell treat with penicillin IM and admit for investigation

• Beware of making a specific diagnosis of measles or rubella clinically. Without serological confirmation 'viral exanthem' should be diagnosed

The exception of course is the development of a maculopapular rash in a pregnant girl when rubella titres should be measured. If a sample is taken for viral titres, a second convalescent sample is required 10 days later, without which a diagnosis cannot be confidently made.

Cultures are required in meningococcaemia but may be negative as most children should have been given intramuscular penicillin prior to admission to hospital.

If the rash is petechial, a platelet count is required to make the diagnosis of thrombocytopenia. Repeated counts are required to monitor the course of the disease.

Management

Prior to the advent of immunization, childhood diseases were a common occurrence with regular epidemics. There was little difficulty in recognizing them, but these clinical skills have now diminished. It is important to recognize the various diseases so that appropriate advice about incubation periods and recommendations for isolation can be made (Table 5.31). In general, children are infective during much of the incubation period and before the specific characteristics of the condition emerge.

Maculopapular rashes are often overdiagnosed clinically as being caused by measles or rubella. As these diagnoses are difficult to make unless in the midst of an epidemic, it is preferable to make the diagnosis of viral exanthem rather than a wrong diagnosis. If accurate diagnosis is required confirmation by serological testing is necessary.

If meningococcaemia (see p. 198) is suspected the child should immediately be given intramuscular penicillin as rapid deterioration can occur, and urgent admission to hospital arranged. The child with suspected ITP also requires urgent hospital evaluation and admission if the platelet count is dangerously low.

Conditions causing acute generalized rashes in childhood

Measles

Measles is a miserable and very infectious viral illness. It is characterized by a distinctive maculopapular rash in conjunction with the three 'C's' (cough, coryza and conjunctivitis). Immunization with a live attenuated vaccine is given at age 12–18 months (see p. 53).

Clinical features After an incubation period of 10–14 days there is a prodromal illness with fever and upper respiratory symptoms, followed by onset of the rash on the third or fourth day. The rash begins on the face and behind the ears and spreads downwards to cover the whole body. In contrast to some of the other childhood infectious diseases the child is ill and irritable. The rash begins to fade after 3 or 4 days and becomes blotchy. During the prodromal period a distinctive exanthem can be visualized. Koplick spots (see Fig. 5.12b) looking like grains of salt on a red background appear on the buccal mucosa of the cheeks. In developing countries there is a high morbidity and mortality and diarrhoea is a common feature.

Complications Acute otitis media and bronchopneumonia are common complications. The serious complication of post-measles encephalitis occurs in one in 5000 cases and causes drowsiness, vomiting, headache and convulsions. The prognosis for normal neurological survival is poor. It

Table 5.31 The course of childhood infectious diseases

Disease	Incubation	Duration of rash	Recommended isolation
Measles*	10–14 days	5 days	From onset of catarrhal stage to day 5 of rash
Rubella*	14–21 days	2–3 days	None, except from non-immune women in first trimester of pregnancy
Roseola	Probably 10 days	1 day	None
Scarlet fever	2–4 days	5 days	1 day after start of treatment
Fifth disease	4–14 days	Weeks	None
Chicken pox	14–17 days	6–10 days	Until all lesions are crusted (usually 5–6 days)
Mumps*†	16–21 days	None	Until swelling subsides (usually 5–10 days)
Pertussis*†	7 days	None	4 weeks or until cough has ceased

* Immunizations against these disease are routinely given (see p. 51).
† Mumps and pertussis are included for completeness although there is no associated rash.

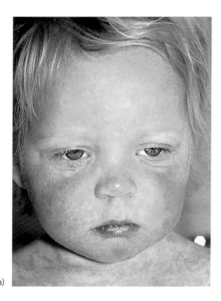

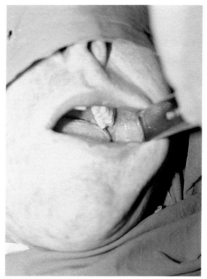

(a)   (b)

Fig. 5.12 (a) A child with measles demonstrating the typical maculopapular rash, conjunctivitis and miserable appearance. (b) Koplick spots.

generally occurs a week after the measles is diagnosed and is probably caused by an immunological cross-reactivity between measles virus and neural tisue. Subacute sclerosing encephalitis (SSPE) is a very rare complication which occurs some 4–10 years after an attack and is characterized by slow progressive neurological degeneration.

Management Treatment of measles is supportive. Antibiotics are required if otitis media or bronchopneumonia develop. The child is contagious prior to the onset of the rash to the fifth day of the rash.

Rubella (german measles)

Rubella is usually a mild illness and the rash may not even be noticed. The importance of the condition does not lie with the effect on the child, but on the devastating effects if rubella is contracted during the first trimester of pregnancy. The fetus may die or develop congenital heart disease, mental retardation, deafness and cataracts. In order to reduce exposure of young mothers to the virus, and to protect girls before they reach childbearing age, rubella immunization is given in early childhood (p. 53). If a rash occurs in pregnancy rubella titres should be measured immediately and after 10 days to determine if recent infection has occurred.

Clinical features After an incubation period of 14–21 days, the rash appears as tiny pink macules on the face and trunk and works its way down the body (Fig. 5.13). The suboccipital lymph nodes are enlarged and there may be generalized lymphadenopathy. Thrombocytopenia, encephalitis and arthritis are rare complications. The rash is quite non-

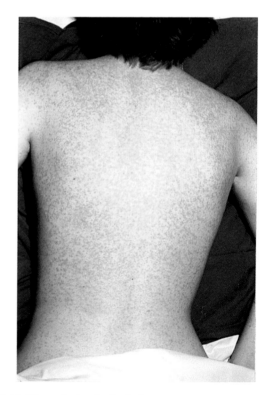

Fig. 5.13 The typical rash of rubella.

specific and the diagnosis of rubella is often erroneously and overconfidently made on clinical grounds.

Management No specific management is required.

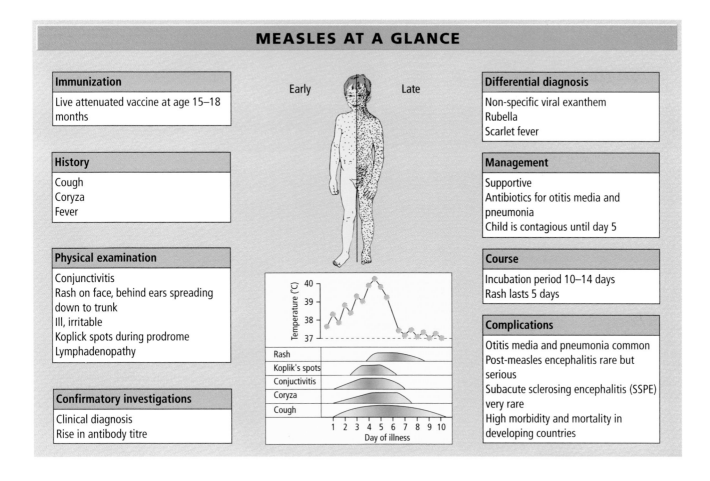

MEASLES AT A GLANCE

Immunization

Live attenuated vaccine at age 15–18 months

History

Cough
Coryza
Fever

Physical examination

Conjunctivitis
Rash on face, behind ears spreading down to trunk
Ill, irritable
Koplick spots during prodrome
Lymphadenopathy

Confirmatory investigations

Clinical diagnosis
Rise in antibody titre

Early   Late

Differential diagnosis

Non-specific viral exanthem
Rubella
Scarlet fever

Management

Supportive
Antibiotics for otitis media and pneumonia
Child is contagious until day 5

Course

Incubation period 10–14 days
Rash lasts 5 days

Complications

Otitis media and pneumonia common
Post-measles encephalitis rare but serious
Subacute sclerosing encephalitis (SSPE) very rare
High morbidity and mortality in developing countries

Roseola

Roseola affects children under the age of 2 years and has a very characteristic course.

Clinical features The child has a pronounced fever reaching to 39° or 40° lasting for 3–4 days. In general, despite the height of the temperature the child does not seem to be particularly unwell, although febrile convulsions may occur on the first day. Occipital lymph nodes are often enlarged. On the fourth day the temperature drops and a faint pink macular rash appears on the trunk, lasting only for a few hours or a day or so. The child then makes an uneventful recovery.

Management The fever needs to be controlled. There are no recommendations to isolate the child.

Scarlet fever

Scarlet fever, which is now uncommon, is the only childhood maculopapular exanthem caused by a bacterium and therefore requiring antibiotic treatment (although children with measles may need antibiotics for complications). It is caused by a strain of group A haemolytic streptococci.

Clinical features After an incubation period of 2–4 days fever, headache and tonsillitis appear. The rash (Fig. 5.14) develops within 12 hours and spreads rapidly over the trunk and neck, with increased density in the neck, axillae and groins. It has a fine punctate erythematous appearance, a 'sandpapery' feel and blanches on pressure. The tongue initially has a white coating, which desquamates leaving a sore 'red strawberry' appearance. The rash lasts about 6 days and is followed by peeling, which is useful in making a retrospective diagnosis.

Management A 10-day course of penicillin or erythromycin eradicates the organism and may prevent other children from being infected.

Complications Sequelae such as rheumatic fever and acute glomerulonephritis (see p. 189) are now rare in developed societies.

RUBELLA AT A GLANCE

Early Late

Immunization

Live attenuated vaccine at age 15–18 months

History

Generally well
Fever*

Physical examination

Tiny pink macules on face and trunk rapidly working downwards
Not ill
Enlarged suboccipital nodes
Generalized lymphadenopathy*

Confirmatory investigations

Rise in rubella titre

NB *Signs and symptoms are variable

Differential diagnosis

Non-specific viral exanthem
Drug rash

Management

None required

Course

Incubation period 14–21 days
Rash lasts 2–3 days

Complications

Devastating effects on fetus if pregnant
Thrombocytopenia
Encephalitis
Arthritis rare

Temperature (°C)

40
39
38
37

Rash
Lymph nodes
Malaise
Conjunctivitis
Coryza

1 2 3 4 5 6 7 8 9 10
Day of illness

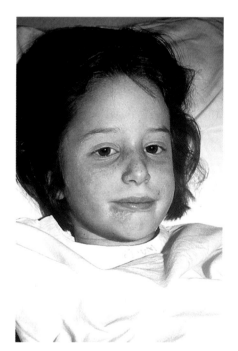

Fig. 5.14 A child with scarlet fever, showing the fine punctate maculopapular rash and perioral pallor.

Fifth disease (erythema infectiosum)

This condition is caused by human parvovirus B19. It is called fifth disease because it was the fifth of five illnesses to be described with somewhat similar rashes. (The other four were rubella, measles, scarlet fever and Filatov–Dukes disease—a mild atypical form of scarlet fever.)

Clinical features The illness usually begins with the sudden appearance of livid erythema of the cheeks, giving the child a 'slapped cheek' appearance. There are usually no prodromal symptoms and fever is absent or low grade. A symmetrical maculopapular lace-like rash (Fig. 5.15) then appears on the arms, trunks, buttocks and thighs. The rash can last up to 6 weeks and may be pruritic. Recrudescences may appear with temperature, exercise and emotional upset. Arthralgia and arthritis occur infrequently.

Management Isolation is not required and as the illness is mild and the duration of the rash may be prolonged, children should be allowed to attend school.

SCARLET FEVER AT A GLANCE

Aetiology

Group A haemolytic streptococcus

Early   Late

History

Fever
Headache
Sore throat

Physical examination

Fine punctate rash with sandpapery
feel, blanches on pressure
Particularly dense in neck, axillae and
groins
In later stages, rash peels
White-coated tongue changing to
'red strawberry' appearance
Tonsillitis

Confirmatory investigations

Group A streptococcus on throat
culture
Rise in ASO titre

Differential diagnosis

Non-specific viral exanthem
Measles

Management

Penicillin or erythromycin for 10 days

Course/complications

Rash lasts 5 days
Rheumatic fever and acute
glomerulonephritis now rare in
Western societies

[Chart: Temperature (°C) vs Day of illness, with rows for Rash and Sore throat; temperature axis 37, 38, 39, 40; day axis 1 2 3 4 5 6 7 8 9 10]

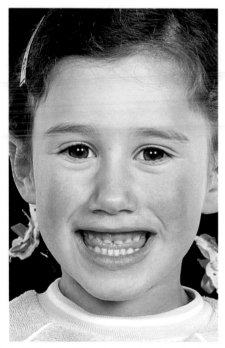

Fig. 5.15 A child with fifth disease showing the 'slapped cheek' rash in a well looking child.

Conditions causing acute vesicular rashes

Chicken pox (varicella)

Chicken pox is a common and highly contagious disease of childhood which is luckily usually mild in this age group. It may be contracted from a patient with shingles. Children who are immunocompromised (such as those on corticosteroids or treated for leukaemia) are at risk for severe, often fatal chicken pox. If such a child comes into contact with chicken pox, prophylaxis with zoster immunoglobulin should be considered. A vaccine against chicken pox is being developed but is not as yet available.

Clinical features After an incubation period of 14–17 days the rash (Fig. 5.16a) appears on the trunk and face. The spots appear in crops, passing rapidly through the stages of macule to papule and then vesicle. The appearance of the vesicles have been likened to 'dewdrops' on an erythematous base. The vesicles rapidly turn into pustules and then crust over. At the height of the illness the lesions simultaneously consist of papules, vesicles and crusts. Itching is constant and annoying. Vesicles in the mucous membranes, particularly in the mouth, rapidly become macerated and form shallow ulcers. The severity of the disease varies from a few lesions in a well child to many hundreds of lesions with severe toxicity.

Complications The commonest complication is secondary infection of the lesions, and scarring. A more severe complication is encephalitis which produces cerebellar signs with ataxia. Thrombocytopenia with haemorrhage into the skin can occur. Varicella pneumonia is uncommon in children.

Management Itching can be alleviated to some extent by cool baths, and application of calamine lotion. If the child is very distressed promethazine syrup can be helpful. Cutting fingernails short and keeping them clean can reduce secondary infection. The child is contagious until all the lesions have crusted over. If the disease develops in an immunocompromised child urgent admission for intravenous acyclovir is indicated.

Hand, foot and mouth disease

Hand, foot and mouth disease is caused by a Coxsackie virus. It occurs in epidemics affecting young children. Vesicular lesions appear on the palms of the hands and fingers, the soles of the feet and in the mouth. The vesicles clear by absorption of the fluid in about a week. There may be a low-grade fever.

Conditions causing purpuric rashes

Meningococcaemia (see also pp. 114, 304)

Meningococcaemia is a rapidly life-threatening condition, and it is vital that every health professional can identify its characteristic rash. Within hours of onset of flu-like symptoms, the rash (Fig. 5.17) appears with morbilliform, petechial or purpuric characteristics. If the septicaemia is fulminant, the purpura rapidly progress with unrelenting shock and coma. As the prognosis is so poor, meningococcal infection must be suspected in any child presenting with a purpuric-like rash and fever, and intravenous or intramuscular penicillin given prior to transfer to hospital. Meningococcaemia is discussed in detail in Chapter 4.

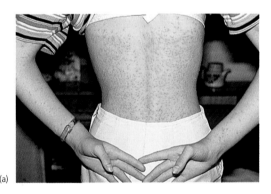

(a)

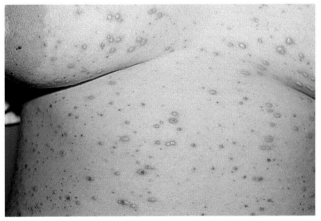

(b)

Fig. 5.16 (a) The very early rash of chicken pox. Many papules are seen, which will all become vesicles in the next few hours. (b) Typical rash showing lesions at all stages of development.

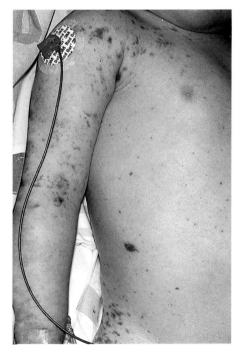

Fig. 5.17 Photograph of a child with the typical purpuric rash of meningococcaemia.

CHICKEN POX AT A GLANCE

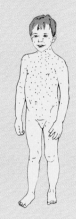

Aetiology

Herpes virus (contracted from chicken pox or shingles)

Immunization

Vaccine being developed
Immunoglobulin indicated for immunocompromised child exposed to chicken pox

History

Fever
Itching lesions
Irritability*

Physical examination

Lesions: a mixture of papules, vesicles, pustules and crusts over the trunk and face
Ulcers in mouth
May look toxic if severely affected*

Confirmatory investigations

Clinical diagnosis

NB *Signs and symptoms are variable

Differential diagnosis

Usually unequivocal

Management

Relieve itching by cool baths, calamine lotion +/– promethazine syrup
Child contagious until all lesions crusted
If child is immunocompromised give IV acyclovir

Course

Incubation period 14–17 days
Lesions last 6–10 days

Complications

Secondary infection of lesions
Encephalitis (cerebellar signs with ataxia)
Thrombocytopenia with skin haemorrhages
Chicken pox is severe or even fatal for the immunocompromised child

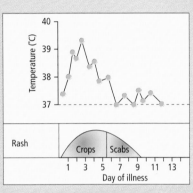

Henoch–Schönlein purpura (anaphylactoid purpura)

Henoch–Schönlein pupura is a form of systemic vasculitis which is presumed to be caused by immune complex mediated disease.

Clinical features The child presents with a purpuric rash in a typical distribution over the buttocks, thighs and legs (Fig. 5.18). The lesions are purple, raised and a few millimetres in diameter. Arthritis or arthralgia and abdominal pain are commonly experienced and occasionally melaena occurs. Seventy per cent of the children develop haematuria and/or proteinuria, but the glomerulonephritis is usually asymptomatic and non-progressive.

Management The diagnosis is usually made by the clinical constellation of the typical rash, and abdominal and joint complaints, with a normal platelet count. Treatment is simply supportive. The rash resolves over a week or two, although microscopic haematuria can persist for over a year.

Children with renal manifestations should continue to have urinary examinations and blood pressure measurements at periodic intervals to detect late development of hypertension and renal impairment.

Idiopathic thrombocytopenic purpura

As its name suggests ITP is caused by thrombocytopenia and presents with petechiae and superficial bruising (Fig. 5.19), but mucosal bleeding from the gums and nose may also occur. It often follows 1 or 2 weeks after a viral infection and is thought to have an immunological basis underlying the destruction of circulating platelets.

Clinical features The onset is frequently acute, and apart from the signs of bleeding the child appears clinically well. The most serious complication is intracranial haemorrhage, which occurs in less than 1% of cases.

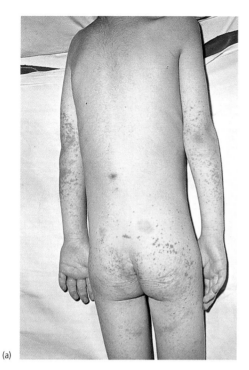

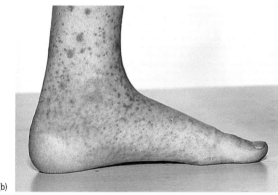

Fig. 5.18 (a) & (b) A child with Henoch–Schönlein purpura.

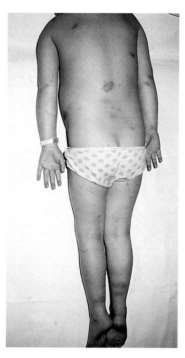

Fig. 5.19 A child with idiopathic thrombocytopenic purpura showing bruising and the petechial rash.

Investigations Diagnosis is made on the finding of a platelet count which is reduced to below 40×10^9/L and may be below 5×10^9/L. The white cell count is normal and there is no anaemia unless significant blood loss has occurred. As the differential diagnosis includes an aplastic or neoplastic process of the bone marrow, bone marrow aspiration is indicated. In ITP a normal or increased number of megakaryocytes is seen, reflecting the increased turnover which occurs as a result of the destruction of platelets peripherally.

Management In those who have only mild symptoms no treatment is necessary, but where there is a risk of severe bleeding a short course of steroids may produce a temporary rise in the platelet count. Platelet transfusion is of little benefit as the transfused platelets survive only briefly. They should be administered, however, if the platelet count falls to less than 20 000 or life-threatening haemorrhage occurs. Infusion of intravenous gammaglobulin causes a sustained rise in the platelet count and may induce remission.

Prognosis Idiopathic thrombocytopenic purpura has an excellent prognosis with 85% having a self-limited course. Severe spontaneous haemorrhage and intracranial bleeding are usually confined to the initial phase of the disease and the majority of children recover spontaneously within 6 months. In a few children ITP becomes chronic. Splenectomy and immunosuppressive therapy may be required in these cases.

Conditions causing acute wheals

Urticaria (hives)

Urticaria is an allergic reaction characterized by well-circumscribed but sometimes coalescent wheals of various sizes (Fig. 5.20). It is usually difficult to identify the allergen. Certain individuals may develop urticaria when exposed to insect bites (papular urticaria), cold, exercise, hot showers and anxiety.

HENOCH–SCHÖNLEIN PURPURA AT A GLANCE

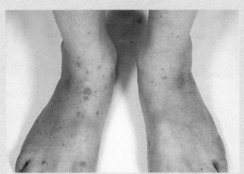

Epidemiology

Any age

Aetiology

Systemic vasculitis presumed to be mediated by immune complexes

History

Arthralgia*
Abdominal pain*
Melaena*

Physical examination

Purple raised lesions
Typical distribution over buttocks, thighs and legs *
Arthritis*

NB *Signs and symptoms are variable

Confirmatory investigations

Clinical diagnosis
Haematuria/proteinuria in 70%
Normal platelet count

Differential diagnosis

Usually unequivocal
(Septicaemia)
(Bleeding diathesis)

Management

Supportive
Urinalysis and blood pressure periodically if renal manifestations are present

Prognosis/complications

Rash lasts 1–2 weeks
Haematuria may persist for many months
Hypertension and renal impairment may occur

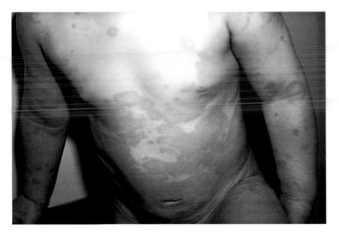

Fig. 5.20 A child with urticaria (hives) demonstrating characteristic, well-circumscribed wheals.

Clinical features The lesions may be intensely pruritic. Each wheal resolves within 2 days but new ones continue to occur, and urticaria may become chronic, persisting for many weeks. In angioneurotic oedema deeper tissues are also involved including the upper respiratory and gastrointestinal tract. Urticaria may also be seen in the child presenting in anaphylactic shock.

Management In most instances urticaria is a self-limited condition requiring no treatment, other than that aimed at reducing itching. Antihistamines are the drug of first choice. The allergen is usually not identified, although it is worth taking a good food and drug history.

CHRONIC SKIN PROBLEMS

Most chronic skin conditions (Table 5.32) in childhood are eczematous. Acute eczema (the generic term used to designate a particular type of skin reaction) is characterized by erythema, weeping and microvesicle formation within the epidermis. Chronic eczema is characterized by thickened, dry, scaly, course skin (lichenification). The commonest type of eczema in children is atopic dermatitis, although contact dermatitis and seborrhoeic dermatitis are also relatively common.

IDIOPATHIC THROMBOCYTOPENIC PURPURA AT A GLANCE

Aetiology

Destruction of circulating platelets by immune mechanism

History

Generally well
Bleeding from nose and gums*
Preceding viral infection 1–2 weeks before*

Physical examination

Petechial rash (**a**)
Superficial bruising (**b**)

Confirmatory investigations

Low platelet count (< 20 x 10^9/L)
Normal white cell count, normal haemoglobin
Bone marrow aspirate shows normal or increased number of megakaryocytes

NB *Signs and symptoms are variable

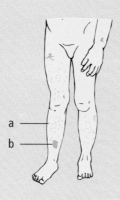

Pathogenesis

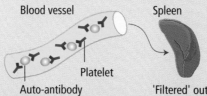

Blood vessel — Spleen
Platelet
Auto-antibody — 'Filtered' out in the spleen

Differential diagnosis

Leukaemia
Aplastic anaemia

Management

Monitor platelet count
No treatment if platelet count is high enough to make severe bleeding unlikely
Short course of steroids or IV gamma globulin for frank bleeding
Platelet transfusion for life-threatening haemorrhage

Prognosis/complications

85% of patients have simple limited course
Spontaneous haemorrhage or intracranial bleeding are the worrying complications
A few patients develop chronic ITP and need splenectomy and immuno-suppressive therapy

Distinguishing features—Acute generalized rashes in childhood

	Type of rash	Characteristics of the rash	Other features
Measles	Maculopapular	Begins on the face and spreads down words	Koplick spots, coryza, cough and conjunctivitis, ill child
Rubella	Macular	Tiny pink macules on the face and trunk, works downwards	Well child, lymphadenopathy sometimes
Roseola	Macular	Faint pink rash on the trunk	Rash occurs after fever defervesces
Scarlet fever	Maculopapular	Fine punctate red rash with sandpapery feel, followed by peeling	Strawberry tongue, perioral pallor, tonsillitis
Fifth disease	Maculopapular	'Slapped cheek' appearance. Lace-like rash on the arms, trunk and thighs	Well child, lasts up to weeks
Chicken pox	Vesicular	Occurs in crops on face and trunk. Papules, vesicles and crusts are present	Shallow ulcers of the mucous membranes
Meningococcaemia	Purpuric	Morbilliform, petechial or purpuric	May progress rapidly to shock and coma
Henoch–Schönlein purpura	Purpuric	Typical rash characteristically distributed over the buttocks, thighs and legs	Abdominal pain, arthralgia, melaena, haematuria
Idiopathic thrombocytopenic purpura	Petechial	Petechial rash over body, with bruising	Bleeding from other sites, e.g. venepuncture, gums, nose
Urticaria	Wheals	Well circumscribed, itchy wheals of different sizes	Rarely accompanied by wheezing or anaphylactic shock

Table 5.32 Common chronic skin conditions in childhood

Atopic dermatitis
Contact dermatitis
Seborrhoeic dermatitis
Psoriasis

Approach to the child with a chronic skin complaint

Most children presenting with a chronic skin rash have atopic dermatitis, but it is important to learn to distinguish other rashes.

History

• *Is the rash itchy?* Itchiness is characteristic of atopic and contact dermatitis. It may also be present in seborrhoeic dermatitis.
• *Are there precipitating factors?* Certain foods such as cow's milk, wheat and eggs may precipitate or exacerbate atopic dermatitis. Saliva, citrus juices, bubble bath, detergents, occlusive synthetic shoes and topical medication are common irritants that cause contact dermatitis.
• *Is there a family history?* Children with eczema often have a family history of atopy. The presence of psoriasis in a parent may support a diagnosis of psoriatic rash in a child. A recent history of scabies in the family or at school would suggest a diagnosis of scabies rather than atopic dermatitis.

Physical examination

• *Characteristics of the rash.* The child needs to be fully undressed in order to examine the rash and its distribution adequately. The pattern of involvement of atopic dermatitis changes during childhood.
• *Other helpful features.* The presence of cradle cap or a rash behind the ears and skin folds is suggestive of seborrhoeic dermatitis. Nail pitting or joint involvement point towards psoriasis.

Management

The skin is visible, so skin disease poses an additional problem not usually found in diseases of other systems. This means that the child and family are subject to the stares and curiosity of others, and the older child may suffer from stigmatization. In managing the child with a chronic skin condition it is important to remember that management should involve not only the skin condition but the whole child too.

Topical corticosteroids form an important part of the management of a variety of chronic skin conditions. They

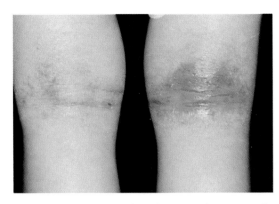

Fig. 5.21 The legs of a child with atopic dermatitis, showing flexural involvement.

must be used with care as long-term use, particularly of the fluorinated variety, leads to atrophy of the skin and an increase in hair growth in some patients. Small amounts of cream applied frequently is more effective than large amounts infrequently. The more potent topical steroids should not be applied to the face, and if applied over the body using occlusive dressings systemic absorption with adrenal suppression can occur.

Common chronic skin conditions in childhood

Atopic dermatitis (eczema) (Fig. 5.21)

Atopic dermatitis is an inflammatory skin condition characterized by erythema, oedema, intense itching, exudation, crusting and scaling. There appears to be a genetically determined predisposition and infants with atopic dermatitis tend to subsequently develop allergic rhinitis and asthma. It most often begins in the first 2–3 months of life, and the onset frequently coincides with the introduction of certain foods such as cow's milk, wheat and eggs into the diet. There is some evidence that genetically susceptible infants are protected from developing eczema if they are exclusively breast-fed. There is often a family history of atopy.

Clinical features The clinical features vary according to the stage of childhood. In infancy the lesions are erythematous, weepy patches on the cheeks which subsequently extend to the rest of the face, neck, wrists, hands and extensor surfaces of the extremities. Pruritus is marked and the infant makes efforts to scratch by face-rubbing on the sheets. This leads to weeping and crusting, and commonly secondary infection.

By preschool age (3–5 years) there is a tendency towards

remission, although some children persist with a mild to moderate dermatitis in the popliteal and antecubital fossae, on the wrists, behind the ears and on the face and neck.

During school years recurrence tends to occur with antecubital and popliteal involvement, and extension to the neck, forehead, eyelids, wrists and dorsa of the hands and feet. The skin becomes dry and thickened and the face can take on a whitish hue. Hyperpigmentation, scaling and lichenification become prominent.

Investigations The diagnosis is a clinical one. Serum IgE levels are often raised and reaginic (RAST) antibodies and eosinophilia may be present. Although skin testing is frequently positive it is rarely helpful clinically.

Management Scratching has a major role in the production of skin lesions, and treatment is directed at trying to interrupt the itch–scratch–itch cycle. Dietary restriction is controversial and generally of limited value. Arbitrary exclusion of a number of foods can lead to malnutrition.

During an acute flare-up wet dressings are helpful as they have an anti-inflammatory and antipruritic effect. Topical steroids are then applied between dressing changes. Antihistamines can be useful for their sedative and antipruritic effect. Scratching often causes infection even if this is not obviously apparent, and so topical or oral antibiotics are often required.

After the acute phase, while the dermatitis is still active, topical steroids are applied in the form of creams or ointments. The more potent steroid creams must be kept to a minimum to control the disease and should not be applied to the face. Systemic corticosteroids are only rarely used.

Lubricants are used after application of steroid creams and continued on a prophylactic basis to keep the skin moist. Bath oils can be added to the bath water after the child has soaked well, so that moisture is sealed into the well-hydrated skin

Prognosis The course of atopic dermatitis is fluctuating and fortunately resolves entirely in some 50% of infants by the age of 2 years. A few continue to be problematic beyond childhood. Reasonable control of this chronic condition can usually be achieved in most children.

Contact dermatitis (Fig. 5.22)

Clinically, contact dermatitis may be indistinguishable from atopic dermatitis, although a detailed history, the sites involved and age of the child often provide clues. It can either be caused by irritants, or allergens in susceptible individuals. It results from prolonged or repetitive contact with a

Advice for children with atopic eczema
• Avoid food and environmental factors known to trigger itching (but arbitrary exclusion of numerous foods from infants' diets is irrational and can lead to malnutrition)
• Avoid extremes of temperature and humidity
• Fingernails should be kept short, to help control scratching
• Clothes should be of smooth cotton and wool should be avoided
• Avoid medicated soap, though a superfatted, simple soap is acceptable
• Bath oils and creams are intended to seal moisture into the skin and should be applied after the child has soaked in the bath for 15 minutes or so
• A pet-free household is advisable given the common development of asthma in atopic children
• Breast-feeding with avoidance of cow's milk protein for the first several months is advisable in subsequent siblings

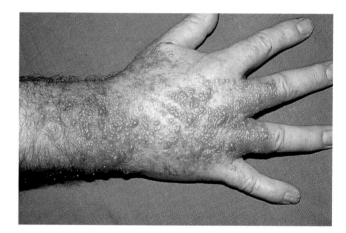

Fig. 5.22 Severe contact dermatitis due to holly.

variety of substances that include saliva, citrus juices, bubble bath, detergents and occlusive synthetic shoes. Topical medications, jewellery and chemicals in manufacture of clothing are all potential allergens.

Clinical features Saliva may cause dermatitis on the face and neckfolds of a drooling child. It also occurs in older children who habitually lick their lips. 'Trainer' or 'sneaker' dermatitis can result from the leaching out of chemicals in the shoe rubber by excessive sweating. Bubble baths can be a cause of severe pruritus.

Management In general, contact dermatitis clears on removal of the irritant or allergen and temporary treatment with a topical corticosteroid preparation.

ATOPIC DERMATITIS AT A GLANCE

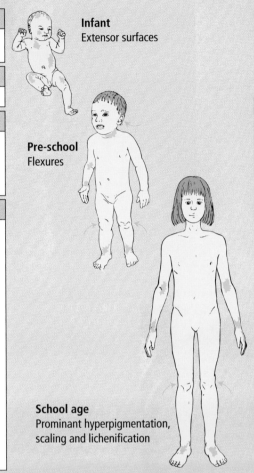

Infant
Extensor surfaces

Pre-school
Flexures

School age
Prominant hyperpigmentation, scaling and lichenification

Epidemiology

Often starts in infancy but clinical picture changes with age

Aetiology

Atopic condition

History

Itchy rash
Often begins at age 2–3 months
Family history of atopy*
Associated allergic rhinitis, asthma*

Physical examination

Infant
Erythematous, weeping, crusting lesions
Sites: patches on cheeks ⟶ rest of face, neck, wrists, hands, extensor surfaces of arms and legs

Preschool
Mild to moderate dermatitis
Sites: popliteal and antecubital fossae, wrists, behind ears, face and neck

School age
More severe, with hyperpigmentation, lichenification, scaling
Sites: popliteal and antecubital fossae, forehead, eyelids, wrists, dorsa of hands and feet

NB *Signs and symptoms are variable

Confirmatory investigations

None
High serum IgE, eosinophilia, RAST antibodies may be found

Differential diagnosis

Scabies
Contact dermatitis
Seborrhoea
Psoriasis

Management

Acute flare-up:
• prevent scratching
• wet dressings
• topical steroids (as least potent as possible)
• antihistamines
• antibiotics for secondary infection (often needed)
Prophylaxis:
• lubricants
• bath oil

Course/prognosis

Fluctuates
Control achieved in most children
Resolves in 50% infants by age 2 years
A few continue to be problematic beyond childhood

Seborrhoeic dermatitis (Fig. 5.23)

Seborrhoeic dermatitis is a chronic inflammatory condition which is commonest during infancy and adolescence. It is often most troublesome in the first year of life.

Clinical features Cradle cap is the commonest manifestation and is seen as diffuse or focal scaling and yellow crusting of the scalp. A dry scaly erythematous dermatitis may also involve the face, neck, axillae and nappy area (see Nappy rash, p. 214) and behind the ears. If the scaling is prominent it may look like psoriasis, and red scaly plaques may appear. Itching may or may not be present.

Management Scalp lesions are usually controlled with anti-seborrhoeic shampoo. Inflamed lesions respond to topical corticosteroid therapy. Secondary bacterial infections and superimposed candidiasis are not uncommon.

Psoriasis (Fig. 5.24)

Psoriasis is a common chronic skin disorder among adults, one third of whom become affected during childhood. Girls are more affected than boys and there is usually a family history.

Clinical features The lesions consist of erythematous papules which coalesce to form plaques of thick silvery or white scales and sharply demarcated borders. They tend to occur on the scalp, knees, elbows, umbilicus and genitalia. Nail involvement, a valuable diagnostic sign, is characterized by pitting of the nail plate. Guttate psoriasis is a variant

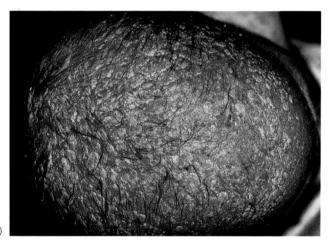

Fig. 5.23 (a) Seborrhoeic dermatitis in a baby. Note the erythematous rash involving the face, neck, chest and nappy area. (b) Severe cradle cap in a baby. There is widespread scaling and crusting of the scalp.

affecting children where multiple small oval or round lesions appear over the body, often following a recent streptococcal infection.

Management Therapy is mainly palliative and should be kept to a minimum. The application of coal tar preparations after a bath is helpful. Salicylic acid ointment is useful in removing scale, but extensive application can result in salicylate poisoning particularly in young children. Topical corticosteroids are effective but must be used with caution.

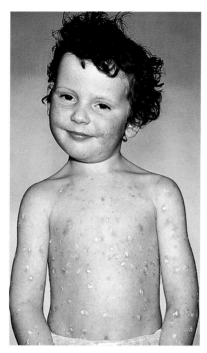

Fig. 5.24 A child with psoriasis showing the characteristic silvery/white plaques over the upper body.

BIRTHMARKS

Common birthmarks

Pigmented naevi (Fig. 5.25)

These naevi are rarely present at birth and start to appear at the age of 2 years. In childhood they are usually flat or only slightly elevated. The risk of malignancy is extremely rare unless they are large congenital naevi.

Café au lait spots (Fig. 5.26)

Café au lait spots are uniformly pigmented, sharply demarcated, macular lesions, which can vary greatly in size. They may be present at birth or develop during childhood. Extensive café au lait spots are a feature of neurofibromatosis (see p. 273).

Strawberry naevus (superficial haemangioma) (Fig. 5.27)

These are bright red, protuberant, compressible, sharply demarcated lesions. Almost all of these lesions, even if large, resolve spontaneously. They may increase in size in the first year of life before fading. Treatment should therefore be

Distinguishing features—Chronic skin conditions

Lesions	**Atopic dermatitis**	**Contact dermatitis**	**Seborrhoeic dermatitis**	**Psoriasis**
Lesions	Erythema, weepiness and crusting leading to dry thickened scaling skin	Erythema and weeping	Dry scaly and erythematous Red plaques may be present	Plaques of thick silvery or white scales with sharp borders
Distribution	See At A Glance Box, p. 205	At sites of contact with the irritant	Face neck, axillae and nappy area	Scalp, knees, elbows and genitalia
Itchiness	+++	+++	+/−	−
Other features	Starts in infancy Family history of atopy		Cradle cap	Nail pitting

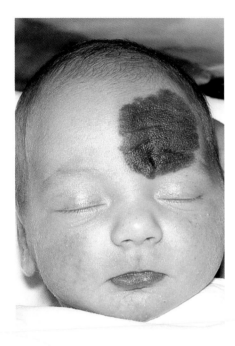

Fig. 5.25 Baby with a large pigmented naevus.

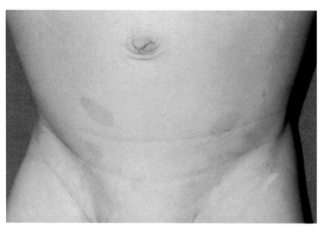

Fig. 5.26 Café au lait spots in a child with neurofibromatosis.

resisted unless the lesion's location interferes with a vital function such as vision.

Naevus flammeus (salmon patch) (Fig. 5.28)

These are small pink flat lesions that occur most commonly on the eyelids, neck and forehead. The lesions on the face usually fade and disappear entirely. They are popularly called storkmarks—signs left by the beak of the stork at delivery!

Mongolian spots (Fig. 5.29)

These are blue or slate grey lesions which occur most commonly in the sacral area. More than 80% of black and Asian babies are born with them. They usually fade during the first few years of life.

Port-wine stain (Fig. 5.30)

Port-wine stains are present at birth. They consist of mature, dilated, dermal capillaries. The lesions are macular, sharply circumscribed, pink to purple in colour and vary in size. If localized to the trigeminal area of the face, the diagnosis of Sturge–Weber syndrome must be considered. In this syndrome there is an underlying meningeal haemangioma and intracranial calcification which can be associated with fits.

DISCRETE SKIN LESIONS

Skin lesions of childhood which occur commonly are shown in Table 5.33.

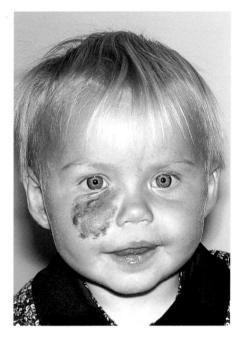

Fig. 5.27 Strawberry naevus on the face of a young child. Note that the naevus is beginning to spontaneously resolve.

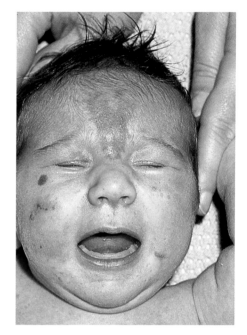

Fig. 5.28 A newborn infant with naevus flammeus (a 'stork mark').

Table 5.33 Common discrete skin lesions

Warts
Impetigo
Molluscum contagiosum
Tinea
Herpes simplex (cold sores)
Birthmarks

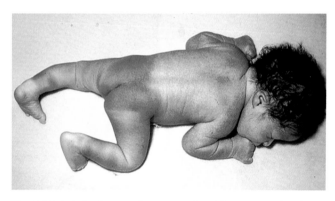

Fig. 5.29 A baby born with a Mongolian blue spot in the classic sacral site and also over the lower legs.

Approach to the child with a discrete skin lesion

Diagnosis of these common lesions demands visual recognition. The student should learn to distinguish them by studying the photographs, and looking for the distinguishing features described at the end of this section.

Common discrete skin lesions

Common warts (Fig. 5.31)

Common warts are harmless and self-limiting. They are transferred by direct contact, but once acquired are spread by autoinoculation.

Clinical features They occur most frequently on the hands, face, knees and elbows, and are well-circumscribed papules with a roughened keratotic, irregular surface. If they are situated on the soles of the feet, they are called verrucas or plantar warts, and are usually flush with the surface of the sole because of the pressure of weight bearing. Plantar warts may be painful.

Management Warts tend to disappear spontaneously within 2 years. No special precautions are indicated for school activities other than swimming, when plantar warts should be covered by a latex sock. If painful, warts can be treated either by the application of a salicylic acid-based wart paint, or frozen using liquid nitrogen.

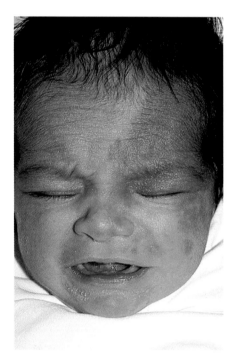

Fig. 5.30 A young baby born with a portwine stain.

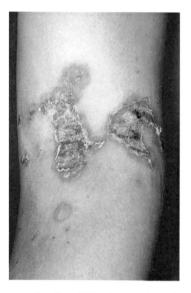

Fig. 5.32 Photograph of a child who has impetigo. Spread has occurred with satellite lesions.

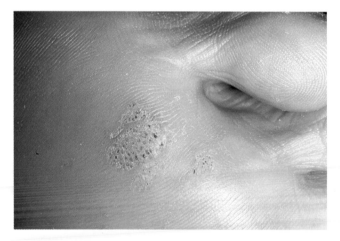

Fig. 5.31 A plantar wart or verruca. Note the roughened irregular keratotic appearance.

Condylomata acuminata

Condylomata acuminata (venereal warts) are moist, fleshy, papillomatous lesions that occur on the perianal mucosa and genitalia. When untreated they proliferate forming large cauliflower-like masses. They can be transmitted with or without sexual contact, and in prepubertal children they suggest sexual abuse. Cervical infections may become latent and are associated with cervical cancer. Condylomata are treated by repeated application of podophyllin in tincture of iodine.

Impetigo (Fig. 5.32)

Impetigo is a skin infection occurring most commonly in children, particularly in the hot humid summer months. The organisms responsible are group A haemolytic streptococci or staphylococci (which commonly also causes a bullous lesion). Infection may spread to other parts of the body by the fingers, clothing and towels. Insect bites, dermatitis and scabies serve as portals of entry for the organism which does not penetrate intact skin.

Clinical features The skin lesions pass rapidly through a vesiculopustular phase, and following rupture sticky, heaped-up, honeycoloured crusts are formed. The sites involved are usually exposed areas.

Management Impetigo can be contagious, and in all cases simple rules of hygiene must be followed to prevent spread. Antibiotic cream is prescribed if the number of lesions are small (fewer than five) and is applied after the crusts have been soaked off with warm water and soap. In more extensive impetigo, oral antibiotics are required, erythromycin being the drug of choice as it covers both streptococcal and staphylococcal infections.

Molluscum contagiosum (Fig. 5.33)

Molluscum contagiosum is a common skin infection caused by a DNA virus. The disease is acquired by direct contact and spread by autoinoculation.

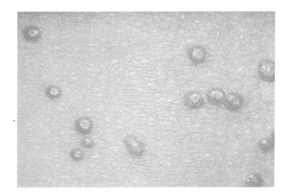

Fig. 5.33 Lesions of molluscum contagiosum. Note the characteristic pearly dome-shaped papules.

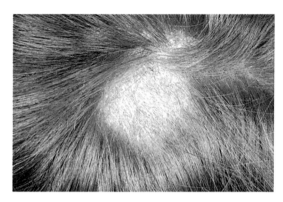

Fig. 5.34 A child with tinea capitis. A circumscribed patch of hair loss is seen with patchy scaling of the scalp.

Clinical features The lesions are discrete, pearly, dome-shaped papules which typically have a central umbilication from which a plug of cheesy material can be expressed. The papules may occur anywhere on the body, but particularly on the face, axillae, neck and thighs.

Management Molluscum contagiosum is a self-limited disease, but can persist for months if not years. Individual lesions can be cleared by pricking the centre with a sharpened stick dipped in liquid phenol. It is important to treat children who also have atopic dermatitis as the infection may spread rapidly.

Ringworm (tinea)

Children can be affected by ringworm which is either anthropophilic (exclusive to humans) or zoophilic (primarily parasites of other animals). Differing organisms cause lesions at different sites.

Tinea capitis

In tinea capitis the child presents with a circumscribed patch of hair loss and patchy scaling of the scalp (Fig. 5.34). Close examination shows the hair to be broken off close to the follicle giving a 'black dot' appearance. It may present as a kerion—a boggy inflammatory mass with local lymphadenopathy. The common form of tinea capitis infection fluoresces brilliant green on Wood's light examination, and can be seen microscopically in a wet mount KOH preparation. Topical therapy alone is ineffective, griseofulvin needs to be taken orally for at least 4 weeks.

Tinea corporis

Tinea corporis can be acquired from infected persons or pets or simply by contact with shed scales or hairs. The typical

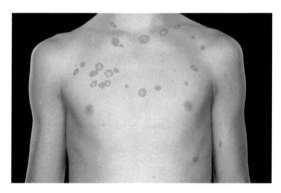

Fig. 5.35 A child with tinea corporis (ring worm) contracted from his pet dog. The typical ring-like patches with central clearing are seen.

lesion (Fig. 5.35) begins as a dry scaly papule which spreads centrifugally, clearing centrally as it does so. The diagnosis can be confirmed by microscopical examination of the scrapings in a KOH wet mount. Lesions usually respond to topical antifungal agents applied for 2–4 weeks, but griseofulvin may be required in extensive cases.

Tinea pedis

Tinea pedis (or athlete's foot) (Fig. 5.36) is uncommon and overdiagnosed in young children, where contact dermatitis is a more likely diagnosis. It does occur with some frequency during adolescence. The interdigital spaces between the toes become macerated, with peeling of the surrounding skin. An odour and severe itching are characteristic. Simple measures such as avoidance of occlusive footwear, drying between the toes and the use of antifungal powder usually suffices for most infections.

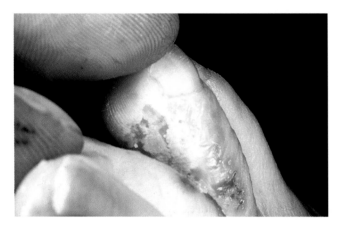

Fig. 5.36 Athlete's foot in a teenage boy. Maceration and peeling are seen in the interdigital space.

Distinguishing features Discrete skin lesions	
Common warts	Roughened keratotic lesions with an irregular surface
Impetigo	Sticky, heaped-up, honey-coloured crusts
Molluscum contagiosum	Pearly, dome-shaped papules, with central umbilicus
Tinea corporis	Dry, scaly papule which spreads centrifugally with central clearing
Cold sore	Single or grouped vesicles/pustules sited periorally

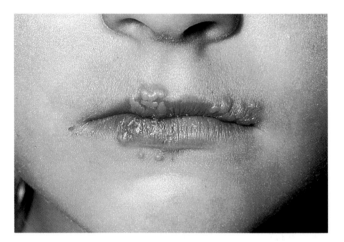

Fig. 5.37 Cold sores caused by herpes simplex infection. The lesions are at the pustular stage prior to crusting.

Cold sore (Fig. 5.37)

Recurrent herpes simplex infections are common as cold sores around the mouth. The virus persists in a latent form after primary infection and appear as single or grouped vesicles periorally. They tend to recur during respiratory tract infections, menstruation and stress. There is minimal therapeutic benefit from the use of topical acyclovir. Children do not need to be excluded from day care or school.

ITCHING

Itching is an unpleasant symptom which, if generalized, is usually associated with a rash. Most of the conditions causing itching (Table 5.34) are covered elsewhere in this chapter.

Table 5.34 Conditions causing itching

Atopic dermatitis (p. 203)
Contact dermatitis (p. 204)
Urticaria (p. 200)
Scabies
Chicken pox (p. 197)
(Seborrhoeic dermatitis)
Head lice
Threadworms

Management of itching

Certain measures can help reduce the discomfort of itching, whatever the cause. Cool baths are soothing, and tight synthetic or woollen clothing should be avoided. It is important to discourage scratching, and finger nails should be kept short and clean to minimize secondary infection. Antihistamines prescribed at night can increase the chances of a more restful night.

Conditions causing itching (not covered elsewhere in this chapter)

Scabies (Fig. 5.38)

Scabies infection is caused by a mite which is transmitted by direct contact.

Clinical features The eruption is intensely pruritic, particularly at night and consists of wheals, papules, vesicles and a superimposed eczematous dermatitis. A characteristic lesion

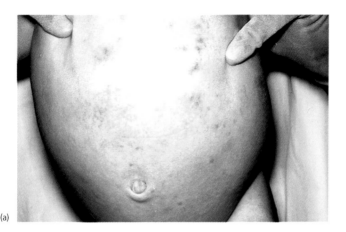

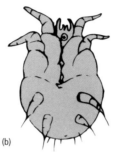

(a)

(b)

Fig. 5.38 (a) Scabies in an infant. (b) The scabies mite.

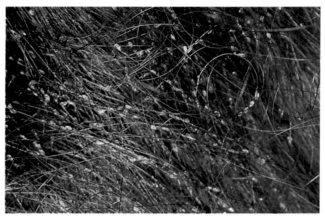

(a)

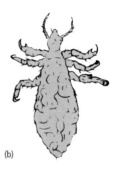

(b)

Fig. 5.39 (a) Nits. (b) A head louse.

occurs which, if seen, is pathognomonic for scabies—the mite burrow appears as a thread-like line commonly seen in the interdigital spaces, but this is often obliterated by scratching. In older children and adults the head, neck, palms and soles are usually spared, but these areas are often affected in babies.

Management The diagnosis is made by microscopic examination of the mites obtained from scrapings. Treatment requires application of scabicides (malathion or permethrin), but these must be used with extreme caution in babies because of their toxic effects. The eczematous reaction and pruritus may persist for some time because of on-going hypersensitivity to dead mites. All the household should be treated and bedding and clothes laundered in hot water.

Head lice (pediculosis capitis) (Fig. 5.39)

Head lice are the only common lice infestation in children. They cause intense itching of the scalp. The lice can be transmitted on infested clothing, combs, brushes or direct human contact. The lice themselves are not always visible, but their eggs (or nits) can be readily identified as white specks adherent to the hair shaft, close to the scalp (Fig 5.39a). The adult louse can be extracted by combing the hair

with a fine tooth comb, particularly if this is carried out after washing with conditioner. Combing in this way provides a good preventative measure. Treatment involves the use of a variety of anti-pediculosis shampoos (e.g. carbaryl). After treatment removal of nits is not necessary to prevent spread.

Threadworms (enterobiasis)

Threadworm infection causes intense itching of the anus and occasionally the vulval area. It is a common infestation particularly affecting preschool children. The threadworms reside in the gut, and the gravid females migrate by night to the perianal region to deposit their eggs. Scratching transmits the eggs to the fingers and the eggs become disseminated and ingested.

Clinical features The infestation may be asymptomatic or may be recognized if a child is seen to be scratching or complains of itching or anal pain.

Management The diagnosis can sometimes be made by examining the anal area during itching, when a tiny (5 mm) white worm may be seen. Alternately the Sellotape test can be applied (Fig. 5.40). Sellotape is applied around the end of a tongue depressor, with the sticky side outermost. This is

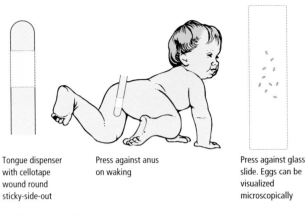

Tongue dispenser with cellotape wound round sticky-side-out

Press against anus on waking

Press against glass slide. Eggs can be visualized microscopically

Fig. 5.40 The Sellotape test for threadworms.

placed against the child's anus on rising in the morning, and then applied to a glass slide. The threadworm eggs can then be visualized microscopically. Examination of stool specimens does not identify threadworms. Treatment consists of a single dose of mebendazole. The whole family may need to be treated. Reinfection is very common.

NAPPY RASH

The nappy area is very prone to rash as it is an area that is warm and moist, usually tightly enclosed in an occlusive waterproof covering, and is in contact with urine, which is an irritant. The common causes of rash are listed in Table 5.35. Mostly the rash is a simple irritative rash, commonly with candidiasis superimposed, but in a prolonged resistant rash, conditions such as seborrhoeic dermatitis and psoriasis should be considered. The baby needs to be examined, paying particular attention to the intertrigenous areas, scalp and mouth.

Ammoniacal (napkin) dermatitis (Fig. 5.41)

Nappy rash can be considered the prototype of irritant contact dermatitis. The rash results as a reaction to overhydration of the skin, friction, maceration, and prolonged contact with urine, faeces, nappy detergents and chemicals. There is some controversy as to whether disposable or cloth nappies are less likely to cause rash.

Clinical features The rash is erythematous, often with papulovesicular or bullous lesions, fissures and erosions. The eruption can be patchy or confluent, but the skinfolds are characteristically spared as they are in less contact with urine than the exposed areas are. Secondary infection with bacteria and yeasts is common.

Table 5.35 Causes of nappy rash

Ammoniacal dermatitis
Candidiasis
Seborrhoeic dermatitis
Psoriasis

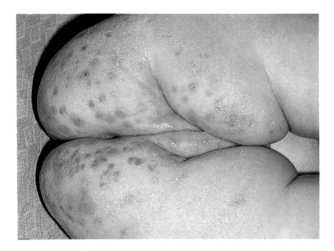

Fig. 5.41 A baby with ammoniacal nappy rash.

Management The rash often responds to simple measures, including regular changing and washing of the genitalia with warm water and mild soap, exposure of the area to air as much as possible, and the application of protective creams such as zinc and castor oil ointment. When these measures do not suffice, limited application of mild hydrocortisone cream can be used. As superimposed candida infection is so common, use of anticandidal agents is also justified.

Candida nappy rash (Fig. 5.42a)

Candida superinfection of other rashes is common. It also commonly follows a course of oral antibiotics as the gut flora is changed so allowing the candida to flourish opportunistically.

Clinical features Candidal dermatitis classically appears as a bright red rash with a sharply demarcated edge and satellite lesions beyond the border. The inguinal folds, in contrast to ammoniacal dermatitis, are usually involved as the warm moist area promotes growth of the yeast.

Thrush (oral candidiasis) may be found on inspection of the mouth. It appears as white 'curds' coating the tongue, gums and buccal mucosa (Fig. 5.42b).

NAPPY RASH AT A GLANCE

Epidemiology

Universal

Aetiology

Prolonged contact with urine, faeces, detergents, chemicals
Candidal superinfection common

Physical examination

Erythema
Patchy or confluent
Sparing of skinfolds (unless candida present too)
Papules, vesicles, bullae, fissures, erosions*
Oral thrush*

NB *Signs and symptoms are variable

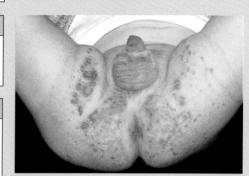

Confirmatory investigations

None

Differential diagnosis

Candida
Seborrhoeic nappy rash
Psoriatic nappy rash

Management

Regular changing and washing area
Exposure to air
Protective creams
Consider use of mild hydrocortisone cream, anticandida creams

---

Management The diagnosis is usually made on clinical grounds, but confirmation can be made on KOH preparation. Treatment consists of application of an anticandidal agent such as nystatin, at each nappy change, until the rash has resolved.

If oral thrush is present oral nystatin suspension should be prescribed.

Seborrhoeic nappy rash (Fig. 5.43)

Seborrhoeic nappy rash is characterized by pink, greasy lesions with a yellow scale. It is most commonly seen in the intertriginous areas. It is commonly associated with seborrhoeic dermatitis of the scalp (cradle cap), face and postauricular areas (see p. 205). The rash usually responds to mild topical corticosteroid cream.

Psoriatic nappy rash (Fig. 5.44)

Psoriasis (p. 205) in the infant can present as a persistent nappy rash, similar to that of seborrhoeic dermatitis. It is worth enquiring into a family history of the condition.

Distinguishing features Nappy rashes

Ammoniacal dermatitis	Erythematous +/− papulovesicular or bullous lesions, fissures and erosions
	Patchy or confluent
	Skinfolds characteristically spared
Candida	Bright red, with sharply demarcated edge and satellite lesions
	Inguinal folds involved
	Oral thrush may be found
Seborrhoeic dermatitis	Pink, greasy lesions with yellow scale
	Often in the skinfolds
	Cradle cap may be found
Psoriatic nappy rash	Like seborrhoeic dermatitis
	Positive family history for psoriasis

viral or reactive causes, but more serious pathology must be excluded.

SWOLLEN JOINTS

Swollen joints from causes other than trauma are not very common in childhood (Table 5.36). These causes include

Approach to the child with swollen joint(s)

In the child with joint swelling, the history and distribution of the joints involved provide clues as to the underlying

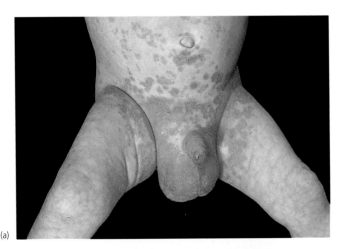

(a)

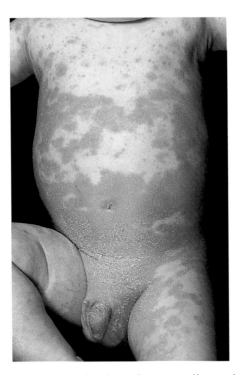

Fig. 5.43 A baby with seborrhoeic dermatitis affecting the nappy area. The lesions are pink and greasy looking. The baby also had severe cradle cap (see Fig. 5.23b).

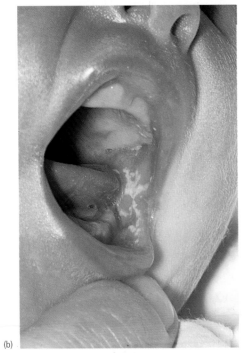

(b)

Fig. 5.42 A baby with candida nappy rash. (a) Note the bright red rash involving the inguinal folds and the satellite lesions. (b) Oral thrush appearing like white curds on the buccal mucosa.

Table 5.36 Causes of swollen, painful joints in childhood

Trauma	
Infection	Septic arthritis, viral
Reactive arthritis	Poststreptococcal or gastrointestinal infections
Vasculitis	Henoch–Schönlein purpura
Collagen vascular disease	Juvenile chronic arthritis, systemic lupus erythematosis
Haematological disease	Leukaemia, haemophilia, sickle cell disease
Gastrointestinal disease	Ulcerative colitis, Crohn's disease
Malignancy	Leukaemia

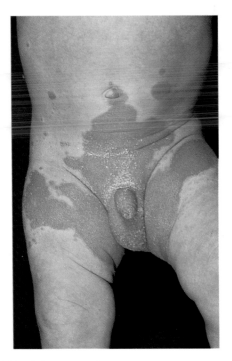

Fig. 5.44 Psoriatic nappy rash.

problem. In a child presenting with an acutely swollen joint, where trauma has not occurred, it is critical that septic arthritis, which demands urgent treatment, is excluded as the diagnosis.

History

- *Joint symptoms*. Stiffness is an important complaint which may be localized or generalized. In most inflammatory arthropathies, the stiffness which occurs in the morning or after periods of inactivity is alleviated by activity, whereas mechanical problems are exacerbated by activity. A history of pain or swelling of other joints is obviously relevant.
- *Systemic symptoms*. Once trauma has been discounted, it must be established whether the child's symptoms are specific to the joint(s) or whether there are clues present such as fever, anorexia, weight loss, rash, weakness and fatigue suggestive of systemic causes.
- *Past medical and family history*. Important information in the past medical and family history includes inflammatory bowel disease, autoimmune conditions, blood dyscrasias and psoriasis, which are all associated with arthritis.

Physical examination

- *Musculoskeletal system*. The musculoskeletal examination should include all four limbs and the spine. The joints affected should be carefully examined by inspection and palpation looking for skin colour changes, heat, tenderness, range of motion and asymmetry. In the young child it is very helpful to observe normal active motion, especially gait, to pinpoint the joints involved.
- *General examination*. Unless there is a clear history of trauma to the joint, the child needs a full physical examination looking for signs such as anaemia, hepatosplenomegaly, cardiac murmurs and rash, which might be associated with systemic disease.

Focal points
Evaluating swollen joints

- Trauma is the commonest cause of an isolated swollen joint
- If the joint is acutely swollen, rule out septic arthritis as the cause
- Clues to the underlying diagnosis are provided by the history and distribution of the joints involved
- Systemic symptoms should be elicited

Investigations

In most children presenting with arthritis or joint swelling investigations are required. These are described in Table 5.37.

Causes of swollen joints in childhood

Trauma

Trauma is a common cause of joint pain and swelling in childhood, and in this case the cause of the swelling is obvious. Two paediatric forms of joint trauma are worthy of particular mention.

Dislocated elbow

Pulled elbow or 'nursemaid's' elbow is a common mishap which occurs in the toddler age group. The child may not complain of pain but refuses to use the arm and holds it in a flexed position. The precipitating cause is sudden forceful traction on the arm, causing dislocation at the elbow. This usually happens when a reluctant child is dragged by the arm, or trips while being held by the hand (Fig. 5.45).

Table 5.37 Useful investigations in the child with swollen joints and their relevance

Full blood count	Elevated white count and shift to the left with bacterial infection Anaemia in collagen vascular diseases, inflammatory bowel disease, malignancy Characteristic features of the haemoglobinopathies
ESR and plasma viscosity	Elevated in bacterial infection, very high in collagen vascular disease and inflammatory bowel disease
Blood culture	Positive in septic arthritis
ASO titre	Indicative of recent streptococcal infection — reactive arthritis or very rarely rheumatic fever
Viral titres	Viral arthritis
Rheumatoid factor and antinuclear antibodies	Negative in most forms of juvenile chronic arthritis
X-ray of the joint	Characteristic depending on the underlying aetiology
Joint aspiration	Microscopy and culture to exclude/confirm septic arthritis. May be helpful in other conditions

The condition is treated by simply supinating the arm fully causing the head of the ulnar to click back into place. No postreduction fixation is necessary. The parents need to be alerted to the cause in order to avoid recurrence.

Growthplate fracture

The other traumatic joint problem peculiar to childhood is fracture of the growthplate. When a child traumatizes a joint, the most vulnerable structure is the growthplate, rather than the ligaments. Children presenting with swelling of a joint following trauma may well have a fracture through the growthplate rather than a ligamentous sprain. The fracture is not easily seen on X-ray. Treatment consists of immobilizing the joint for some weeks.

Septic arthritis

Septic arthritis is a serious cause of joint swelling (see also p. 154) which if untreated rapidly leads to destruction of the joint.

Clinical features The joint is usually hot, swollen and acutely tender, and more than one joint may be involved. Fever may or may not be present. Movement of the affected joint is limited and extremely painful.

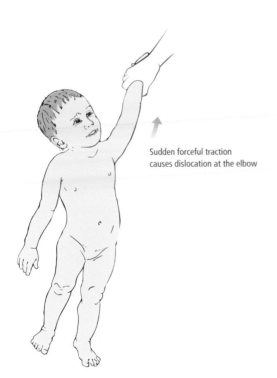

Sudden forceful traction causes dislocation at the elbow

Fig. 5.45 Nursemaid's elbow. Sudden forceful traction dislocates the elbow joint.

Investigations Supportive evidence of bacterial infection may be found in the white cell count and elevated ESR. X-ray of the hip may show widening of the joint space caused by fluid accumulation, and in some cases signs of an adjacent osteomyelitis.

Management If septic arthritis is suspected, aspiration of the joint should be carried out urgently for microscopy and culture. The joint fluid is purulent with organisms found on Gram stain. *Staphylococcus aureus* is the commonest organism and intravenous flucloxacillin the treatment of choice. The joint should be splinted in the acute stage, and mobilization and physiotherapy given during convalescence to prevent joint flexion deformities.

Viral infections

Viral infections, notably rubella, may be associated with an arthritis that can resemble chronic rheumatic disease.

Reactive arthritis

Following infection with streptococcus or bacterial gastroenteritis there may be a sterile arthritis which may affect one or more joints. The arthritis is generally transient and the outcome good.

Vasculitis

Henoch–Schönlein purpura is a diffuse allergic vasculitis characterized by a distinctive rash (p. 199). It is often accompanied by pain in the joints with or without swelling. The joint manifestations resolve fairly rapidly.

Juvenile chronic (rheumatoid) arthritis

Juvenile chronic arthritis (JCA) has three main patterns of presentation—systemic, poly- and pauciarticular arthritis. Each form has distinctive clinical features and differing prognoses. The various features are summarized in Table 5.38.

Systemic juvenile chronic arthritis (Stills' disease)
This is the rarest form of JCA. It often presents as a diagnostic puzzle as there may not be any joint symptoms at the outset. The child looks ill with features of a remitting fever, variable rash, hepatosplenomegaly, anaemia, weight loss or abdominal pain. Joint manifestations may be overlooked in view of the other features. Sepsis and malignancy are often considered in the diagnosis. There are no characteristic laboratory findings, and rheumatoid factor is negative.

Type	Characteristics	Sex ratio	Rhesus factor/ANA*	Iridocyclitis	Severe arthritis
Systemic	Large and small joints affected	M > F	Negative	No	25%
Polyarticular	Large and small joints affected	F > M	RhF neg, ANA may be positive	No	12%
Pauciarticular	<5 joints usually large	F > M	RhF neg, ANA may be positive	High risk	No usually

Table 5.38 Features of juvenile chronic arthritis

* ANA, antinuclear antibody.

Polyarticular juvenile chronic arthritis
Children with polyarticular JCA present with painful swelling and restricted movement of both large and small joints, which is commonly symmetrically distributed. Systemic features are not prominent although poor weight gain and mild anaemia may be found. Morning stiffness is common and young children may be quite irritable. Rheumatoid factor is usually negative, although antinuclear antibodies may be positive. The prognosis is generally good.

Pauciarticular juvenile chronic arthritis (Fig. 5.46)
This condition commonly affects girls under the age of 4 years. By definition pauciarticular arthritis involves few (fewer than five) joints, commonly knees, ankles and elbows. Systemic symptoms are minimal and the appearance of the joints is identical to those in the polyarticular form. Rheumatoid factor is again negative, although antinuclear antibodies may be positive.

The important distinction between the two conditions, apart from the number of joints involved, is the risk of chronic iridocyclitis. In this condition inflammation of the inner structures of the eye may lead to loss of vision and even permanent blindness. The changes are only detectable by slit lamp examination and for this reason regular ophthalmological examinations are necessary.

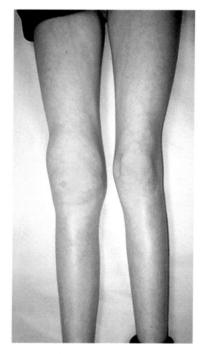

Fig. 5.46 A 10-year-old girl with pauciarticular juvenile chronic arthritis affecting the right knee.

Management

The aims of management are twofold:
• to preserve joint function;
• to help the child to achieve optimal psychosocial adjustment.

The goals of medical treatment are to reduce joint inflammation, maintain function and prevent deformity. Non-steroidal anti-inflammatory drugs are used to suppress the inflammation. Corticosteroids are indicated for severe systemic disease unresponsive to other therapies. Steroid injection into selected joints may be helpful, but should not be used repeatedly. Hydroxychloroquine, penicillamine, gold injections, methotrexate and immune regulatory drugs are used in severe disease.

Physical and occupational therapy are important to improve movement and physical strength, affected joints and to maintain the function of the child as a whole. Treatment consists of daily exercises, hydrotherapy, and day and night splints.

The family needs support and children should be encouraged to lead as normal and self-sufficient lives as possible. Unpredictable exacerbations are disheartening, and families need encouragement to work at maintaining joint mobility. The prognosis in the various subgroups differs, but overall most children have a good prognosis with no or only minor

JUVENILE CHRONIC ARTHRITIS AT A GLANCE

Epidemiology

Three patterns occur: systemic (Still's disease) and pauciarticular in young children; polyarticular in older children

Aetiology

Immune disorder

Clinical features

A. SYSTEMIC JCA:
History
• fever and shaking chills
• malaise
• weight loss
• arthralgia*
Physical examination
• ill child
• high, spiking fever
• hepatosplenomegaly,
Lymphadenopathy
• salmon pink rash*
• arthritis at onset*

B. POLYARTICULAR JCA:
History
• painful swollen joints
• poor weight gain
Physical examination
• swollen, tender large and small joints

C. PAUCIARTICULAR JCA:
History
• painful swollen joints
Physical examination
• < 5 swollen joints (knees, ankles or elbows)

NB *Signs and symptoms are variable

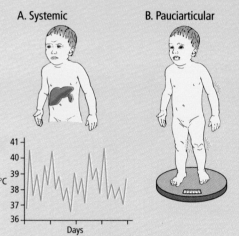

A. Systemic   B. Pauciarticular

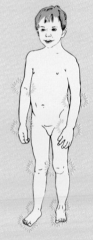

C. Polyarticular

NB Rule out sepsis

Confirmatory investigations

High erythrocyte sedimentation rate
Anaemia with high white cell count
Rheumatoid factor-negative
ANA may be positive in pauci- and polyarticular types
X-ray: soft tissue swelling, periostitis, early-loss of cartilage, bone destruction and fusion

Differential diagnosis

Sepsis and malignancy in systemic type
Other causes of swollen joints in pauci- and polyarticular types
(Table 5.38)

Management

Reduction of inflammation using non-steroidal anti-inflammatory drugs
Steroids for severe disease
Physio- and occupational therapy
Psychosocial support

Prognosis/complications

• Generally good, with eventual resolution of arthritis in most
• 25% of systemic type develop chronic disabling arthritis
• Pauciarticular form at high risk for chronic iridocyclitis

---

disability in adulthood. Children with residual handicaps need help in vocational planning.

Haematological and malignant disease

Leukaemia

Leukaemia and other malignancies occasionally present with pain (which is often severe) and swelling of one or more joints. These diagnoses should be considered when onset is recent, particularly if severe anaemia, thrombocytopenia or other abnormalities of peripheral white blood cells are present.

Haemophilia

A hallmark of haemophilia is haemarthrosis affecting elbows, knees and ankles. The bleeding often seems to be spontaneous. It does not form a diagnostic problem as the child will have presented earlier in life with obvious bleeding. Repeated haemorrhages into a joint can produce degenerative changes and ultimately a fixed unusable joint.

Sickle cell disease

Children with sickle cell disease may have symmetrical, painful swelling of the hands and feet as a result of vaso-occlusive crises. This may be the initial manifestation in infancy. In older patients the large joints too may swell. The diagnosis is indicated by anaemia with characteristic sickle cells on the smear, and a positive sickle test.

Gastrointestinal disease

Both ulcerative colitis and Crohn's disease can be associated with arthritis, with about 10% of children experiencing arthritis at some time. Swellings of the joints follow a pauciarticular pattern and tend to coincide with periods of active bowel disease. The prognosis of the joint condition is good unless the child is HLA B27 positive when ankylosing spondylitis may occur.

PYREXIA OF UNKNOWN ORIGIN

In most children presenting initially with fever and no apparent site of infection, the diagnosis becomes apparent or the fever resolves within a short period of time. Pyrexia of unknown origin (PUO) refers to prolonged fever which is defined as more than 1 week in young children and 2–3 weeks in the adolescent.

The underlying cause in most cases of PUO is infection (Table 5.39). Usually it is an atypical presentation of one of the common illnesses such as UTI or pneumonia, although endocarditis is an important consideration in a child with congenital heart disease. Other significant causes include the collagen vascular diseases, malignancy, and inflammatory bowel disease in the adolescent.

Approach to the child with pyrexia of unknown origin

A thorough history and repeated physical examinations are paticularly important as clues may emerge which can lead to a diagnosis.

History

- *Review of systems.* A thorough review of all organ systems is imperative as symptoms may be elicited which provide a lead to the aetiology.

Table 5.39 Causes of pyrexia of unknown origin

Bacterial infection
Urinary tract infection
Pneumonia
Endocarditis
Occult abscesses (NB dental)
Tuberculosis
Osteomyelitis
Viral infection
Infectious mononucleosis
Hepatitis
HIV infection
Collagen vascular disease
Inflammatory bowel disease
Neoplastic disease
Factitious fever

Focal points
Evaluating pyrexia of unknown origin

- A thorough history and repeated physical examinations are required and may save the child from multiple, unpleasant investigations

- Hospitalization is needed to confirm and observe the pattern of the fever

- The characteristics of the fever may give a clue to diagnosis

- Samples for culture should be taken at the peak of fever

- *Contact with infectious diseases.* Clues may be found on identifying someone in the family or school who is ill.
- *Travel.* A history of travel reaching back to birth should be sought, as re-emergence of disease may occur years after visiting an endemic area.
- *Exposure to animals.* Zoonotic infections can be acquired from pets or wild animals.
- *Genetic origin.* Tuberculosis is still prevalent in Asian communities. Some rare genetic disorders can cause PUO.

Physical examination

An assiduous physical examination, including all organ systems, may lead to diagnostic clues and so save the child from a battery of investigations. The physical examination needs to be repeated to look for the emergence of new signs.

Table 5.40 Investigations and their relevance in pyrexia of unknown origin

Investigation	Relevance
Full blood count	Elevated white cell count and shift to the left in bacterial infection. Very high white cell count in leukaemia
Urinalysis and culture	Occult urinary tract infection
Examination of blood smear	Parasitic infections, e.g. malaria
ESR or plasma viscosity	Elevated in bacterial infection. Highly elevated in collagen vascular disease and malignancy
Blood cultures (aerobic and anaerobic)	Bacterial infection. Repeated samples needed to diagnose endocarditis, osteomyelitis and occult abscesses
Liver function tests	Hepatitis
TB skin test	Tuberculosis
X-rays: chest, bones, sinuses, gastrointestinal tract	Characteristic findings with bacterial infection
Bone marrow aspirate	Leukaemia, metastatic neoplasms, rare infections
Serological tests	Infectious mononucleosis, other infections, rarely helpful in collagen vascular disease
Radioactive scans	Helpful in detecting osteomyelitis and abdominal masses, tumours, abscesses
Echocardiography	In endocarditis vegetations can be seen on the leaflets of heart valves
Ultrasonography	Identification of intra-abdominal abscesses
Total body CT or MRI scanning	Detection of neoplasms and abscesses

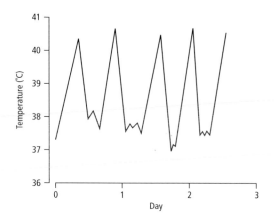

Fig. 5.47 A temperature chart showing swings suggestive of septicaemia.

- *Temperature chart* (Fig. 5.47). Repetitive chills and temperature spikes are common in children with septicaemia from any cause, but particularly suggest an abscess, pyelonephritis or endocarditis. Factitious fever should be suspected if there is an absence of tachycardia and sweating associated with peaks of fever.
- *The mouth and sinuses.* Tenderness to tapping over the sinuses and teeth should be sought and the sinuses transilluminated. The finding of candida in the mouth may be a clue to a disorder of the immune system. Hyperaemia of the pharynx may suggest infectious mononucleosis.
- *Muscles and bones.* The muscles and bones should be palpated. Point tenderness suggests either osteomyelitis or bone marrow invasion from neoplastic disease. Generalized muscle tenderness occurs in collagen vascular disease.
- *Heart.* The finding of a pathological murmur (see p. 81) or a change in character of a murmur should raise concern that infective endocarditis has developed.

Investigations (Table 5.40)

The number of investigations that can and often are performed are legion. Ordering of investigations, beyond those commonly available should be made cautiously. It is important to obtain blood cultures at fever peaks as the yield at that time is much higher. At least three specimens should be obtained. In general, radiological tests should be guided by clues obtained on the clinical evaluation. Ultrasound, CT or MRI can be used to guide aspiration or biopsy of suspicious lesions.

Management

In general, the child should be hospitalized for careful observation as much as for investigation. This may also provide relief of parental anxiety. Antipyretics should not at first be given as they obscure the pattern of fever. Antibiotics should never be used as antipyretics, and empirical trials should in general be avoided, as they are dangerous and can obscure the diagnosis of infections such as endocarditis and osteomyelitis.

It is helpful to know that the child with PUO has a better prognosis than that reported for adults, and that the cause is usually an atypical presentation of a common childhood illness. In many cases no diagnosis is established but the fever abates spontaneously.

Specific causes of pyrexia of unknown origin in childhood

Infective endocarditis

Infective endocarditis occurs as a complication of congenital heart disease. The risk is highest with those lesions that result in a turbulent jet of blood, such as ventricular septal defect, coarctation, patent ductus arteriosus and aortic stenosis.

The commonest organism is *Streptococcus viridans* which may be introduced during dental or other surgery. Because of the risk of endocarditis, prophylactic antibiotics are needed to cover any dental or surgical procedure in a child with congenital heart disease (see p. 338).

Clinical features The child usually presents with fever, malaise and anorexia. Signs include clubbing and splinter haemorrhages in the nails, and splenomegaly. The pre-existing heart murmur may change in character. Microscopic haematuria may be found.

Management The diagnosis is made on blood culture (arterial samples are particularly helpful) which may need to be repeated on several occasions. Echocardiography reveals vegetations on the heart valves. Intravenous antibiotics are required for a period of 6 weeks, with monitoring of serum levels to ensure that bacteriocidal levels are maintained.

Osteomyelitis

Osteomyelitis affects the metaphyses of long bones and is usually haematogenous in origin. The commonest organisms are *Staphylococcus pyogenes*, *Haemophilus influenzae* and *Streptococcus pyogenes*.

Clinical features Although children may present with PUO, more usually the infected limb is obviously painful and held immobile. Swelling and redness eventually appear. The adjacent joint may contain a sterile 'sympathetic' effusion.

Management Repeated blood culture determines the causative organism. X-rays are not of any diagnostic help in the first 10 days as it takes time for the radiological changes of the subperiosteum to develop. Bone scans, however, are useful early in the course of the disease. High dose intravenous antibiotics are required for 6 weeks. If there is no immediate response, surgical exploration and drainage is required. If the infection is inadequately treated, irreversible bone necrosis, draining sinuses and limb deformity can occur.

Collagen vascular disease

The collagen vascular diseases may present with PUO and must be considered as a diagnosis once infection has been excluded. The disease that is most responsible for being a diagnostic puzzle is systemic juvenile chronic arthritis (Still's disease) which often presents as a remitting fever (see p. 217). Unfortunately, serological tests in childhood collagen vascular disease are less helpful than in adults as they are more commonly negative (see p. 218).

Inflammatory bowel disease

Crohn's disease and ulcerative colitis are conditions of adolescence. They may present as PUO, although often a careful history reveals abnormalities in bowel patterns, which have been accepted by the child as being normal.

Neoplastic disease

Leukaemia may present as PUO, but it is less usual for other malignancies to do so.

Factitious fever

Factitious fever usually results from manipulation of the thermometer, by patient (often adolescent) or parent, although rarely may result from inoculation of pyrogenic material. If factitious fever is in any way suspected, temperatures must be documented in hospital by an individual who stays with the patient while the temperature is being taken.

RECURRENT INFECTION

Most children experience recurrent infections. These are commonly respiratory infections, colds and tonsillitis which

OSTEOMYELITIS AT A GLANCE

Aetiology

Infection of the metaphysis (usually bloodborne)
Organisms: *Staphylococcus pyogenes*
Haemophilus influenzae,
Streptococcus pyogenes

History

Fever
Painful limb

Physical examination

Swelling and redness at site
Sympathetic effusion of adjacent joint*

NB *Signs and symptoms are variable

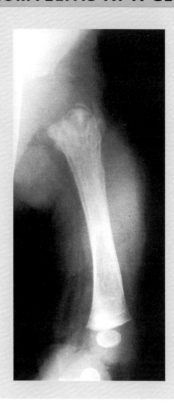

Confirmatory investigations

High white cell count and erythrocyte sedimentation rate
Blood culture (repeat samples needed)
Bone scan to detect early changes
Subperiosteal changes on X-ray seen only after 10 days

Differential diagnosis

Soft tissue infection
Trauma
Malignancy
Septic arthritis

Management

High dose antibiotics for 6 weeks
Surgical exploration and drainage

Prognosis/complications

If inadequately treated may lead to bone necrosis, draining sinuses, limb deformity

---

peak when the child starts school or nursery, or when an older sibling brings infections home. Poor nutrition, poverty, poor housing and inadequate hygeine may be contributing factors. Breast-feeding provides some protection during infancy, at least from otitis media and gastroenteritis.

The common recurrent infections of childhood may cause great parental concern, but should not initiate a diagnostic exploration. However, the child who experiences recurrent serious infections needs to be thoroughly evaluated for the underlying cause (Table 5.41). Details of the investigation of immune deficiency states are beyond the scope of this book.

Causes of serious recurrent infection

HIV infection and AIDS

Paediatric acquired immunodeficiency syndrome (AIDS) is caused by human immunodeficiency virus (HIV) type 1. The two paediatric populations at risk are:
1 infants born to infected mothers;

Table 5.41 Causes of recurrent serious infections

Defective white cell function

Immunoglobulin deficiency
   Congenital deficiency
   HIV

Splenectomy

Chest
   Foreign bodies
   Cystic fibrosis

Urinary tract
   Reflux

Meningitis
   Congenital dermal sinus

2 adolescents who acquire infection sexually or by the intravenous use of drugs.

There is essentially no risk of being infected by casual

contact with an HIV infected child in the family, at nursery or at school. Most children with HIV are diagnosed before the age of 3 years.

Clinical features Infected infants are usually diagnosed because they have features of immunodeficiency, namely failure to thrive, diarrhoea, candidiasis or hepatosplenomegaly, or because they develop severe bacterial infections. Severe life-threatening infections include pneumonia, septicaemia, persistent pulmonary infiltrates, pneumocystis carinii pneumonia (PCP), tuberculosis and systemic candida.

Diagnosis Diagnosis is made by the detection of HIV antibody, which is very specific and sensitive. However, passive maternal transplacental IgG obscures the diagnosis in young infants, as the antibody may still be measurable up to the age of 18 months in uninfected clinically well infants. A positive test prior to this age must not therefore be taken to be diagnostic of infection, particularly in the absence of clinical disease.

Management At present the goals of intervention in HIV infected patients focuses on the use of antiviral drugs, prophylactic antibiotics, viral vaccines and, where necessary, immune serum globulin. The psychosocial and emotional needs of the family must also be addressed.

Prognosis Of babies born to HIV-positive mothers 20–30% become HIV positive themselves. In children with clinical HIV infection the prognosis is very variable, but in general the earlier and more severe the presentation the worse the prognosis.

Prevention The administration of the antiviral drug, zidovudine (AZT), to HIV infected pregnant women, and delivery by Caesarean section reduces the transmission of

HIV INFECTION AND AIDS AT A GLANCE

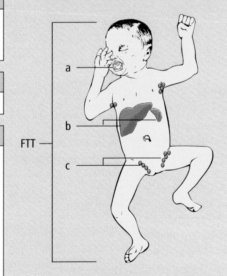

Epidemiology

Infants born to infected mothers *or* adolescents: acquired sexually or by IV drug use

Aetiology

Human immunodeficiency virus type 1

Prevention

Perinatal management:
• zidovudine (AZT) to HIV-positive pregnant women
• delivery by caesarean section
• zidovudine at birth
• avoidance of breast-feeding (Western countries)
Other ages:
• universal precautions for body fluids
• safe sex

History

Severe bacterial infections
Poor weight gain
Diarrhoea*
Loss of developmental milestones*

NB *Signs and symptoms are variable

Physical examination

Failure to thrive (FTT)
Candidiasis (a)
Hepatosplenomegaly (b)
Lymphadenopathy (c)
Chest signs*
Other specific signs relating to organs involved*

FTT

Confirmatory investigations

HIV antibody detection (*but* in infants this may have been passively acquired and is not necessarily a sign of infection)
Immunological testing

Differential diagnosis

Depends on organ systems involved
Other immunodeficiency disorders

Management

Antiviral drugs
Prophylactic antibiotics
Viral vaccine
Immune serum globulin
Psychosocial/emotional support

Prognosis/complications

20–30% babies born to HIV-positive mothers become infected
High risk for pneumonia, septicaemia, persistent pulmonary infiltrates, *Pneumocystis carinii* pneumonia, tuberculosis, systemic candida
Variable prognosis: earlier and more severe presentation have worse prognosis

the virus to infants. The infant at birth should also receive zidovudine for some weeks. In developed countries where the risks of bottle feeding are low, HIV-positive mothers should not breast-feed, as the virus may be transmitted in breast milk. For the adolescent and adult, prevention of HIV includes precautions in coming into contact with bodily fluids and the practice of safe sex, with the use of condoms.

Splenectomy and hyposplenism

Children who lack an effective spleen are at increased risk of sepsis. Hyposplenism may occur as a result of sickle cell disease, splenectomy for trauma and some metabolic and haematological conditions.

Clinical features The major risk of hyposplenism is infection, including an increased risk of overwhelming sepsis or meningitis. This is especially high in children under 5 years old. As the spleen is responsible for filtering the blood and early antibody responses, sepsis can progress rapidly, leading to death within 24 hours.

Treatment and prevention Penicillin reduces the risk of infection in hyposplenic children. Other measures include prompt evaluation and treatment of fevers.

SWELLINGS IN THE NECK

Swellings in the neck may arise from one of four sites: the cervical lymph nodes, the thyroid gland, the parotid glands and the mastoid process (Table 5.42).

Cervical lymph glands

The commonest glands to enlarge in the neck are the anterior cervical nodes which drain the tonsils and pharynx. This may occur with any URTI and, if the child is afebrile and the glands not obviously tender, they are of little significance. Acute enlargement with fever is usually a result of streptococcal infection with the differential diagnosis including infectious mononucleosis. Cytomegalovirus, toxoplasmosis and rubella cause generalized lymphadenopathy. Leukaemia and lymphoma are sometimes accompanied by striking degrees of lymph node enlargement, and other malignant tumours occasionally metastasize to lymph nodes.

Thyroid gland

The finding of a goitre usually indicates autoimmune thyroiditis, although the manifestation of congenital defects (see p. 26) can be delayed and present with goitre in childhood. Thyroid cancer is rare and causes a nodular rather than smooth swelling. Since the iodization of salt, goitre secondary to iodine deficiency no longer exists in Britain.

Parotid glands

The commonest cause of parotid swelling, whether unilateral or bilateral is mumps (p. 227).

The mastoid

Swelling of the mastoid process is included in this discussion although it is not strictly part of the neck. Infection can spread from the adjacent ear, and cause serious morbidity.

Approach to the child with a swelling in the neck

The first aspect of the clinical evaluation is to identify the site of origin of the enlarged gland(s). This can usually be distinguished on clinical examination (Table 5.43, Fig. 5.48).

History and physical examination

The history and physical examination depend on the gland involved. In suspected infection of the lymph glands, parotids and mastoid, enquiry must be made into fever,

Table 5.42 Causes of swellings in the neck

Cervical lymph nodes	Upper respiratory tract infection
	Cervical adenitis
	Infectious mononucleosis
	Neoplastic processes (Table 10.11, p. 341)
Parotid gland	Mumps
Thyroid gland	Thyroiditis
	Congenital hypothyroidism (p. 272)
	(Cancer)
Mastoid	Mastoiditis

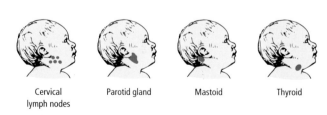

Cervical lymph nodes   Parotid gland   Mastoid   Thyroid

Fig. 5.48 Common swellings in the neck.

Table 5.43 Clinical distinction of enlarged glands in the neck

Cervical lymph nodes	May swell unilaterally or bilaterally along the anterior cervical chain
Parotid glands	Overlie the angle of the jaw. When enlarged they may be distinguished from the cervical lymph glands as they obscure the bony angle of the jaw and displace the ear upward and outward
Thyroid gland	Midline anterior structure overlying the trachea at the level of the thyroid cartilage. Best palpated by standing behind the child with hands encircling the neck (Fig. 5.49). Examination helped by asking the child to drink water—the gland can be seen and felt to move on swallowing
Mastoid process	When enlarged is seen as a tender, inflamed swelling behind the ear which pushes the ear outward

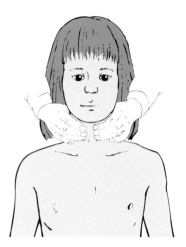

Fig. 5.49 Palpation of the thyroid gland.

Focal points
Evaluating swelling in the neck

• Identify the gland involved

• If the process is thought to be infective, assess how sick the child is, and the state of hydration

• If cervical lymphadenopathy is identified, look for generalized lymphadenopathy and hepatosplenomegaly

• If a goitre is found assess whether the child is hypothyroid, hyperthyroid or euthyroid

• If mastoiditis is found admit the child as a surgical emergency

Table 5.44 Signs of hypo- and hyperthyroidism

Hypothyroidism
Sluggishness
Constipation
Dry skin
Poor growth
Underachievement at school
Bradycardia, hypotension
Delayed tendon reflexes

Hyperthyroidism
Nervousness
Hyperactivity
Increased appetite
Tremor
Increased sweating
Tachycardia and hypertension
Lid lag and retraction

malaise and fluid intake. Physical examination should focus on identifying other sites of infection such as tonsillitis and otitis media, and an assessment of the child's hydration, as fluid intake is likely to be reduced. If cervical lymphadenopathy is identified, it is important to examine the child for generalized lymphadenopathy by examining the axillae, groins, liver and spleen.

If a goitre is found the thyroid status must be clinically assessed as being euthyroid, hypothyroid or hyperthyroid. The signs of hypothyroidism and hyperthyroidism are shown in the Table 5.44.

Investigations (Table 5.45)

In the primary care setting it is usually acceptable to treat cervical adenitis without laboratory confirmation of an organism. If infectious mononucleosis is suspected a full blood count and Epstein–Barr virus screen are advisable. Mumps does not require investigation, but a serum or urine amylase is helpful if it is not clear if the swelling is sited in the parotid or lymph glands. Thyroid function tests and antibodies are indicated in a child with goitre.

Conditions causing swellings in the neck

Cervical adenitis

Cervical adenitis results from infection by the group A beta-haemolytic streptococcus. The child presents as acutely unwell with tender swollen cervical lymph glands, with or without signs of tonsillitis. Bacterial infection is indicated by an elevated white cell count with a shift to the left, and the organism confirmed by positive throat or blood culture. In the primary care setting it is acceptable to pre-

Table 5.45 Investigations which may be indicated for a swelling in the neck

	Investigation	Significance
Cervical lymph nodes	Full blood count	Elevated white cell count and shift to the left in bacterial infection, atypical lymphocytes in infectious mononucleosis
	Epstein–Barr virus screen	Positive in infectious mononucleosis
	Throat culture	Group A haemolytic streptococcal infection needs antibiotics
Parotid glands	Serum or urine amylase	Elevated in mumps, and therefore distinguishes the parotid from the lymph glands
Thyroid gland	Thyroxine thyroid-stimulating hormone	To confirm whether the child is hypo-, hyper- or euthyroid
	Thyroid antibodies	Often positive in thyroiditis
Mastoid process	Tympanocentesis	To identify responsible organism and drain infection

scribe penicillin on a clinical basis without laboratory confirmation.

Infectious mononucleosis (glandular fever)
(see also p. 228)

The Epstein–Barr virus is the cause of this infection. When tonsillitis is prominent the differential diagnosis includes streptococcal infection and diphtheria.

Clinical features Infectious mononucleosis usually presents in the child, as in the adult, with marked cervical lymphadenopathy, fever, sore throat and enlarged purulent tonsils. Generalized lymphadenopathy and splenomegaly are commonly found, and a macular rash occurs in 10–20% of cases, especially if ampicillin is inadvertently given. Hepatitis often occurs with jaundice.

Investigations The diagnosis is supported by the presence of atypical lymphocytes in the blood film which may account for 10–25% of the total white cell count. The test for heterophile antibodies is positive in 60% of cases in the first week of the illness and Epstein–Barr virus IgM is present in the early stages. Liver function tests may be abnormal.

Management and prognosis Infectious mononucleosis is a self-limiting disease. The course of the condition is variable. The throat may be so inflamed as to preclude drinking and if so the young child particularly must be examined repeatedly to ensure that dehydration is not developing. Children often recover from infectious mononucleosis without the prolonged fatigue and depression which characterize adolescent and adult infection.

Mumps

Mumps remains the commonest cause of parotitis despite the introduction of immunization (see p. 53). It is, in general, a mild illness in childhood. The child is contagious until the swelling has resolved.

Clinical features After a long incubation period of 16–21 days, the child presents with fever and malaise, and enlargement of the parotid glands, which may be bilateral or unilateral. The child can usually drink but may experience pain on swallowing particularly sweet or sour liquids. The swelling lasts for 5–10 days.

Management The diagnosis is usually obvious clinically, particularly during an epidemic. However, if in doubt as to whether the swelling is parotid, confirmation can be obtained by measuring serum or urinary amylase which will be raised.

Complications The importance of mumps lies in its complications, principally deafness and meningoencephalitis. The incidence of post-mumps deafness is one in 15 000. The virus attacks the eighth nerve causing sensorineural deafness which is usually severe and unilateral. Meningoencephalitis is very common, but is usually mild and characterized by headache, neck stiffness and photophobia. The cerebrospinal fluid contains an increased number of lymphocytes and raised protein. Orchitis does occur, but very rarely in the prepubertal boy. Mumps has been implicated in the development of diabetes.

Thyroiditis (Fig. 5.50)

Thyroiditis is more common in girls than boys.

Clinical features In thyroiditis the gland is diffusely enlarged, smooth and non-tender, although nodules may occur. The onset is usually insidious, with the goitre noticed as an incidental finding or observation. The child may be

INFECTIOUS MONONUCLEOSIS AT A GLANCE

Aetiology

Epstein–Barr virus

History

Fever (**a**)
Sore throat

Physical examination

Large purulent tonsils (**b**)
Generalized lymphadenopathy,
particularly cervical (**c**)
Splenomegaly (**d**)
Hepatomegaly*
Macular rash*

Confirmatory investigations

Atypical lymphocytes (10–25% of
white cell count) on blood smear
Positive heterophile antibody test in
60%
Epstein–Barr virus IgM-positive early
Abnormal liver function tests

NB *Signs and symptoms are variable

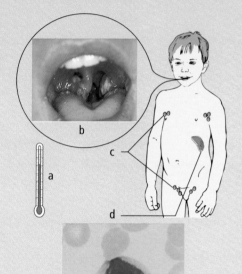

Differential diagnosis

Streptococcal tonsillitis
(Diphtheria now rare)
Leukaemia
Lymphoma
Toxoplasmosis
Cytomegalovirus
Hepatitis

Management

Supportive
Consider steroids if symptoms very
severe

Prognosis/complications

Self-limiting disease
Dehydration may develop in the
young child
Fatigue/depression are rare in children

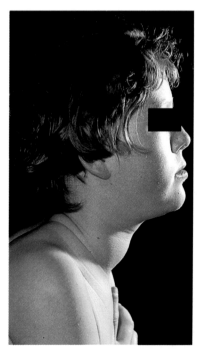

Fig. 5.50 A girl with a goitre due to thyroiditis.

clinically euthyroid or hypothyroid (see Table 5.44), although thyroid overactivity (tremor, palpitations, diarrhoea, sweating) is sometimes seen at the onset. Hypothyroidism is manifested by deceleration of growth with a marked delay in bone age (see p. 58), lethargy, constipation, dry skin and sluggish deep tendon reflexes. Surprisingly, school work does not appear to suffer, although following treatment the child is often transformed from a quiet personality to a spirited child.

Investigations Laboratory investigations show either normal thyroid function tests, or evidence of primary hypothyroidism with a normal or low T4 and elevated thyroid-stimulating hormone (TSH) Antithyroid antibodies (antimicrosomal and antithyroglobulin) may be present.

Management If there is evidence of hypothyroidism, replacement treatment with thyroxine is indicated. The goitre usually shows some decrease in size. Even if untreated all children require follow-up of their thyroid status. If nodules persist despite treatment biopsy should be performed as thyroid cancer can develop.

MUMPS AT A GLANCE

Immunization

Live attenuated virus given at 12–18 months

Aetiology

Mumps virus

History

Fever (a)
Malaise
Neck swelling
Pain on swallowing sweet/sour liquids

Physical examination

Unilateral or bilateral parotid swelling (b)
10% Meningoencephalitis (c)

c ———— Headache/meningitis
b ————
a

Incubation period   Parotid gland swelling

Infectious period

16–21 days   2 4 6 8
Exposure   Day 0 Clinical onset
Time frame for mumps infection

NB • Subclinical meningitis often present (>50% have a CSF pleocytosis)
• Orchitis is rare; only in pubertal boys

Confirmatory investigations

None required
(Serum/urinary amylase raised)

Differential diagnosis

Cervical lymphadenopathy

Management

Supportive

Course

Incubation period 16–21 days
Contagious until swelling subsides

Complications

Sensorineural deafness
Meningoencephalitis
Orchitis rare in prepubertal boy

Mastoiditis

Mastoiditis is now a rare, but serious infection of childhood which demands emergency treatment. The infection usually extends from otitis media, and the responsible bacteria is *Haemophilus influenzae*. Treatment is by surgical drainage and intravenous antibiotics.

OEDEMA

Generalized oedema is an uncommon problem and invariably results from some form of the nephrotic syndrome. It is important to remember that peripheral oedema is not a feature of congestive heart failure in childhood, which is manifested by liver enlargement rather than oedema.

Nephrotic syndrome

The nephrotic syndrome is characterized by proteinuria, hypoproteinaemia, oedema and hyperlipidaemia. The underlying pathology is an increase in glomerular capillary wall permeability, which leads to urinary protein loss, and as a result of hypoalbuminaemia oedema develops. Three histological patterns are seen in nephrotic syndrome, the

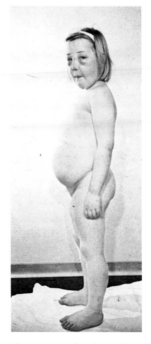

Fig. 5.51 A girl with severe nephrotic syndrome, showing periorbital oedema, gross oedema of the legs and an abdomen distended with ascites.

commonest being 'minimal change', which is seen in 85% of cases.

Clinical features (Fig. 5.51) Nephrotic episodes may follow a viral URTI. Periorbital or pitting oedema of the legs is usually noticed first. With time it becomes more generalized and is associated with weight gain, ascites, pleural effusion and declining urinary output. Symptoms of anorexia, abdominal pain and diarrhoea are common, but hypertension is rare. An increased susceptibility to infection occurs.

Investigations Typical results of investigations are shown in Table 5.46. Renal biopsy is only necessary if the clinical picture does not appear to be typical of minimal change nephrotic syndrome, or if the child does not respond to steroids within a month.

Management It is usual to hospitalize the child for diagnostic, therapeutic and educational purposes. Excessive fluid intake is discouraged and sodium intake is limited to 'no added salt'. Steroid treatment (prednisone) is given to induce remission, which may take 2 weeks to occur. Recovery is monitored by daily weights and proteinuria. Low dose steroids are continued for 4–6 weeks. During steroid treat-

Table 5.46 Typical investigations in nephrotic syndrome

Urinalysis	3+ or 4+ protein +/– microscopic haematuria
Serum albumin	Low
Serum cholesterol and triglycerides	High
C3 levels	Normal

NEPHROTIC SYNDROME AT A GLANCE

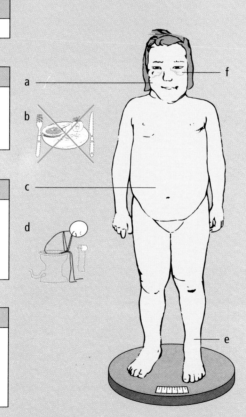

Epidemiology

'Minimal change' form most common

Aetiology

Idiopathic
Increase in glomerular permeability leads to proteinuria, hypoalbuminaemia and oedema

History

Puffiness (a)
Anorexia (b)
Abdominal pain* (c)
Diarrhoea* (d)
Preceding URTI*

Physical examination

Pitting oedema of the legs (e)
Periorbital oedema (f)
Weight gain
Ascites and pleural effusion*
Reduced urine output

NB *Signs and symptoms are variable

Confirmatory investigations

Proteinuria +/– haematuria
Low serum albumin
High cholesterol
High triglycerides
Normal C3
Renal biopsy if presentation atypical or poor response to steroids

Differential diagnosis

Other causes of oedema are extremely rare

Management

Hospitalize, monitor weight and urinary protein loss
Moderate fluid and salt intake
Steroids to induce remission
Low dose steroids for 3–6 months (NB child at risk for severe chicken pox)
Prophylactic penicillin
Cyclophosphamide if steroids ineffective

Prognosis/complications

Relapses are common
Long-term prognosis good for minimal change
Other forms can lead to renal impairment

ment children are at risk if exposed to chicken pox or live vaccine. Prophylactic penicillin is given because of the risk of infection when hypoproteinaemic (antibodies are lost in the urine).

Approximately 75% of children who initially respond to steroids experience a subsequent relapse with proteinuria. Children who frequently relapse or who show signs of steroid toxicity should be treated with cyclophosphamide. A renal biopsy is not necessary unless the child is resistant to steroid treatment.

Prognosis Most children experience relapses over the subsequent 10 years or so, which must be treated in the same way as the initial episode. The long-term prognosis for minimal change nephrotic syndrome is good and residual renal impairment is rare. The prognosis for other forms of nephrotic syndrome is more guarded.

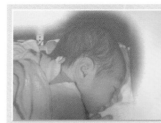

6 The Newborn

Introduction, 232
Resuscitation and asphyxia, 232
The newborn examination, 234
Specific congenital abnormalities, 240
The small baby, 241
Problems of the small baby, 244

Respiratory distress, 246
Specific causes of respiratory distress, 247
Neonatal jaundice, 250
Specific causes of neonatal jaundice, 252
Cyanosis in the neonatal period, 253

Specific causes of cyanosis, 254
Convulsions, 255
Specific causes of neonatal convulsions, 256
Apnoea, 258
Specific causes of apnoea, 258

My mother groan'd, my father wept;
Into the dangerous world I leapt,
Helpless, naked, piping loud,
Like a fiend hid in a cloud.

Struggling in my father's hands,
Striving against my swaddling bands,
Bound and weary, I thought best
To sulk upon my mother's breast.

Blake, 1793

Introduction

Care of the newborn infant is a very important part of paediatrics. Routine examination for occult, but treatable, abnormalities must be undertaken in all newborn infants to prevent long-term disability. Intensive care of the sick preterm and ill full-term infant has significantly improved mortality and morbidity.

Improvement in care of the newborn over recent years can be monitored by observing changes in perinatal and neonatal mortality rates (see below for definitions). The perinatal mortality rate has halved in Britain over the last 20 years and is now approximately eight per 1000 live births.

The improvement in perinatal mortality rates (which includes stillbirths) is largely a result of improvements in obstetric care. Reduction in neonatal mortality rate (now below five per 1000 liveborn infants) has been mainly a result of more effective management of congenital abnormalities by safer surgical techniques and improvements in supporting premature infants with lung disease.

This chapter is arranged in the sequence most appropriate to the way newborn babies present to paediatricians. Only a minority of babies require resuscitation, but for those who do, this must be undertaken immediately after birth and in an efficient and safe manner. All babies should be seen and examined by a doctor in the first 24 hours of life to detect occult congenital abnormalities. Medical students should become familiar with the newborn examination and undertake at least five such examinations on their own. The common congenital abnormalities described in this section must be known. Only 7% of babies are born premature, but these constitute the vast majority of the time that paediatricians spend caring for the newborn. The small baby and his or her problems are the final and major section of this chapter.

Definitions and terminology

It is important to know the definitions of a number of widely used terms in perinatal statistics shown in Table 6.1.

Resuscitation and asphyxia

Resuscitation

Rapid and effective resuscitation must be available for every newborn baby wherever birth takes place. The need for resuscitation can be anticipated in many cases. Table 6.2 lists risk factors predisposing to the need for resuscitation. However, despite careful fetal surveillance in labour, babies may be born in poor condition and unexpectedly require resuscitation.

The infant's condition after birth can be described by the Apgar score (Table 6.3). This records five features, each of which can be scored as either 0, 1 or 2 points. The baby can obtain a maximum of 10 points or a minimum of 0 (no signs of life).

A normal score at 1 minute is 7–10, a score of 4–6 at 1 minute represents a moderately depressed baby and an Apgar score of 0–3 at 1 minute indicates severe depression.

Babies who require active resuscitation at birth can be divided broadly into one of two groups on the basis of their appearance.
• *Primary apnoea.* In this group the babies are blue as a

Table 6.1 Definitions used in perinatal statistics

Term	Definition
Full-term	An infant born between 37 and 42 weeks of gestation
Preterm	An infant born before 37 completed weeks of gestation
Post-term (postmature)	An infant born after 42 completed weeks of gestation
Low birthweight	This is an old fashioned term which has little value in modern terminology. It refers to infants whose birthweight is 2500 g or less. This term makes no distinction between prematurity and intrauterine growth retardation as the cause for the baby being of low birthweight (see below)
Very low birthweight	A baby born with a birthweight of 1500 g or less
Extremely low birthweight	A baby born with a birthweight of 1000 g or less
Small for gestational age	A baby of birthweight below the 10th centile for the duration of gestation
Stillborn infant	A baby who shows no signs of life (including no heart beat) after delivery. Stillbirth is a term used only if the infant is of 24 weeks of gestation or above
Perinatal mortality rate	The number of stillbirths and neonatal deaths in the first week of life per 1000 liveborn and stillborn infants
Neonatal mortality rate	The number of deaths of liveborn infants in the first 28 days of life per 1000 liveborn infants
Infant mortality rate	The number of deaths of all liveborn infants in the first year of life per 1000 liveborn infants

Table 6.2 High-risk situations where a paediatrician needs to be present at delivery

Prematurity
Fetal distress
Thick meconium staining of the amniotic fluid
Emergency caesarean section
Vacuum, mid or high forceps delivery
Abnormal fetus
Multiple birth
Prolonged rupture of the membranes

Table 6.3 The Apgar score

Sign	0	1	2
Heart rate	Absent	<100/min	>100/min
Respiratory rate	Absent	Weak cry	Strong cry
Muscle tone	Limp	Some flexion	Good flexion
Reflex irritability (suctioning pharynx)	No response	Some motion	Cry
Colour	White	Blue periphery	Pink all over

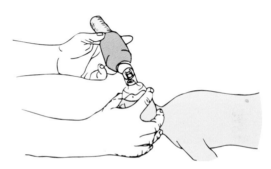

Fig. 6.1 Bag and mask resuscitation.

result of failure to establish spontaneous respiration, but their cardiovascular system is intact with good circulation. This corresponds to an Apgar score at 1 minute of 4–6.
• *Secondary apnoea.* These babies appear white at birth as a result of failure of the circulation as well as of respiration. Without vigorous resuscitation these babies will die. This group corresponds to a 1 minute Apgar score of 0–3.

Resuscitation of the baby with moderate depression (Apgar 4–6)

The baby will require respiratory assistance. The following measures should be undertaken:
• Suction of the infant's airway.
• Mask applied over the baby's mouth and nose and air or oxygen given to inflate the lungs. This is carried out by squeezing a self-inflating bag attached to the mask (Fig. 6.1).

• If the baby fails to respond, intubation with intermittent positive pressure ventilation is necessary.
• Administration of naloxone (a specific opiate antagonist) if the mother has received opiates for pain relief in the 4 hours prior to delivery.

Resuscitation of the baby with severe depression (Apgar 0–3)

The baby with severe depression requires both respiratory and cardiovascular support. The priorities in the emergency treatment can be summarized as the following.
• *Airway.* First establish an adequate airway by tracheal intubation.
• *Breathing.* Next give intermittent positive pressure ventilation.
• *Circulation.* Give external cardiac massage to ensure cardiac output.

Further methods to support the circulation of a severely depressed baby include:
• Sodium bicarbonate to correct metabolic acidosis.
• Adrenaline given down the endotracheal tube if poor cardiac output persists.

Asphyxia

Physiologically asphyxia is caused by tissue hypoxia with the production of lactic acid and carbon dioxide. This results in tissue acidosis. The healthy fetus can withstand asphyxia for some time, but eventually physiological compensatory mechanisms become exhausted and the fetus decompensates with potential irreversible injury to a number of organ systems, most importantly the brain.

Diagnosis

There is no generally accepted clinical definition of asphyxia. The following are commonly used:
• cord blood acidosis with pH <7.05;
• severe depression of Apgar scores (0–5 at 10 minutes);
• delay in establishing spontaneous respiration (>10 minutes);
• hypoxic–ischaemic encephalopathy (a sequence of abnormal neurological signs including convulsions lasting for more than 2 days).

Management

Rapid and effective resuscitation must be available wherever babies are born. Measures are taken to avoid cerebral oedema and to treat ensuing convulsions.

Prognosis

Death and severe handicap occur in approximately 25% of all severely asphyxiated full-term infants. There is no treatment that has been shown to improve outcome.

Principles of management
Resuscitation and asphyxia

• Rapid and effective resuscitation

• Circulatory support if the baby is hypotensive

• Ventilatory support if the baby fails to establish adequate spontaneous respiration

• Fluid restriction to prevent cerebral oedema

• Anticonvulsants to treat severe convulsions

The newborn examination

Every newborn baby should be carefully examined in the first 24 hours of life. The newborn is closely inspected by his or her mother and many congenital abnormalities will be detected by her and brought to medical attention. It is the purpose of the physician's examination to detect occult abnormalities not obvious to the mother or where the significance of the apparently minor deviation from normal is unrecognized.

Technique of neonatal examination

The reason for the neonatal examination must be explained to the parents and they should be present during the examination if at all possible. The baby should be fully undressed in a warm room prior to examination.

History

Ask the mother whether the baby is feeding well and if she has any worries about the baby.

Observation

• *Respiratory rate.* Respiratory rate should be counted. A rate above 60 breaths per minute (tachypnoea) may be abnormal, but is normal after a feed or if the baby has been crying.
• *Colour.* Central cyanosis (involving the tongue) is always abnormal and if present the baby must be rapidly investigated (see p. 253). Jaundice in the first 24 hours is always abnormal and suggests haemolytic disease (see p. 253).
• *Spontaneous movements.* Normally full-term babies have frequent smooth movements. They are often reciprocal so that when a leg extends the other flexes.
• *Jitteriness.* This refers to spontaneous movements which are stimulus independent and jitteriness is not necessarily abnormal, but hypocalcaemia and hypoglycaemia should be excluded as a cause.
• *Irritability* Irritability is a stimulus-sensitive phenomenon and is always abnormal, suggesting a neurological problem.

Measurement

Careful measurement of head circumference, length and birthweight must be made and recorded in the notes. These measurements are plotted onto centile charts to ensure that the baby has grown symmetrically.

Accurate measurements of occipitofrontal head circumference and length in the newborn are not easy to make and require some training. These techniques are discussed in Chapter 2, p. 17.

Physical examination

The physical examination must be systematic so that nothing is omitted. It is traditional to start at the head and work down to the toes. Particular attention should be paid to the following potentially treatable abnormalities which, if missed, may cause irreversible damage to the baby. Figure 6.2 summarizes the main features of the newborn examination.

Cataracts

The earliest detection and treatment of cataracts is essential for normal visual development. Examination of cataracts is an important part of the newborn examination and is described in detail on p. 47.

Cleft palate and lip (Fig. 6.3)

The most reliable method to detect a cleft palate is for the examiner to insert his or her *clean* little finger into the baby's mouth with the soft part of the finger palpating the palate. A cleft of the palate is easily felt and this method may also detect the rare submucous cleft with a bony defect but intact mucosa.

Aetiology Cleft lip, a distressing congenital abnormality in view of the cosmetic implications, occurs in one in 1000 children and tends to recur in families although there is no autosomal inheritance. Cleft palate is seen in association with a cleft lip in 70% of cases.

Clinical implications The parents of children with cleft palate must be seen as soon after birth as possible and the nature of the condition discussed with them. Cleft palate is associated with the problems listed in Table 6.4.

Management The cosmetic appearance is excellent following plastic surgery and photographs of treated cases are particularly helpful in allaying parents' anxieties (see Fig. 6.3). Surgical correction is usually undertaken at about 9 months of age. The parents may need specialized advice to ensure effective feeding. It is important to involve speech therapists, an orthodontic and plastic surgeon and to arrange regular audiology assessment to prevent sequelae of the disorder.

Syndromes and dysmorphic features

A **dysmorphic feature** is a variation from normal and is often subtle. Many normal people have at least one or two dysmorphic features, but the more that such features coexist, the more likely that a recognizable dysmorphic syndrome is present. A **syndrome** is a consistent pattern of dysmorphic features which is usually recognized to be of genetic origin. The commonest syndrome recognizable in the neonatal period is Down's syndrome (p. 270).

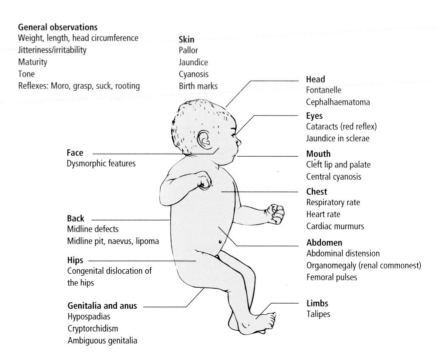

General observations
Weight, length, head circumference
Jitteriness/irritability
Maturity
Tone
Reflexes: Moro, grasp, suck, rooting

Skin
Pallor
Jaundice
Cyanosis
Birth marks

Head
Fontanelle
Cephalhaematoma

Eyes
Cataracts (red reflex)
Jaundice in sclerae

Face
Dysmorphic features

Mouth
Cleft lip and palate
Central cyanosis

Chest
Respiratory rate
Heart rate
Cardiac murmurs

Back
Midline defects
Midline pit, naevus, lipoma

Hips
Congenital dislocation of the hips

Abdomen
Abdominal distension
Organomegaly (renal commonest)
Femoral pulses

Genitalia and anus
Hypospadias
Cryptorchidism
Ambiguous genitalia

Limbs
Talipes

Fig. 6.2 Main features of newborn examination.

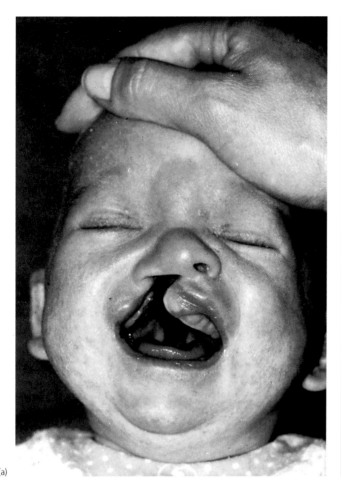
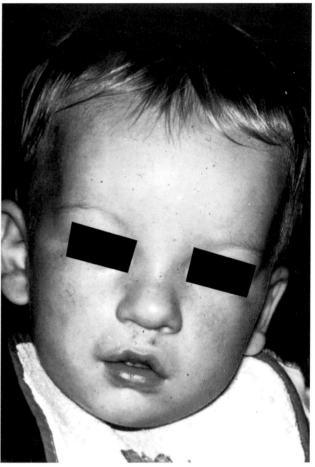

(a)   (b)

Fig. 6.3 (a) Photograph of baby with cleft lip and (b) the same baby after plastic surgical repair.

Table 6.4 Problems to be anticipated in babies with cleft palate

Difficulties in establishing milk feeding
Milk aspiration
Speech difficulties caused by nasal escape
Conductive hearing loss as a result of eustachian tube dysfunction
Dental problems as a result of gingival margin maldevelopment

Cardiac murmur

Cardiac murmurs are commonly heard in the neonatal period and are usually innocent. In contrast, some very severe cardiac anomalies may not be associated with a murmur at the 24 hour examination. The following features suggest that a murmur is more likely to indicate cardiac pathology:
• diastolic or gallop murmur;
• an active praecordium;

• the presence of cyanosis or breathlessness;
• absence of femoral pulses (see below).

Femoral pulses and coarctation of the aorta

The femoral pulse should be palpated at the groin. Absence of a femoral pulse suggests severe coarctation of the aorta. Less severe coarctation which leads to hypertension in later life is not associated with absent pulses at the neonatal examination.

Coarctation of the aorta refers to the severe narrowing usually at the site of the ductus arteriosus with the resulting impairment in the arterial blood flow to the lower half of the body. Babies who have a severe coarctation can only perfuse the majority of the systemic circulation by blood from the pulmonary artery flowing through the patent ductus arteriosus (Fig. 6.4). Closure of the ductus precipitates a low output state and a severe deterioration. Intravenous prostaglandin

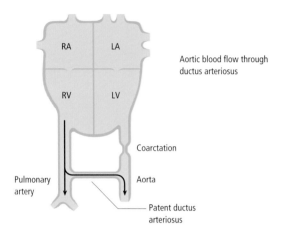

Fig. 6.4 Blood flow in coarctation of aorta.

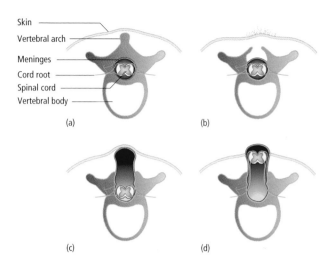

Fig. 6.5 Varieties of neural tube disorders: (a) normal; (b) spina bifida occulta; (c) meningocoele with intact cord; (d) meningo-myelocoele.

- loss or asymmetry of the Moro reflex;
- feeding problems.

Neural tube defects (spina bifida)

Spina bifida is a very important cause of severe disability and is a result of the failure of the neural tube to close normally in early pregnancy. The introduction of periconceptual folic acid supplementation has reduced the incidence of spina bifida lesions by 75%. Routine screening of almost all women in early pregnancy by either ultrasound or alpha fetoprotein with selective termination of pregnancy has made open spina bifida a rare condition.

Various degrees of severity of neural tube disorder exist and are illustrated in Fig. 6.5.

- *Anencephaly.* This is the most severe form of neural tube disorder where there is complete failure of the development of the cranial part of the neural tube and the brain does not develop.
- *Myelomeningocoele.* This refers to an open lesion with the malformed and exposed spinal cord (myelocoele) being covered by a thin membrane of meninges (meningocoele). This is associated with severe neurological abnormality of the lower limbs, bladder and anal innervation together with hydrocephalus. Surviving children have major disabilities requiring life-long supervision.
- *Meningocoele.* In this condition the spinal cord is intact and functions normally, but the defect involves an exposed bag of meningeal membranes which ruptures easily. Meningitis and hydrocephalus are a major risk in these cases. Rapid surgical closure is necessary to avoid infection.
- *Spina bifida occulta.* This refers to a 'hidden' abnormality of the developing neural tube which, if unrecognized and untreated, may later cause serious neurological disability.

will reopen the ductus and this is a life-saving treatment until surgery can be organized. The diagnosis is confirmed by cardiac ultrasound scan or cardiac catheterization. Surgical correction carries a good prognosis.

Abdominal distension

A distended abdomen suggests bowel obstruction. Bile-stained vomiting must always be rapidly investigated as it is often the first sign of obstruction. The causes of bowel obstruction are discussed at the end of this section (p. 240).

Organomegaly is detected by careful abdominal examination. Enlargement of a single kidney as a result of pyelou-reteric junction obstruction is the most common cause of a mass in the abdomen. Hepatosplenomegaly is not a common finding in the newborn infant. The causes of organomegaly are discussed at the end of this section (p. 241).

Umbilical hernias

Umbilical hernias are not seen until the umbilical cord separates and the cord stump heals. It is particularly common in low birthweight infants and in black infants. It appears as a soft swelling that protrudes during crying, coughing or straining and is usually easily reducible. Strangulation is very rare and most disappear spontaneously by 1 year of age.

Abnormal neurological behaviour

Abnormal findings on neurological examination are rarely specific for particular forms of central nervous system pathology. The main features suggestive of serious neurological abnormality are the following:

- hypotonia (floppiness) or hypertonia (stiffness);
- irritability;

The first three conditions are very obvious at birth and the mother will draw them immediately to medical attention. Spina bifida occulta may be missed on cursory examination and have very severe implications.

Spina bifida occulta

Spina bifida occulta (SBO) may be the only visible feature of tethering of the spinal cord within the spinal canal with eventual stretching of the cord. This is associated with the development of bladder dysfunction and pyramidal tract signs in the lower limbs as the child grows. Spina bifida occulta is suggested by a subtle abnormality of the midline over the spine. In particular these include:
- a deep pit over the lower back;
- a tuft of hair;
- a naevus;
- a fatty tumour (lipoma) at or near the midline.

Ultrasound is the best investigative technique to exclude tethering of the spinal cord and all babies with the possibility of SBO should be referred for scanning.

Hypospadias (Fig. 6.6)

Hypospadias is a condition where the urethra is abnormally sited. It occurs in approximately one in 500 boys. The meatus may be sited anywhere from the ventral aspect of the

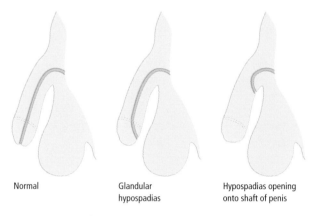

Normal

Glandular hypospadias

Hypospadias opening onto shaft of penis

Fig. 6.6 Hypospadias.

NEURAL TUBE DEFECTS (SPINA BIFIDA) AT A GLANCE

Epidemiology

Now rare as a result of antenatal screening and folic acid supplementation preconceptually

Aetiology/pathophysiology

Failure of neural tube closure early in pregnancy. The defects range from anencephaly to spina bifida occulta (Fig. 6.5), with complications related to the severity of the lesion

Clinical features

Open midline lesion with malformed and exposed spinal cord and meninges
Variable paralysis and sensory loss of legs
In spina bifida occulta a pit, hair tuft, naevus or lipoma may be found in the midline of the back (**a**)

Confirmatory investigations

Ultrasound can detect significant spina bifida occulta

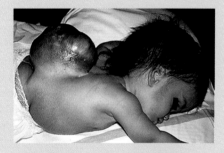

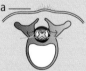

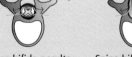

a

Spina bifida occulta

Spina bifida with meningomyelocele

Complications

(Vary according to severity of lesion)
Neurogenic bladder
Neurogenic bowel
Hydrocephalus (in 90% with meningomyelocoele)
Scoliosis

Management

Immediate surgical closure
Mobility:
Physiotherapy to prevent joint contractures
Walking aids
Bladder and bowel:
Intermittent urinary catheterization to allow regular, complete emptying of the bladder
Prophylactic antibiotics for UTI
Regular toiletting, laxatives, suppositories
Hydrocephalus:
Ventriculoperitoneal shunt
Skin care:
Avoidance of ulceration due to sensory loss

Prognosis

If the defect is severe there is likely to be significant physical and some intellectual impairment

glans penis (the commonest type) to the penoscrotal junction or even the perineum. With increasing degrees of severity the penis is curved ventrally (chordee).

Severe cases require repair to allow the boy to void standing, to allow future sexual function and to avoid the psychological consequences of malformed genitalia. Management is surgical reconstruction before the age of 2 years. Severe cases require reconstruction using the foreskin and the parents must be given strict instructions not to have the child circumcised.

Undescended testicles (see p. 87)

The testes are present in the scrotum in 95% of full-term male infants. Most undescended testicles enter the scrotum during the first year of life with no treatment.

Ambiguous genitalia

Babies are rarely born with ambiguous genitalia and indeterminate sex. This should be considered to be a medical emergency as it may be associated with major electrolyte imbalance. A decision should be made as soon as possible as to which sex the baby should be raised. This depends as much on the surgical possibility of producing a functional penis as the genetic sex. The diagnostic approach to the baby with ambiguous genitalia is beyond the scope of this book.

Congenital dislocation of the hip

Congenital dislocation of the hip (CDH) is diagnosed at birth and occurs in 0.2% of neonates. Factors associated with increased risk of CDH are shown in Table 6.5. Routine examination of the hips at birth will detect babies in whom the hips are either dislocated or dislocatable and both these abnormalities require early treatment to prevent permanent maldevelopment of the hip joints with severe impairment in walking. The hips are also routinely checked at 6 weeks and 6–9 months (p. 47).

Examination of the hips should be left to the end as it usually causes the baby to cry. There are three components of hip examination.

Table 6.5 Factors associated with increased risk of congenital dislocation of the hip

Family history
Breech delivery increases risk 10-fold
Female sex
Neurological defects associated with impaired lower limb movement, e.g. spina bifida

1 *Observation.* Is there any asymmetry of gluteal folds around the buttocks? Is there any difference in leg length or posture?

2 *The Ortolani test* (Fig. 6.7). This is a test to see whether the hip is already dislocated. The baby is examined on his or her back with the knees flexed. The infant's thigh is grasped with the examiner's middle finger on the greater trochanter and the thumb on the lesser trochanter and the hip is gently abducted. If the hip is dislocated the examiner will be unable to abduct the hip. The Ortolani test attempts to relocate the already dislocated hip by lifting the thigh upwards and gently abducting it to bring the hip from its dislocated position back into the acetabulum. This is associated with a 'clunk' as the head of the femur is relocated in the acetabulum.

3 *The Barlow test* (Fig. 6.8). This test detects the hip that is in joint but is dislocatable because of underdevelopment of the acetabulum. The baby is placed in the same position as for the Ortolani test and the baby's thigh is grasped by the examiner's hands in a similar manner. The hip is placed in an adducted position and the aim of the test is to use downward and lateral force via the examiner's thumb to attempt to dislocate the hip posteriorly. Dislocation is palpable as the femoral head slips over the posterior lip of the acetabulum.

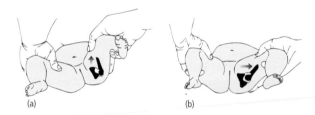

(a)   (b)

Fig. 6.7 The Ortolani test.

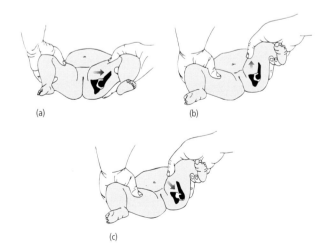

(a)   (b)

(c)

Fig. 6.8 The Barlow test.

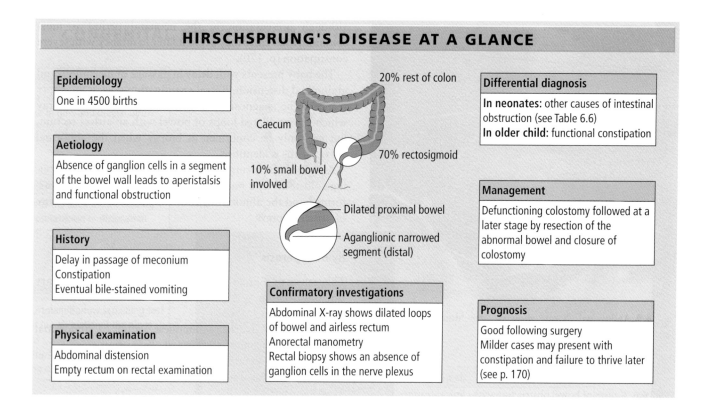

HIRSCHSPRUNG'S DISEASE AT A GLANCE

Epidemiology

One in 4500 births

Aetiology

Absence of ganglion cells in a segment of the bowel wall leads to aperistalsis and functional obstruction

History

Delay in passage of meconium
Constipation
Eventual bile-stained vomiting

Physical examination

Abdominal distension
Empty rectum on rectal examination

20% rest of colon

Caecum

10% small bowel involved

70% rectosigmoid

Dilated proximal bowel

Aganglionic narrowed segment (distal)

Confirmatory investigations

Abdominal X-ray shows dilated loops of bowel and airless rectum
Anorectal manometry
Rectal biopsy shows an absence of ganglion cells in the nerve plexus

Differential diagnosis

In neonates: other causes of intestinal obstruction (see Table 6.6)
In older child: functional constipation

Management

Defunctioning colostomy followed at a later stage by resection of the abnormal bowel and closure of colostomy

Prognosis

Good following surgery
Milder cases may present with constipation and failure to thrive later (see p. 170)

As the causes, management and prognosis of these conditions are different it is important to determine into which of these three categories any small baby falls.

Prematurity

A premature baby is one whose gestation falls short of 37 completed weeks. Approximately 7% of all babies are premature and 1% of births are severely premature with birthweight <1500 g (very low birthweight).

Assessment of gestation

Gestational age is determined by the following techniques.
• Calculation of gestational age from the maternal last menstrual period.
• Assessment of fetal maturity from early antenatal ultrasound scans.
• Assessment of neonatal maturity by clinical assessment of gestation after birth. This is based on observation of both external physical criteria and neurological criteria. External criteria include skin development, nipple and genitalia appearance and ear form. Neurological criteria include posture, neck and limb tone and joint mobility.

Disorders of prematurity

Table 6.7 lists the conditions most likely to occur in premature infants. It is generally the case that the more severe the prematurity, the more likely it will be that these complications will occur and the more severe they are likely to be.

Intrauterine growth retardation

Impaired fetal growth will cause the baby to be born smaller than expected for the duration of gestation. These babies are referred to as being 'small for gestational age' (SGA). In order to make the diagnosis of an SGA baby it is necessary to make a careful assessment of gestational age and to plot the baby's weight on a centile chart to determine whether the baby's weight is below the 10th centile for the gestational age. SGA infants can be described as symmetrically or asymmetrically small.

Symmetrical growth retardation

A symmetrically small infant is one whose weight, head circumference and length all fall below the 10th centile in the

PREMATURITY AT A GLANCE

Definition

Birth at less than 37 weeks gestation

Epidemiology

7% of births are premature
1% are severely premature

Clinical features

Thin, transparent skin
Immature nipples, genitalia and ear-shape
Hypotonic posture with limbs in extension
Increased joint mobility

Management

Maintain environmental temperature
Non-oral feeding if too immature or sick
Management of complications as indicated

Related to immature organs

Complications

- Hypothermia
- **Metabolic:** hypoglycaemia, hypocalcaemia, jaundice (**f**)
- **Respiratory:** respiratory distress (**e**) syndrome, apnoea and bradycardia
- Feeding problems (**g**)
- Intracranial haemorrhage (**a**)
- Infection
- Retinopathy of prematurity (**b**)
- Patent ductus arteriosus (**c**)
- Necrotizing enterocolitis (**d**)

Prognosis

Excellent if born beyond 32 weeks gestation
Premature babies are now viable from 24 weeks gestation
Babies weighing less than 1500 g are at risk for neurodevelopmental problems; 5–10% have serious disability

Table 6.7 Relative risk of various forms of pathology in premature babies and those who suffered intrauterine growth retardation (IUGR)

	Prematurity	Intrauterine growth retardation
Hypothermia	++	+++
Hypoglycaemia	++	+++
Jaundice	++	
Infection	++	+
Respiratory distress syndrome	+++	Reduced risk
Necrotizing enterocolitis	++	++
Retinopathy of prematurity	+++	−
Intracranial haemorrhage	+++	−
Feeding difficulties	+++	−

same proportion (Fig. 6.10). It is possible that a symmetrically small baby is simply a normal baby whose measurements happens to fall below the 10th centile: by definition, 10% of normal babies will have weight and other measurements below the 10th centile. The further the measurements are below the 10th centile, the more likely it is that the baby has a pathological reason for being small. The baby who is symmetrically growth retarded suggests that an insult causing impaired growth of both body and head occurred early in gestation. The commonest cause for this is infection in early pregnancy. Other causes for symmetrical intrauterine growth retardation (IUGR) are shown in Table 6.8.

Prenatal infection
Prenatal infection occurs as the result of a number of organisms. These are usually described by the acronym TORCH infection:

Toxoplasma
Other (syphilis)
Rubella
Cytomegalovirus
Herpes.

Toxoplasma, syphilis and rubella are now very rare in Britain as causes of significant illness in the newborn. Cytomegalovirus is much more common, but rarely causes severe disabling sequelae. Babies present in the neonatal period with hepatosplenomegaly, purpura (caused by thrombocytopenia) and conjugated hyperbilirubinaemia.

of necrotizing enterocolitis and gastric feeding may be contraindicated. Growth retarded and asphyxiated premature infants may also be at additional risk because of impaired blood flow to the bowel prior to delivery. These babies may benefit from delayed onset of milk-feeding.

Infection

Both premature and growth retarded newborn infants have impairment of their immune function and are more prone to infection than full-term and appropriately grown infants. Great attention must be paid to avoidance of cross infection and broad spectrum antibiotics used if infection is suspected (see p. 258).

Necrotizing enterocolitis

This is a rare complication of newborn infants. It is caused by impaired blood flow through the bowel which predisposes the mucosa to invasion by enteric organisms.

Clinical features The babies present with acute deterioration, apnoea, abdominal distension and bloody diarrhoea. In 20% of cases bowel perforation occurs followed by signs of peritonitis.

The diagnosis is confirmed on abdominal X-ray when gas produced by the invading organisms can be seen in the bowel.

Management This is initially expectant. Enteral feeds are stopped for at least 10 days and broad spectrum antibiotics started. If bowel perforation has occurred, laparotomy is indicated.

Prognosis Most babies make a full recovery but 10% later develop bowel stricture in the area of necrotizing enterocolitis involvement.

Retinopathy of prematurity

This is a common condition of very premature infants. It occurs in 50% of babies with birthweight <1500g, but resolves spontaneously in the vast majority of cases. In Britain retinopathy of prematurity (ROP) causes blindness in 1% of severely immature infants.

The cause of ROP is incompletely understood, but oxygen toxicity is a factor although in premature infants probably not a major factor. The retina becomes ischaemic and if this is severe, fibrosis and eventually retinal detachment occur with resulting blindness.

Clinical features Developing ROP can only be recognized by regular ophthalmoscopy.

Management and prognosis Retinal detachment can be avoided by cryotherapy to the back of the eye if the condition appears to be rapidly progressive. Most babies require no treatment and the prognosis is good.

RESPIRATORY DISTRESS

Respiratory disease is a very common symptom in premature infants and requires careful assessment in all cases in order to determine the diagnosis and whether specific treatment is required. Respiratory distress occurs in approximately 5% of full-term infants and in over 50% of very low birthweight infants.

Aetiology

The commoner causes are listed in Table 6.9. In prematurely born infants respiratory distress syndrome is the most common diagnosis although infection must be considered in all infants because if treatment is delayed the baby may die very rapidly of overwhelming infection. The commonest surgical cause is diaphragmatic hernia (p. 250).

Clinical evaluation

The clinical features of respiratory distress include the following:
- tachypnoea;
- recession (subcostal, intercostal, sternal);
- cyanosis;
- expiratory grunting.

Chest X-ray is the best method to distinguish between the various causes and to make a definitive diagnosis. Respiratory distress syndrome has a characteristic radiological appearance (Fig. 6.11) and an X-ray will distinguish it from a number of other common causes.

Management

Management depends on the diagnosis, but there are general principles of management of the baby with respiratory distress. These include:

Table 6.9 Commoner causes of acute respiratory distress in premature infants

Respiratory distress syndrome
Pneumonia (congenital or acquired)
Pneumothorax
Surgical conditions (diaphragmatic hernia)
Cardiac causes

• *Monitoring vital signs.* Babies with respiratory distress are potentially if not actually very ill. Early deterioration may be detected by monitoring respiratory rate, heart rate and blood pressure. Maintenance of normal blood pressure is particularly important in avoiding cerebral complications.

• *Monitoring blood gases.* This is essential in all infants with respiratory distress. It is only possible to determine what the appropriate oxygen concentration is for an individual baby by measuring the partial pressure of oxygen in arterial blood (Pa_{O_2}) and titrating the inspired oxygen to maintain the arterial oxygen concentration in the normal range. The decision as to whether a baby requires respiratory support is determined by the blood pH and by the partial pressure of carbon dioxide in arterial blood (Pa_{CO_2}).

• *Respiratory support.* Babies with deteriorating lung disease, particularly those who are very small and weak, require respiratory support. This takes the form of either continuous positive airway pressure (CPAP) or intermittent positive pressure ventilation (IPPV).

• *Treat infection.* The possibility of infection must always be considered. Blood cultures and antibiotics are given until the cultures are known to be negative.

Specific causes of respiratory distress

Respiratory distress syndrome

Respiratory distress syndrome (RDS) has in the past been referred to as hyaline membrane disease (HMD), a condition recognized on histological examination. The condition is caused by surfactant deficiency in the immature lung. It is the commonest cause of death in premature infants and disability as a result of complications of the respiratory disease in the infants who survive the condition.

NEONATAL RESPIRATORY DISTRESS AT A GLANCE

Epidemiology

50% premature infants
5% full-term infants

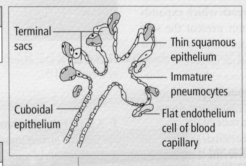

Terminal sacs
Cuboidal epithelium
Thin squamous epithelium
Immature pneumocytes
Flat endothelium cell of blood capillary

Confirmatory investigations

Chest X-ray
Infection screen
Blood gases

Aetiology

• Respiratory distress syndrome (surfactant deficiency) in premature infants (**a**)
• Pneumonia (**b**)
• Pneumothorax (**c**)
• Diaphragmatic hernia (**d**)
• Cardiac causes (**e**)
• Meconium aspiration

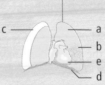

Management

Monitor vital signs
Titrate inspired O_2 concentration against arterial O_2
Surfactant in respiratory distress syndrome
CPAP and/or IPPV for respiratory failure
Antibiotics for infection
Monitor function of other organ systems

Clinical features

• Tachypnoea
• Recession (intercostal, subcostal, sternal)
• Cyanosis
• Expiratory grunting

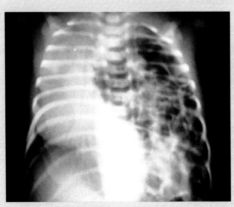

Diaphragmatic hernia

Prognosis

Depends on underlying causes and infant's maturity

NEONATAL JAUNDICE AT A GLANCE

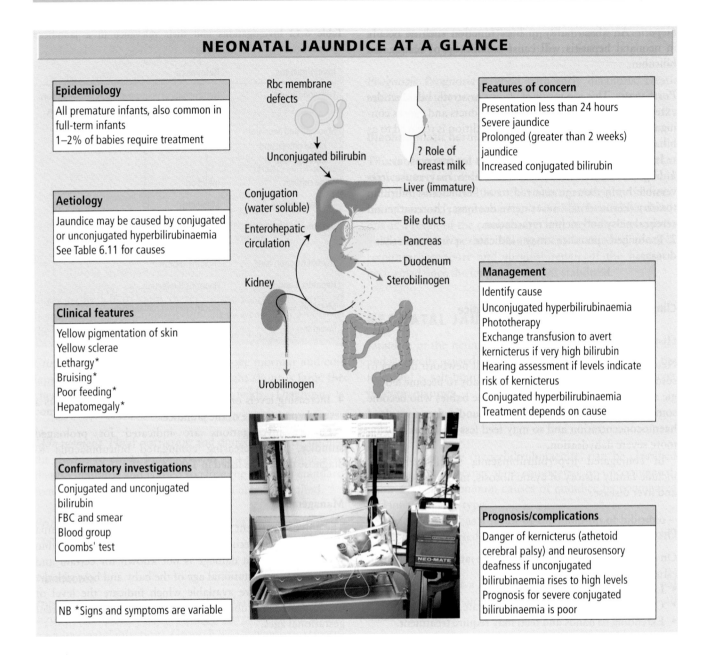

Epidemiology

All premature infants, also common in full-term infants
1–2% of babies require treatment

Aetiology

Jaundice may be caused by conjugated or unconjugated hyperbilirubinaemia
See Table 6.11 for causes

Clinical features

Yellow pigmentation of skin
Yellow sclerae
Lethargy*
Bruising*
Poor feeding*
Hepatomegaly*

Confirmatory investigations

Conjugated and unconjugated bilirubin
FBC and smear
Blood group
Coombs' test

NB *Signs and symptoms are variable

Rbc membrane defects

Unconjugated bilirubin

? Role of breast milk

Conjugation (water soluble)

Enterohepatic circulation

Kidney

Liver (immature)

Bile ducts

Pancreas

Duodenum

Sterobilinogen

Urobilinogen

Features of concern

Presentation less than 24 hours
Severe jaundice
Prolonged (greater than 2 weeks) jaundice
Increased conjugated bilirubin

Management

Identify cause
Unconjugated hyperbilirubinaemia
Phototherapy
Exchange transfusion to avert kernicterus if very high bilirubin
Hearing assessment if levels indicate risk of kernicterus
Conjugated hyperbilirubinaemia
Treatment depends on cause

Prognosis/complications

Danger of kernicterus (athetoid cerebral palsy) and neurosensory deafness if unconjugated bilirubinaemia rises to high levels
Prognosis for severe conjugated bilirubinaemia is poor

unconjugated bilirubin to non-toxic soluble compounds and these are excreted in the urine. If levels continue to rise to a potentially toxic level a series of exchange transfusions are necessary.

The management of conjugated hyperbilirubinaemia depends on the underlying cause.

Specific causes of neonatal jaundice

Jaundice of prematurity

All premature infants become visibly jaundiced in the few days after birth. This is caused by immaturity of the liver and failure of the hepatocytes to conjugate the bilirubin adequately.

Clinical features The babies are well. Jaundice of prematurity never reaches levels high enough to consider an exchange transfusion. The diagnosis is made by excluding other conditions.

Management This is a self-limiting condition. Moderately high levels of bilirubin may require phototherapy, but no other treatment is necessary.

Haemolytic disease of the newborn

Haemolysis occurs in the fetus as a result of maternal anti-bodies reacting with antigen on the fetal red blood cell. The two commonest reasons for this are rhesus incompatibility and ABO blood group incompatibility.

In rhesus disease the mother is rhesus negative and the fetus rhesus positive. The mother has been sensitized to rhesus positive cells in earlier pregnancies when fetal cells cross into the maternal circulation. This causes the mother to develop anti-rhesus antibodies which cross the placenta and cause haemolysis of fetal red blood cells. This tends to be worse in successive pregnancies.

In ABO blood group incompatibility the mother is most commonly blood group O and the baby is blood group A. The mother's natural anti-A antibodies react with the fetal cells causing haemolysis and jaundice. This condition cannot be detected antenatally.

Clinical features Fetal haemolysis causes the fetus to be anaemic initially and if untreated, severe oedema (hydrops) occurs. At birth the severely affected baby is very oe-dematous and anaemic with rapid development of jaundice. Less severely affected infants show anaemia at birth with development of jaundice in the first 24 hours after birth. Babies with rhesus disease are more likely to develop RDS.

Management The aim of management is to deliver the baby before severe haemolysis has occurred and then undertake a series of exchange transfusions to wash out the antibodies as well as the toxic bilirubin. Rhesus-negative women are now immunized with anti-D antibody and consequently rhesus haemolytic disease is now very rare.

The treatment of infants with ABO incompatibility is similar and is aimed at preventing dangerously high levels of unconjugated hyperbilirubinaemia.

Late anaemia (6–8 weeks after birth) is common in haemolytic conditions and the baby may require a top-up blood transfusion.

Prognosis If kernicterus is avoided the prognosis is excel-lent. Sensorineural hearing impairment may be the only sign of bilirubin toxicity.

Breast-milk jaundice

This is a benign condition and requires no treatment. It is generally diagnosed by excluding other more serious condi-tions. In this condition the baby is being breast-fed, develops mild to moderate hyperbilirubinaemia in the second week of life and remains well. Breast-feeding should continue with appropriate reassurance for the parents.

Systemic infection

Neonatal jaundice caused by infection occurs as a result of prenatal infection acquired in early pregnancy (p. 243) or bacterial infection in the neonatal period (most commonly affecting the urinary tract). This condition is discussed fully on p. 258.

Neonatal hepatitis

This is a rare condition. It is usually caused by either a virus (hepatitis B, cytomegalovirus), cystic fibrosis or a metabolic cause. There is no specific treatment.

An avoidable cause of morbidity from hepatitis B is when the baby contracts the infection from the mother. The baby is most at risk if the mother contracts hepatitis B in the last trimester of pregnancy. The baby should be immunized immediately after birth with hepatitis B vaccine and again at 6 months as well as receiving hepatitis immunoglobulin at birth and again at 3 and 6 months of age.

Biliary atresia

Biliary atresia is an important but rare condition and is caused by atresia of intrahepatic or extrahepatic bile ducts. The babies present with increasing conjugated hyperbiliru-binaemia from 4 weeks of life. If undiagnosed, there is rapid progression to liver failure and death, but if the diagnosis is made within 3 months of birth, surgery may restore liver function to near normal.

CYANOSIS IN THE NEONATAL PERIOD

Peripheral cyanosis involving hands and feet is very common in the neonatal period and is referred to as acrocyanosis. This is of no clinical significance providing the baby has no central cyanosis (tongue involvement). Central cyanosis is always significant and indicates respiratory or cardiac disease. It must be rapidly investigated.

Aetiology

The major causes of cyanosis are listed in Table 6.13.

The commonest cardiac cause of cyanosis presenting in the neonatal period is transposition of the great vessels. This is a surgically remediable condition with a good prognosis. Cardiac failure rarely presents in the neonatal period other than in premature infants with patent ductus arteriosus (p. 249). They are not cyanosed.

Fallot's tetralogy (p. 255), the commonest cause of cyan-otic heart disease in childhood, rarely presents with cyanosis in the neonatal period.

Table 6.13 Causes of cyanosis in the neonatal period and associated features on clinical evaluation

Causes of cyanosis	Features on clinical evaluation
Cardiac	
Transposition of the great vessels	Murmur
	Characteristic chest X-ray
	Echocardiogram
Other congenital cardiac lesions with right to left shunt	Murmur
	Echocardiography
	Chest X-ray may be diagnostic
Respiratory	
Respiratory distress syndrome	Signs of respiratory distress
	Characteristic chest X-ray
Other causes of respiratory distress (see Table 6.9)	Chest X-ray
	Blood cultures

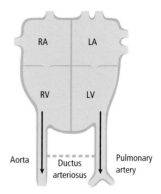

Fig. 6.13 Transposition of the great vessels.

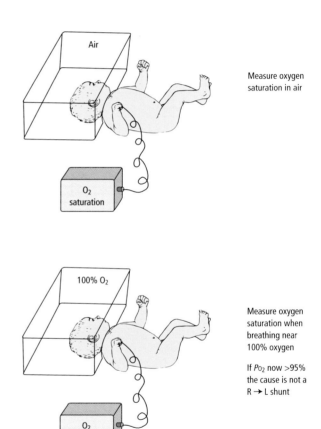

Measure oxygen saturation in air

Measure oxygen saturation when breathing near 100% oxygen

If Po_2 now >95% the cause is not a R → L shunt

Fig. 6.14 The nitrogen washout test.

Clinical evaluation

Cyanosis caused by respiratory disease can be differentiated in most cases from that caused by cardiac disease by the presence of respiratory distress which suggests the presence of lung disease. Occasionally babies (particularly those born prematurely) may have both respiratory and cardiac disease.

The helpful clinical distinguishing features between cardiac and lung disease are shown in Table 6.13.

A nitrogen wash-out test is sometimes used to determine whether the baby has cyanotic heart disease or lung disease where diagnosis is difficult (Fig. 6.14). This involves monitoring oxygen saturation while the baby is breathing oxygen as close to 100% as possible. If the oxygen saturation exceeds 95% there cannot be a significant right to left shunt.

Investigations of a child with suspected cyanotic heart disease include chest X-ray, electrocardiogram (ECG) and echocardiography which should define the structural anatomy.

Management

The management of cyanotic lesions depends on the underlying diagnosis. Oxygen, CPAP and mechanical ventilation (p. 247) may be of considerable benefit for respiratory disease, but is usually of little benefit in cardiac disease. Prostaglandin infusion to maintain the ductus arteriosus open may be life-saving in infants with a duct dependent cyanotic cardiac lesion.

Specific causes of cyanosis

Transposition of the great vessels (Fig. 6.13)

This is the commonest cause of congenital cyanotic heart disease presenting in the neonatal period. In transposition of

CYANOSIS IN THE NEWBORN PERIOD AT A GLANCE

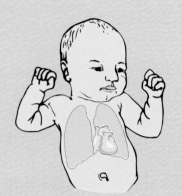

Epidemiology

Cyanosis due to respiratory disease is common; due to cardiac disease is rare. See Table 6.13 for causes

Clinical features

Cyanosis of the lips and tongue (distinguish from acrocyanosis)
Respiratory distress if cyanosis is respiratory
Heart murmur if cyanosis is cardiac*

NB *Signs and symptoms are variable

Confirmatory investigations

Blood gases — low arterial O_2
Nitrogen washout to distinguish cardiac from respiratory disease
Chest X-rays
ECG and echocardiography if cardiac cyanosis is suspected

Management

Oxygen, CPAP and ventilation for respiratory cyanosis
Investigate cardiac disease
Cardiac surgery usually required for cyanotic heart disease

Prognosis

Good for most respiratory causes and operable cardiac lesion

---

the great vessels, the aorta arises from the right ventricular outflow tract and the pulmonary artery from the left ventricle. Mixing of venous and arterial blood occurs through the ductus arteriosus and often through a septal defect which may accompany this condition. The less mixing of blood occurs between the two circulations, the more intensely cyanosed the baby appears.

Clinical features The condition is diagnosed by X-ray (a narrow cardiac pedicle) and by echocardiography.

Management Surgery offers the opportunity of cure by switching the origins of the pulmonary artery and aorta. Emergency treatment of a severely cyanosed child with poor systemic circulation is by an infusion of prostaglandin to maintain the ductus.

Fallot's tetralogy (Fig. 6.15)

This refers to a cardiac anomaly involving four characteristic features:
1 ventricular septal defect;
2 overriding of the aorta;
3 infundibular pulmonary stenosis;
4 right ventricular hypertrophy.
This condition, unusual in the newborn, presents with cyanosis at about 3 months of age. The treatment is surgical and the prognosis is good.

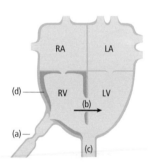

Fig. 6.15 Fallot's tetralogy. (a) Pulmonary stenosis. (b) Ventricular septal defect with shunt. (c) Over-riding aorta. (d) Right ventricular hypertrophy.

Respiratory causes of cyanosis

These are discussed in detail on p. 246.

CONVULSIONS

Neonatal convulsions are very common and occur in 0.5–1.0% of all babies. It is sometimes very difficult to interpret whether unusual movements in premature infants are convulsive in nature. Jitteriness is not a sign of cerebral dysfunction and is described on p. 234. Neonatal convulsions are usually clonic and fragmentary, often involving different limbs for a short time. Less commonly, neonatal convulsions may be tonic or myoclonic.

Aetiology

The causes of neonatal convulsions are listed in Table 6.14. Idiopathic epilepsy (p. 331) does not occur in the neonatal period.

Clinical approach to the child with convulsions

History

A careful maternal and perinatal history is required in all cases. Particular attention should be paid to maternal illness (diabetes predisposes the baby to hypoglycaemia), evidence of fetal distress, symptoms of neurological abnormality prior to the convulsion (feeding problems, irritability, stiffness) and whether there is a family history of neonatal convulsions.

Physical examination

- *Extensive bruising*. This is suggestive of birth trauma.
- *Dysmorphic features*. These are suggestive of an underlying brain anomaly.
- *Intrauterine growth retardation*. If the baby is SGA this increases the risk of hypoglycaemia and hypocalcaemia.
- *Hepatosplenomegaly and purpura*. These suggest prenatal infection (TORCH).

Investigations

The investigations listed in Table 6.15 should be undertaken in all neonates with convulsions. These include:
- metabolic tests;
- infection;
- brain imaging.

Management

Management should be directed towards treating the under-

Table 6.14 Commoner causes of neonatal convulsions

Asphyxia
Hypoglycaemia
Hypocalcaemia
Meningitis
Congenital brain anomalies
Intracranial haemorrhage
Unknown (idiopathic)

lying cause of the convulsions (meningitis, hypoglycaemia, etc.) as well as therapy to prevent further convulsions if a specific cause cannot be found.

Phenobarbitone is the first line anticonvulsant used in the neonatal period.

Prognosis

The prognosis depends on the underlying cause for the convulsions. A very poor prognosis is likely if a major congenital brain anomaly is detected and there is a 50% chance of poor outcome if the fits are caused by meningitis, asphyxia or major intracranial haemorrhage.

Specific causes of neonatal convulsions

Neonatal meningitis

Meningitis occurring in the neonatal period is sufficiently different from meningitis in older children to be considered separately. The incidence of neonatal meningitis is 1 in 4000 babies.

The neonate is relatively immunocompromised by immaturity which predisposes to meningitis. Any organism may cause neonatal meningitis, but the most common are group B beta-haemolytic streptococci and *Escherichia coli*.

Table 6.15 Investigations and their significance in neonates with convulsions

Investigations	Significance
Full blood count	Abnormal white cell count suggestive of infection
Blood cultures	Infection
Lumbar puncture	Meningitis
Blood glucose	Hypoglycaemia
Serum calcium	Hypocalcaemia
Ultrasound brain imaging	Intracranial haemorrhage Periventricular leukomalacia Congenital anomaly
Metabolic screen	Inborn error of metabolism

Neonatal meningitis

- There are often no specific signs of neonatal meningitis
- Cyanosis and apnoea are common early signs of meningitis
- Irritability indicates the need for lumbar puncture

Clinical features The neonate does not develop specific symptoms of meningitis such as a stiff neck and the signs of infection are often very non-specific. This is why meningitis must be considered in any baby with unexpected deterioration. Signs include cyanotic and apnoeic spells, unstable temperature, irritability and convulsions. Lumbar puncture is essential in any neonate with unexplained deterioration to confirm or exclude the diagnosis.

Management Treatment is directed towards the causal organisms. Broad spectrum antibiotics should be given prior to isolation of the infecting bacterium.

Prognosis This depends on how quickly the diagnosis is made and appropriate antibiotic treatment started. In general, prognosis is not good. Approximately 25% of babies die and a further 25% become severely handicapped. Hydrocephalus is a common complication after neonatal meningitis.

Intracranial haemorrhage

Intracranial haemorrhage is very common in premature newborn infants. In particular, intraventricular haemorrhage (IVH) occurs in up to 40% of very low birthweight infants. Intracranial haemorrhage develops in the floor of the lateral ventricle and usually ruptures into the lateral ventricle. In only 25% of cases does further rupture occur into the periventricular white matter. This form of parenchymal haemorrhage is the most severe and if the child survives there is a high risk of cerebral palsy (p. 277).

Periventricular leukomalacia (PVL) is caused by cerebral ischaemia and frequently occurs in babies with IVH. It is less common than IVH, but PVL is the commonest cause of cerebral palsy in surviving premature infants. Poor outcome is particularly likely if the baby develops cystic PVL.

Clinical features Many babies who develop IVH show no symptoms, but convulsions are not uncommon in babies

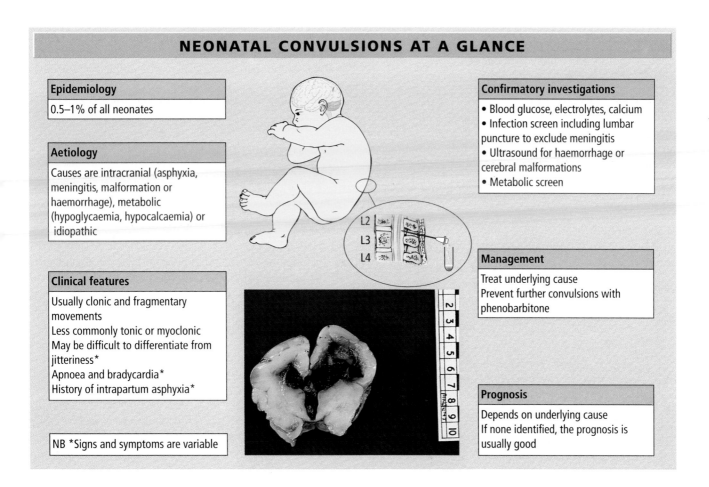

NEONATAL CONVULSIONS AT A GLANCE

Epidemiology

0.5–1% of all neonates

Aetiology

Causes are intracranial (asphyxia, meningitis, malformation or haemorrhage), metabolic (hypoglycaemia, hypocalcaemia) or idiopathic

Clinical features

Usually clonic and fragmentary movements
Less commonly tonic or myoclonic
May be difficult to differentiate from jitteriness*
Apnoea and bradycardia*
History of intrapartum asphyxia*

NB *Signs and symptoms are variable

Confirmatory investigations

• Blood glucose, electrolytes, calcium
• Infection screen including lumbar puncture to exclude meningitis
• Ultrasound for haemorrhage or cerebral malformations
• Metabolic screen

Management

Treat underlying cause
Prevent further convulsions with phenobarbitone

Prognosis

Depends on underlying cause
If none identified, the prognosis is usually good

with parenchymal haemorrhage. The diagnosis is made by ultrasound examination.

Management There is no specific treatment, but posthaemorrhagic hydrocephalus occurs in 15–20% of babies following IVH.

Prognosis Cerebral palsy (see p. 277) occurs in 80% of babies with cystic PVL, and is usually severe. Cerebral palsy may also occur in infants with parenchymal haemorrhage but this is usually less severe than that seen with PVL.

APNOEA

Apnoea is a very common symptom in the neonatal period and is particularly seen in premature infants. The definition of apnoea is a pause in respiration lasting for 20 seconds or more. It is a non-specific symptom and the baby requires careful assessment to discover the underlying cause.

Apnoea may be central or obstructive in origin (Table 6.16). Central causes may involve the brainstem or higher cortical structures. Obstructive causes occur as a result of airway obstruction and can sometimes be recognized by observing the episode.

Clinical approach to a baby with apnoea

Obstructive apnoea

The baby continues to make respiratory efforts despite increasing cyanosis or bradycardia suggesting that the airway is becoming blocked and the baby is fighting to overcome this effect.

Central apnoea

In this condition the baby usually shows periodic respiration with slowing in the respiratory rate until apnoea occurs.

Table 6.16 Causes of apnoea in the neonate

Central apnoea
Apnoea of prematurity
Hypoglycaemia
Infection
Intracranial haemorrhage
Necrotizing enterocolitis
Convulsions
Obstructive apnoea
Small jaw
Thick oropharyngeal secretions
Congenital blockage of the posterior nares (very rare)

It is always important to consider infection as the cause of apnoeic episodes and to investigate this rapidly and institute treatment as early as possible. Other investigations should be performed to exclude or confirm the causes of the apnoea.

Obstructive apnoea can be excluded by passing a cannula through the nares and evaluating whether the baby has a small jaw (see below).

Management

The acute apnoeic episode should be treated rapidly. The management depends on the severity and frequency of the attacks. Initially, tactile stimulation is effective and nasopharyngeal suction may be necessary in obstructive causes. Severe apnoeic episodes may require bag and mask resuscitation.

Treatment should also be directed towards the cause of the condition if this is known. Where the cause is thought to be apnoea of prematurity non-specific therapy involves administration of a xanthine-based drug to stimulate the respiratory system. Aminophylline, theophylline and caffeine are most widely used. Continuous positive airway pressure may be useful in more refractory cases and the most severe cases require mechanical ventilation.

Rarely, the baby will have severe apnoea which is sometimes referred to as acute life-threatening events of no known cause. This is associated with sudden infant death syndrome which is considered in detail on p. 312. In these cases sending the baby home on an apnoea monitor is indicated.

Specific causes of apnoea

Infection

The newborn, and particularly the premature infant, is particularly susceptible to infection resulting from immaturity of the immune system. An important factor in the integrity of the immune response is maternal IgG which crosses the placenta to the fetus in the last 3 months of pregnancy. Babies who are born severely preterm miss the maternal IgG contribution.

Aetiology Infection in the newborn is usually bacterial and may be acquired either at birth from the maternal genital tract during delivery (perinatally) or by cross-infection (nosocomial) from medical and nursing staff. Perinatally acquired early infection is most commonly caused by group B beta-haemolytic streptococcus and *E. coli*. Nosocomial infection is most commonly caused by *staphylococcus epidermidis* and *Pseudomonas*.

Clinical features There are no specific signs of infection in the newborn and infection must always be considered to be a possible cause of any compromise in all newborn infants. Signs of infection are listed in Table 6.17.

Investigations Infection must be considered to be a cause of almost any acute symptom or sign in the neonate and requires rapid investigation. Infection screen includes the following:
- full blood count;
- blood and urine cultures;
- swabs from skin, throat, trachea and rectum;
- lumbar puncture.

Management Antibiotic treatment is most effective if started early. Bacteriological confirmation of infection will take 24–48 hours from taking the specimens and consequently, if infection is suspected, broad spectrum antibiotics should be started immediately. They can be stopped if microbiological surveillance is negative. If positive a full course should be given for 5–7 days.

Apnoea of prematurity

This results from immaturity of the respiratory system. It is diagnosed by excluding other causes of apnoea in otherwise well premature infants. The management is with a xanthine-based drug (caffeine, aminophylline or theophylline). The prognosis is excellent.

The baby with this condition usually shows a periodic pattern of respiration with periods of hyperventilation alternating with periods of hypoventilation leading to eventual brief apnoeic episodes.

Obstructive apnoea

This condition occurs in babies with either anatomical or functional problems.

Table 6.17 Clinical signs suggestive of acquired neonatal infection

Unstable temperature
Lethargy
Apnoeic or bradycardic episodes
Hypotonia
Irritability
Convulsions
Poor feeding
Respiratory distress
Jaundice
Vomiting
Abdominal distension

APNOEA AT A GLANCE

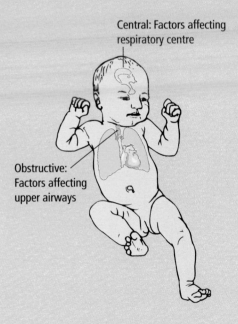

Epidemiology

Common symptom, particularly in premature infants

Aetiology

Apnoea may be due to partial obstruction of the airway or central causes (see Table 6.16)

Clinical features

Pause in breathing lasting longer than 20 seconds
Often associated with periodic breathing
Bradycardia
Cyanosis*

NB *Signs and symptoms are variable

Central: Factors affecting respiratory centre

Obstructive: Factors affecting upper airways

Confirmatory investigations

Infection screen in all cases
Assess for anatomic problems of upper airway
Assess for brain pathology

Management

Treat all apnoeic episodes with stimulation
Treat underlying cause where possible
Xanthine derivatives if apnoea is persistent
CPAP or IPPV if apnoea is very severe
Home apnoea monitors are rarely indicated except for severe life-threatening apnoeic episodes (see p. 312)

Prognosis

Good except where there is major central pathology

Anatomical obstruction Anatomical obstruction of upper airway structures occurs, for example, in posterior nasal obstruction (choanal atresia). Babies born with a small jaw (micrognathia) are subject to obstructive apnoea when the tongue falls back and causes the upper airway to be occluded.

Functional obstruction Functional obstruction occurs in premature infants who may have hypotonia of the oropharyngeal musculature which predisposes to collapse of the upper airway structures during breathing.

Clinical features Obstructive apnoea may be recognized by the effort of breathing that the baby makes to overcome upper airway obstruction. Anatomical obstruction caused by choanal atresia is diagnosed by an inability to pass a cannula through both nostrils. Evaluate whether the child has micrognathia by looking at the face in profile.

Management Anatomical obstruction requires surgical correction. Obstruction in premature infants is best treated by nasal CPAP. This improves the patency of the upper airway until the baby grows and the tone improves spontaneously.

Prognosis With surgical correction of anatomical obstruction the prognosis is good. Premature babies with functional obstruction usually grow out of the problem.

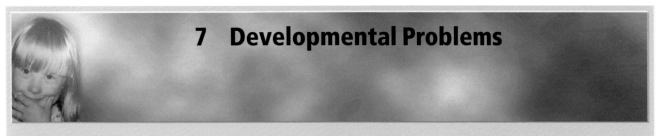

7 Developmental Problems

Introduction, 261
THE CHILD WITH ABNORMAL OR DELAYED
DEVELOPMENT, 261
Delay or difficulty in talking, 263
Common causes of language delay and
   difficulties, 265

The child who is delayed in walking, 266
Conditions associated with delayed walking,
   267
Global developmental delay, 269
Conditions associated with global
   developmental delay, 270

THE CHILD WITH A DISABILITY, 273
Cerebral palsy, 277
Learning disability (mental retardation), 281
The deaf child, 284
The blind or partially sighted child, 286

There are some who hear a different drummer
And who march a different pace.

Henry David Thoreau

Introduction

Psychomotor development and growth are issues unique to paediatrics. As in growth, children progress developmentally at different rates and, as in growth, a slower rate of development may be a variation of normal or may be an indicator of serious concern. This chapter discusses the problem of the child presenting with delayed or abnormal development, and then goes on to address the management of the child who has a recognized disability.

In order to approach the child with either possible or proven developmental problems, a good understanding of normal development must be acquired along with skill in evaluating a child's developmental progress (Table 7.1).

Given the wide range of normality that occurs in acquiring developmental milestones, it is important to decide when delays should arouse concern. In general, if the skills attained are of good quality and the child continues to progress, somewhat delayed or advanced acquisition is unimportant. Table 7.2 gives guidelines as to when one should become concerned that a child's development is significantly delayed.

The child with abnormal or delayed development

Causes of abnormal or delayed development

It is not always possible to identify the factors underlying a child's delayed or abnormal development. However, it is important to attempt to do so. Important factors underlying

some developmental problems are shown in Table 7.3 with examples.

How the child presents

Delayed or abnormal development may affect individual areas of development or the child's overall development, in which case it is known as global delay.

Unusual development is commonly identified by the parents, or is detected during child health surveillance, when routine examinations are carried out by the health visitor. In certain circumstances, when a child is known to be at high risk for developmental difficulties, such as after neonatal problems, head injury or meningitis, routine medical follow-up is arranged in order to identify problems early.

Clinical evaluation

The clinical evaluation of a child's development requires time and skill. It is highly dependent on the child's cooperation and often requires evaluation over a period of time. The developmental area in question has to be accurately assessed, and all other developmental areas evaluated too, so that a complete picture of the child's development is obtained. In addition it is important to look for an aetiology for the difficulties so that when possible a diagnosis can be made.

History

The history is of paramount importance. Children are quite likely to be uncooperative when relating to an unfamiliar person and in unfamiliar surroundings, and a reliable parent's report can provide much information.

The history should include an assessment of the following:
- current developmental skills;
- history of developmental milestones;
- birth history;
- past medical history;

Table 7.1 Skills required in development paediatrics

A grasp of normal development (p. 2)
Ability to conduct a developmental evaluation (p. 39)
Recognition of delay
Recognition of abnormal patterns of development

Table 7.2 Developmental warning signs

At any age
Maternal concern
Regression in previously acquired skills

At 10 weeks
Not smiling

At 6 months
Persistent primitive reflexes
Persistent squint
Hand preference
Little interest in people, toys, noises

At 10–12 months
No sitting
No double syllable babble
No pincer grasp

At 18 months
Not walking independently
Fewer than six words
Persistent mouthing and drooling

At 2½ years
No two to three word sentences

At 4 years
Unintelligible speech

Table 7.3 Aetiological factors underlying developmental problems

Factor	Example
Genetic	Chromosomal anomalies
	Inborn errors of metabolism
Environmental	Deprivation/neglect
	Lead poisoning
Injury	
Prenatal	Intrauterine infections
	Toxins: alcohol, anticonvulsants, etc.
At birth	Birth trauma/asphyxia
Postnatal	Meningitis
	Head trauma
Idiopathic	Autism

Focal points
Evaluating abnormal or delayed development

- Accurately assess the developmental area which is delayed

- Assess all other developmental areas

- Attempt to make a diagnosis or identify the aetiology for the difficulties

- Remember to correct for prematurity in the first 2 years

- Make sure that the child's developmental skills are not regressing

- family history;
- parental anxieties.

Allowances for prematurity must be made during the first 2 years, but beyond that period catch-up in development rarely occurs. Parents often find it difficult to recall their child's developmental milestones, but in the event of delay they are likely to be more accurate. Of particular importance in taking a history is the identification of any regression in skills.

Physical examination

- *Developmental skills.* It is prudent to attempt to evaluate development before carrying out any other part of the physical examination, as undressing the child is likely to arouse some antagonism. Each developmental area—gross motor, fine motor/adaptive, language and social skills—should be assessed in turn, and an attempt made to evaluate the child's vision and hearing.

Check-lists of developmental skills can be helpful (see p. 40). In addition, it is also important to assess factors such as alertness, responsiveness, interest in surroundings, determination and concentration, which all have positive influences on a child's attainments.

The child may well not respond to a demand to cooperate with particular tasks, particularly if they are tired, shy or at the stage of stranger anxiety. Much information can be obtained from simply observing the child at play while taking the history.

- *General examination.* A complete physical examination is required in order to identify medical problems. Of particular relevance are dysmorphic signs, microcephaly, poor growth and signs of neglect.

- *Neurological examination.* This needs to be thorough, looking for abnormalities in tone, strength and coordination, deep tendon reflexes, clonus, cranial nerves and primitive reflexes.

Investigations

Investigations may be required, depending on the nature of the problem.

Management

Whether a particular problem has been identified or not, the parents' concerns must be properly addressed, as on-going parental anxiety in itself can be damaging to the child. If simple developmental delay alone is identified, reassurance is required. In any event the child is likely to require follow-up to ensure that developmental progress is maintained. Referral to an appropriate therapist may be required, either to carry out a more detailed assessment or to provide the child and family with guidance in how to encourage the development of skills. Caution is always required in developmental predictions, and repeat examinations over time are often required to predict outcome with any confidence.

Complex developmental problems

When developmental difficulties are complex, the paediatrician alone is unlikely to be able to make a sufficiently detailed assessment of the child's abilities and to advise on appropriate management. In this circumstance the child should be referred to a child development team (see p. 275).

DELAY OR DIFFICULTY IN TALKING

Language is the most highly developed of all human skills.

GENERAL ISSUES FOR THE CHILD WITH DELAYED/ABNORMAL DEVELOPMENT AT A GLANCE

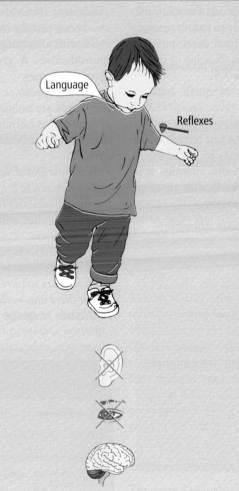

Causes
Often no cause is found, but cerebral insults and genetic and environmental factors should be considered

How the child presents
Delay may be global or affect individual areas of development
Identified by parents, during child health surveillance, or in medical follow-up of high risk problems

Clinical evaluation
Time, skill and co-operation are required
Assess all developmental areas — gross motor, fine motor/adaptive, language and social skills
Correction for prematurity should be made until 2 years of age

History
Current developmental skills
History of developmental milestones
Birth, medical and family history
Parental concerns
Regression in skills

Physical examination

Development
Observation of the child in free play, assessment of specific skills, vision and hearing, and identification of positive features such as alertness, determination and concentration

General examination
Dysmorphic signs, microcephaly, poor growth, signs of neglect

Neurological examination
Abnormalities in tone, strength and co-ordination, deep tendon reflexes, clonus, cranial nerves and primitive reflexes

Investigations
Sometimes required

Management
Follow-up and reassurance for simple delay
If a developmental problem is identified:
• full discussion with the parents
• consider referral to a therapist
• referral to a Child Development Team if the problems are complex
Caution is needed in predicting outcome

Distinguishing features — Children with language delay and difficulties

	Language development	Other developmental areas	Ability to form interpersonal relationships
Stammer	Comprehension and expressive language is normal, but speech is immature, stuttered or unintelligible	Normal	Normal
Hearing deficit	Comprehension and expressive language delayed	Normal	Normal
Maturational delay	Comprehension and expressive language delayed	Normal	Normal
Learning disabilities	Comprehension and expressive language delayed	Delayed	Often normal
Autism	Comprehension and expressive language delayed	Usually delayed	Abnormal
Language disorders	Language delayed but also disordered	Usually delayed	Normal

than being simply delayed. Receptive or expressive language may be affected. These children are at risk for specific learning difficulties such as dyslexia, and may even require special education. Speech therapy is important.

THE CHILD WHO IS DELAYED IN WALKING

Independent walking is acquired on average at the age of 13 months, although many children walk some months before this. Black babies tend to walk earlier than white. Walking is considered to be delayed if it has not been achieved by the age of 18 months.

Delay in walking can result either from delay in maturation of the neuromuscular system or as a result of pathology affecting muscle tone or strength (Table 7.5).

Clinical evaluation

The importance of the clinical evaluation lies in determining whether the delay is isolated to gross motor skills, or whether there is a more global developmental problem. The quality of the child's motor development to date and

Table 7.5 Commoner causes of delayed walking*

Delay in motor maturation
Delayed motor maturation (often familial)
Severe learning disabilities (mental retardation)
Environmental factors

Abnormalities of muscle tone or power
Hypertonia—cerebral palsy
Hypotonia of any cause
Muscular dystrophy

* Obesity and congenital dislocation of the hip are not causes of delayed walking.

the neurological examination should give an indication as to whether the problem is one of simple delay, or whether neurological or neuromuscular pathology is present. Aetiological factors may be identified to account for the delay.

History

The history should follow the pattern outlined for the presentation of any developmental problem (see p. 261). A clear assessment of all four developmental areas must be made. A careful history of motor skills should include the baby's ability to sit supported or unsupported, roll over from both front and back, get to the sitting position independently, crawl, pull to stand and cruise.

A family history of late walking is important as this provides support for the benign diagnosis of maturational delay. It is also important to identify environmental factors such as deprivation or lack of opportunity to exercise gross motor skills.

Physical examination

The physical examination should confirm the developmental history, and also identify any abnormal neuromuscular signs. A good assessment of developmental skills should be

Focal points
Evaluating delayed walking

• Determine whether the delay is isolated to gross motor skills or whether there is a more global developmental problem

• Look for abnormal neurological findings

• Identify any responsible aetiological factors

attempted to clarify whether the delay is generalized or isolated to gross motor skills. A great deal of information can be obtained by placing the child on the floor with some toys in easy reach, while the history is being obtained. The child can then be observed in natural activity. A more formal evaluation should then be attempted.

The neurological examination should be thorough, and look for abnormalities in tone, deep tendon reflexes, strength, asymmetry of movements and the presence of primitive reflexes.

Investigations

If the delay in walking is isolated and the child in other respects has normal development, the only investigation required is a creatinine phosphokinase level (CPK or CK) as late walking may be the earliest manifestation of muscular dystrophy (see later).

If signs of cerebral palsy or hypotonia are demonstrated, investigations may be required (see p. 278).

Conditions associated with delayed walking

Delayed motor maturation

Delayed motor maturation is simply a descriptive term for the child who acquires the skill of walking late, but who is normal in other respects. There is often a family history of late walking.

Clinical features The delay is generally obvious as walking is probably the milestone that receives most attention. Motor skills are normal in terms of quality, but are simply delayed. Mild hypotonia may be present. Other developmental skills are normal. The diagnosis is made on clinical grounds, and by exclusion of pathology.

Management Parents should be reassured that the child will eventually walk. Intervention is not generally required, although if there is anxiety, advice from a physiotherapist can be helpful.

Prognosis The prognosis is good. Acquisition of other gross motor skills such as running and cycling are likely to be delayed.

Severe learning disabilities (mental retardation)

Severe learning disabilities are covered in detail on page 281.

Clinical features Severe learning disability is to be suspected if there is delay in all developmental areas. In general, gross motor development is often less affected than language, fine motor and social skills. Obvious dysmorphic features may be noted, and hypotonia is often present.

Management Multidisciplinary involvement is usually required. Physiotherapy may be helpful to address gross motor development, particularly if hypotonia is marked.

Prognosis This depends on the underlying cause.

Environmental factors

Environmental factors can delay the onset of walking. In the past, institutionalized children were restricted to their cots, and delay in gross motor skills caused by lack of opportunity was commonly observed. A similar process is seen in children who have been ill and confined to bed for an extended period. Emotional deprivation tends to affect gross motor skills less than other developmental skills.

Clinical features A careful history may give clues as to environmental factors which may be slowing the acquisition of skills. In some cases signs of neglect may be evident.

Management and prognosis Provided children are given the opportunity to exercise their gross motor skills, catch-up is seen.

Cerebral palsy

Cerebral palsy is covered in detail on page 277.

Clinical features Delayed walking may be the presenting feature of the milder forms of cerebral palsy: hemiplegia and spastic diplegia. In the more severe forms concern regarding developmental progress is likely to have been aroused long before the child is expected to walk.

Management Physiotherapy is an essential part of the child's treatment.

Prognosis This depends on the degree of spasticity. Most children with hemiplegia or diplegia eventually learn to walk, although the gait is not normal.

Duchenne muscular dystrophy

Duchenne muscular dystrophy is the commonest hereditary neuromuscular disease. It is a progressive disorder resulting in death in the early twenties. It is inherited as an X-linked recessive trait.

Clinical features Baby boys are normal at birth, and delayed walking is usually only identified retrospectively. Symptoms

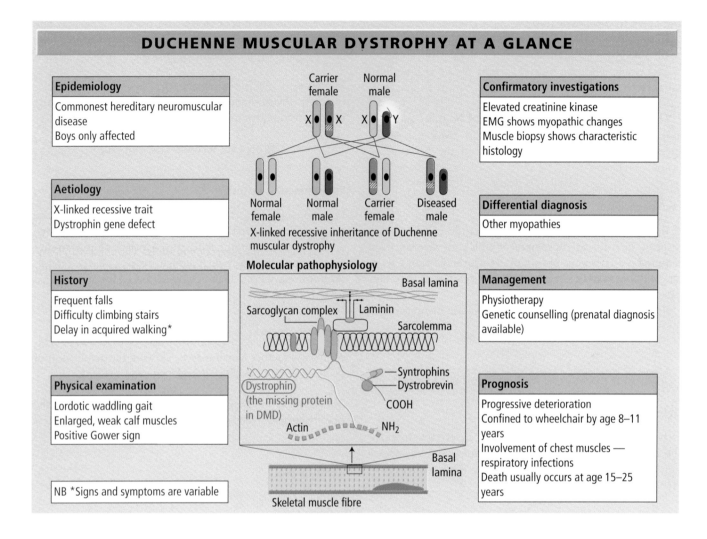

DUCHENNE MUSCULAR DYSTROPHY AT A GLANCE

Epidemiology

Commonest hereditary neuromuscular disease
Boys only affected

Aetiology

X-linked recessive trait
Dystrophin gene defect

History

Frequent falls
Difficulty climbing stairs
Delay in acquired walking*

Physical examination

Lordotic waddling gait
Enlarged, weak calf muscles
Positive Gower sign

NB *Signs and symptoms are variable

Carrier female   Normal male

X-linked recessive inheritance of Duchenne muscular dystrophy

Normal female   Normal male   Carrier female   Diseased male

Molecular pathophysiology

Basal lamina
Sarcoglycan complex   Laminin
Sarcolemma
Syntrophins
Dystrobevin
Dystrophin (the missing protein in DMD)
COOH
Actin   NH₂
Basal lamina
Skeletal muscle fibre

Confirmatory investigations

Elevated creatinine kinase
EMG shows myopathic changes
Muscle biopsy shows characteristic histology

Differential diagnosis

Other myopathies

Management

Physiotherapy
Genetic counselling (prenatal diagnosis available)

Prognosis

Progressive deterioration
Confined to wheelchair by age 8–11 years
Involvement of chest muscles — respiratory infections
Death usually occurs at age 15–25 years

appear between the ages of 4 and 6 years and are progressive. They consist of frequent falls, a lordotic waddling gait and difficulty climbing stairs. On examination the child has enlarged but weak calf muscles. The Gower sign is characteristic (Fig. 7.1); on rising from a lying position the boy uses his hands to 'climb up' his legs to get to an upright posture.

Distinguishing features—Conditions associated with delayed walking

Cause	History	General physical examination	Other developmental milestones	Neurological signs
Delayed motor maturation	Family history of delayed walking	Normal	Normal	Normal (or mildly decreased tone)
Severe learning disabilities (mental retardation)		Dysmorphic features, microcephaly, etc. may be found	Delayed usually to a greater degree than gross motor	Normal (or decreased tone)
Environmental factors	Lack of opportunity	Normal	May be delayed	Normal
Hypertonia–cerebral palsy			Often delayed	Increased tone and decreased tendon reflexes in affected limb
Muscular dystrophy	Other family members affected	Later on large but weak calf muscles	Normal	Later on weakness of the hip girdle muscles

On investigation the creatine kinase level is elevated by at least 10 times the normal level.

Management The child needs physiotherapy, support and help through school. Genetic counselling is extremely important for the family as 50% of sons will be affected. Early detection by finding an elevated CPK level in boys late in starting to walk allows the family to plan future pregnancies, as prenatal diagnosis is now possible.

Prognosis Most of these boys are unable to walk by the age of 8–11 years and become confined to a wheelchair. Chest muscles are also affected and death is precipitated by respiratory infections by the age of 15–25 years.

GLOBAL DEVELOPMENTAL DELAY

The term global developmental delay refers to a delay in acquiring all developmental milestones, but particularly language, fine motor and social skills. It is extremely worrying when this occurs as it usually indicates learning disabilities (mental retardation). Gross motor skills may also be delayed, though they do not reflect intellectual capacity in the same way as the other skills, and are sometimes spared. Causes of global developmental delay are shown in Table 7.6.

Clinical evaluation

The purpose of the clinical evaluation is first of all to ascertain whether the child truly has global developmental delay, and to what extent each area is affected. The next stage is to attempt to find the underlying cause. The history and physical examination may provide an explanation, and should give indications as to whether investigations are likely to contribute in any way.

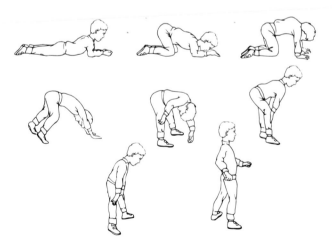

Fig. 7.1 Gower's sign.

History

The guidelines given in the previous section (p. 261) are particularly relevant to the child with overall developmental delay. The history needs to cover the following structure.
• *What are the child's current skills?* A detailed history of the child's current abilities in all four areas must be obtained. The parents should be asked if they have any concerns about the child's hearing or vision.
• *When did the child achieve earlier milestones?* It is important to identify whether development was initially appropriate or whether there were concerns from birth. Developmental difficulties may have followed trauma or an illness.
• *Has there been a regression in skills?* The child with learning disabilities tends to have a slow but steady acquisition of skills. Regression of skills would suggest a neurodegenerative disorder.

Table 7.6 Causes of global developmental delay

Cause	Example
Chromosomal abnormalities	Down's syndrome
	Fragile X
Dysmorphic syndromes	
Injury	
Prenatal	Fetal alcohol syndrome
	TORCH infection (see p. 243)
Perinatal	Hypoxic–ischaemic insult
Postnatal	Meningitis
	Non-accidental injury
	Neglect
Central nervous malformations	Neural tube defects
	Hydrocephalus
Endocrine and metabolic defects	Hypothyroidism
Neurodegenerative disorders	
Neurocutaneous syndromes	
Idiopathic	

Focal points
Evaluating global developmental delay

• Correct for prematurity if the child is less than 2 years old

• Confirm the delay is global

• Assess the extent of the delay in each area

• Determine if there is regression of skills

• Attempt to identify a cause for the delay

• *Past medical history*. A detailed perinatal history is particularly important and enquiry into alcohol consumption, medications, prematurity and neonatal complications should be made. The link between developmental difficulties and postnatal events such as meningitis or head trauma are usually obvious.

• *Family history*. A family history of learning disabilities or consanguinity is important as it suggests a possible genetic cause for the problem.

Physical examination

The physical assessment involves a detailed developmental evaluation, followed by a complete physical examination focusing on neurological findings.

Developmental assessment

All four developmental areas must be assessed. This assessment described in detail on pp. 39–43.

General examination

The physical examination may be informative, but is often unremarkable. The following features are of relevance.

• *Growth*. Many children with developmental problems are short. If actual fall off in growth has occurred, hypothyroidism and non-organic failure to thrive should be considered.

• *Microcephaly*. Microcephaly is a common, often non-specific finding, but if present at birth it suggests intrauterine infections or fetal alcohol syndrome and if it develops over time it suggests a neurodegenerative disorder.

• *Dysmorphic signs*. Not uncommonly global developmental delay is associated with congenital anomalies and dysmorphic features. If present they are suggestive of a genetic defect, chromosomal anomaly or teratogenic effect.

• *General appearance*. Signs of neglect such as an undernourished appearance, skin and hair in poor condition, uncleanliness and irritative rashes in the skinfolds may indicate psychosocial factors responsible for the delay.

• *Skin*. The skin should be examined for signs such as café au lait spots, depigmented patches and port-wine stains which are indicative of neurocutaneous syndromes.

• *Hepatosplenomegaly*. The finding of an enlarged liver or spleen are suggestive of a metabolic disorder.

Neurological examination

Features of particular importance are the following.

• *Hypotonia*. This is often a non-specific finding. It occurs in Down's syndrome.

• *Signs of cerebral palsy* (see p. 277). Cerebral palsy affects motor skills but learning disabilities also commonly occur.

• *Hearing and vision*.

• *Ocular abnormalities*. The finding of ocular abnormalities such as cataracts suggests the presence of a metabolic disorder.

Investigations

Chromosomal analysis and thyroid function tests should be performed in every child with global developmental delay. More sophisticated investigation of metabolic function or brain imaging may be indicated in some.

Management

Every attempt should be made to identify an underlying cause for the delay. Although there is rarely specific treatment, parents are helped by being given a diagnosis, and there may be genetic implications for subsequent pregnancies.

The term developmental delay is sometimes used euphemistically as a diagnosis in itself. This is inappropriate. A child should be described as being delayed only up to the point when the diagnosis of learning disabilities becomes clear (usually well before the age of 3 years). The management of the child with global developmental delay is covered in detail in the section on The child with severe learning disabilities (see p. 281).

Conditions associated with global developmental delay

Down's syndrome

Down's syndrome is the commonest congenital anomaly associated with global developmental delay. The underlying chromosomal abnormality is trisomy of chromosome 21. The extra chromosome is usually of maternal origin, and the incidence of Down's syndrome increases with maternal age (2% at age 38 years).

Clinical features The features of Down's syndrome are easily recognized—upward sloping palpable fissures, epicanthal folds, Brushfield spots (speckled iris), a protruding tongue, flat occiput, single palmar creases and mild to moderate developmental delay where social skills often exceed the other milestones (Fig. 7.2). One third of babies with Down's syndrome are born with gastrointestinal problems, most commonly duodenal atresia, and one third have cardiac anomalies (most commonly atrioventricular canal defects). Secretory otitis media, strabismus, hypothyroidism, atlantoaxial instability and leukaemia occur more commonly than in normal children.

DOWN'S SYNDROME AT A GLANCE

Epidemiology

Commonest congenital anomaly associated with learning disability
Incidence (1 per 650 births) increases with maternal age

Aetiology

Trisomy of chromosome 21

Antenatal diagnosis

Triple test early in pregnancy, followed by amniocentesis for those at high risk

Clinical features

Mild to moderate developmental delay
Upward sloping palpebral fissures
Epicanthal folds
Brushfield spots
Protruding tongue
Flat occiput
Single palmar creases
Hypotonia
Small stature

Confirmatory investigations

Chromosome analysis shows trisomy 21 with non-dysjunction, translocation or mosaicism

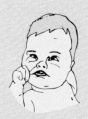

Maternal age	Incidence
20	1 in 1700 births
40	1 in 100 births
44	1 in 40 births

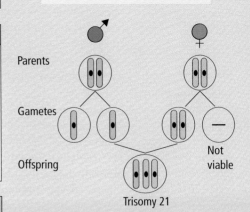

Parents
Gametes
Offspring
Not viable
Trisomy 21

Genetics: extra chromosome 21
(Translocation between chromosome 14 and 21 is rarer)

Differential diagnosis

Facial features are usually clinically evident from birth

Management

Cardiac evaluation at birth
Referral to ophthalmology if squint is present
Routine audiological and thyroid tests
Genetic counselling for family
Arranging for special educational needs

Complications

Cardiac anomalies
Duodenal atresia
Secretory otitis media
Strabismus
Hypothyroidism
Atlantoaxial instability
Leukaemia

Prognosis

Individuals have varying degrees of learning disability
Children can usually be integrated into mainstream primary school
At risk from Alzheimer's disease in adult life

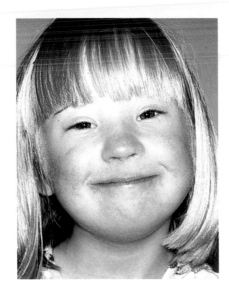

Fig. 7.2 A 5-year-old girl with Down's syndrome.

Management The medical management of Down's syndrome demands a routine cardiac evaluation at birth. In view of the incidence of hypothyroidism and hearing difficulties, routine audiological and thyroid tests are needed throughout childhood and ophthalmological assessment if there is any evidence of a squint. The child's growth needs to be followed on special Down's growth charts. The family requires genetic counselling.

Prognosis Children with Down's syndrome have varying degrees of learning disability. They can usually be integrated into a mainstream primary school with extra provision made for their educational needs. Individuals with Down's syndrome are at risk for early onset Alzheimer's disease.

Fragile X

Fragile X is an important and the most common genetic cause of learning disabilities among boys. The chromosomal anomaly consists of a 'fragile site' at the end of one of the long arms of the X-chromosome. The diagnosis should be sought in any boy who has unexplained moderate or severe learning disability. Some girls carrying the chromosome have mild learning disabilities.

Fetal alcohol syndrome

The fetal alcohol syndrome is a common cause of learning disabilities. It is caused by a moderate to high intake of alcohol during pregnancy, with the severity of the features related to the quantity of alcohol consumed. The clinical features are characterized by poor growth and microcephaly, a characteristic facial appearance and cardiac defects.

Other dysmorphic syndromes

Not uncommonly congenital anomalies and dysmorphic features are found in children with learning disabilities. In some, particularly those with significant anomalies, a specific diagnosis can be made. The diagnostic process has been helped by the development of computerized databases.

It is always worth taking blood for a karyotype in children with delay and dysmorphism as chromosomal anomalies are not uncommonly found.

Abuse and neglect

Emotional abuse and neglect can have serious consequences for a child's developmental progress.

Clinical features The developmental delay is often associated with failure to thrive (see pp. 61, 67). On presentation the child may be apathetic, and show evidence of physical neglect such as dirty clothing, unkempt hair and nappy rash. There may be signs of non-accidental injury, and if there is any suggestion of regression of developmental skills, the diagnosis of chronic subdural haematomas (which can occur as a result of shaking injuries) should be considered.

Management Intensive input and support is required. Day nursery placement can provide good stimulation, nutrition and care. If the child continues to be at risk for on-going abuse or neglect he or she must be removed from the home (see pp. 56, 97).

Prognosis The prognosis depends on the degree of the damage incurred and how early the intervention is provided.

Children who require removal from the home often have irreversible learning and emotional difficulties.

Inborn errors of metabolism

This group of disorders are caused by single gene mutations, which are inherited in an autosomal recessive manner. They may present in a variety of ways of which developmental delay is one. As individual conditions they are very rare. Phenylketonuria is the commonest and is routinely screened for in all neonates (p. 47).

Congenital hypothyroidism

Lack of thyroid hormone in the first years of life has a devastating effect on both growth and development. However, since neonatal screening has been introduced (see p. 46), congenital hypothyroidism is a rare cause of developmental delay. The underlying pathological defect is either abnormal development of the thyroid gland or inborn errors of thyroxine metabolism.

Clinical features Babies usually appear normal at birth, and rarely have the characteristic features of cretinism. These include coarse facies, hypotonia, a large tongue, an umbilical hernia, constipation, prolonged jaundice and a hoarse cry. In the older baby or child delayed development, lethargy and short stature are found. Thyroid function tests reveal low T4 and high thyroid-stimulating hormone levels.

Management Congenital hypothyroidism is one of the few treatable causes of learning disabilities. Thyroid replacement is required throughout life and must be monitored carefully as the child grows.

Prognosis If therapy is started in the first few weeks of life and if compliance is good, the prognosis for normal growth and development is excellent.

Neurodegenerative disorders

A neurodegenerative disease is one where there is progressive deterioration of neurological function. The causes are heterogeneous and include biochemical defects, chronic viral infections and toxic substances, although many remain of unknown aetiology. The course for all of these conditions is one of relentless and inevitable neurological deterioration.

Distinguishing features — Conditions associated with global development delay

Condition	History	Physical examination	Other features
Down's syndrome	Older maternal age is common	Characteristic facial features, single palmar crease, Brushfield spots, hypotonia	Congenital heart disease, anal/duodenal atresia, growth should be followed on Down's charts
Fragile X	Other boys in the family affected	Long face, prominent ears, large jaw, large testes at puberty	Fits, behaviour problems
Fetal alcohol syndrome	Possible history of alcohol in pregnancy, intrauterine growth retardation	Short palpebral fissures, maxillary hypoplasia, thin upper lip, microcephaly	Cardiac defects, minor joint and limb abnormalities
Dysmorphic syndromes		Dysmorphic features, +/− congenital anomalies	Poor growth common
Abuse and neglect	Family possibly known to social services	Possible signs of neglect or old injuries	Failure to thrive common
Inborn errors of metabolism	Consanguinity, neonatal seizures, hypoglycaemia, vomiting, coma	Sometimes coarse features, hepatosplenomegaly, microcephaly, failure to thrive	Developmental regression may occur
Congenital hypothyroidism		May have features of cretinism Plateauing of growth	
Neurodegenerative disorders*	Developmental regression	May have coarse features, microcephaly develops	Fits, visual and intellectual deterioration
Idiopathic learning difficulties		Mild dysmorphic features common	
Intrauterine infections*	Possible history of contact in pregnancy, intrauterine growth retardation	Visual or hearing deficits common, microcephaly	
Neurocutaneous syndromes	Often familial	Characteristic skin lesions	

* Features vary according to the type of disorder.

Idiopathic severe learning disabilities (mental retardation)

In about one third of children with global developmental delay no specific cause is identified. However, this picture is changing as a result of advances in the field of genetics. Diagnoses are now being made in children who in the past were thought to have idiopathic learning disabilities.

Intrauterine infections (see p. 243)

The best known intrauterine infections are rubella, cytomegalovirus (CMV) and toxoplasmosis. If infection with these agents occurs for the first time during pregnancy severe fetal damage can result, leading to multiple handicaps.

Neurocutaneous syndromes

The neurocutaneous syndromes are a heterogeneous group of disorders characterized by neurological dysfunction and skin lesions. In some individuals there may be severe learning disabilities and in others intelligence is normal. Examples of neurocutaneous syndromes include Sturge–Weber syndrome, neurofibromatosis and tuberous sclerosis. The aetiology of these problems is not known, but most are familial.

The child with a disability

The prevalence of physical and multiple disabilities in children is approximately 10–20 per 1000. In this section the child with long-lasting and complex needs is considered. The commoner causes of disability are shown in Table 7.7.

Presentation and how the diagnosis is made

Children with disabilities are identified either as a result of parental suspicion, concern by health professionals or child

Table 7.7 Commoner causes of disability among school children

Physical and multiple disabilities	
Cerebral palsy	2.5 per 1000
Spina bifida	0.3 per 1000
Muscular dystrophy	0.2 per 1000
Severe learning difficulties	
Chromosomal abnormalities	4.0 per 1000
Central nervous system abnormality	0.2 per 1000
Idiopathic	0.5 per 1000
Special senses	
Severe visual handicap	1.0 per 2500
Severe hearing loss	1.0 per 1000

health surveillance. Recognition of the disability occurs at different stages, depending on the problem. A syndrome or central nervous system abnormality may be identified in the antenatal period or at birth. Deafness, motor handicaps and severe learning disabilities often become apparent during the first year. Moderate or even severe learning disabilities, language disorder and autism may not be recognized until the child is in the second or third year when family or health visitors question the child's developmental progress. Finally, children may present after life-threatening events such as head injury or encephalopathy.

Assessment of the disability

Recognition of the child's underlying medical problem is only one aspect of the child's diagnosis. A detailed assessment of the child's development and how the difficulties are likely to impinge on his or her life is required. When the difficulties are complex, the paediatrician alone is unlikely to be able to make a sufficiently detailed assessment or advise on appropriate management. In this circumstance the child should be referred to a child development team.

The child development team (Table 7.8)

The child development team is a multidisciplinary team comprising all professionals who are likely to be required in the assessment and management of children with complex difficulties. The members of the team and the manner in which they work may vary from centre to centre, and their roles may considerably overlap in practice.

Principles of management

Management of the child with a disability goes beyond diagnosis, explanation of the nature of the problem and the pro-

vision of specific therapeutic input. It involves supporting the family while they come to terms with the child's difficulties and learn how to cope. It also involves a great deal of liaison work with other professionals both medical and non-medical.

The major benefits of the team approach lie in the co-ordination of a child's care, so ensuring that the family does not receive a mixture of contradictory advice and that the various professionals communicate with each other well.

Practical aspects of management

Breaking the news

The diagnosis of a disability is usually devastating and the way that the news is initially broken is of long-lasting importance to the family. The session should be conducted in private by a senior doctor in the presence of both parents. There should be plenty of opportunity for questions, and a follow-up session should be arranged shortly thereafter. If the problem is one of congenital anomalies it should take place directly after birth, when possible with the baby present.

Medical management

Once a detailed assessment of the child's difficulties has been made, appropriate therapeutic input is required. This may be delivered in the child development centre, at home or in a nursery setting. Once the child is in full-time school, the services are delivered there by community therapists whose task is not only to work with the child but also to advise school staff.

Genetic counselling

When a child has been diagnosed as having a disability the family will want to know the genetic implications for themselves and their relatives. Many disabilities have a genetic basis and in this circumstance informed advice must be provided. However, even if no specific underlying genetic cause is identified, the family will need to discuss the risks of further children being affected.

Provision of services

Agencies other than Health are involved in providing services to the family.

Education services Education services are responsible for assessing learning difficulties, providing preschool home teaching, nursery schooling and education both in mainstream and special schools.

Table 7.8 The child development team

Professional	Role
Developmental paediatrician	Diagnosis of medical problems Advice on medical issues
Physiotherapist	Assessment and management of gross motor difficulties, abnormal tone and prevention of deformities in cerebral palsy Provision of special equipment
Occupational therapist	Assessment and management of fine motor difficulties Advice on toys, play and appliances to aid daily living
Speech and language therapist	Advice on feeding Assessment and management of speech, language and all aspects of communication
Psychologist	Support and counselling of family and team
Special needs teacher	Advice on special educational needs
Social worker	Support for the family Advice on social service benefits, respite care, etc.
Health visitor	Support for the family Liaison with local health visitor

Social services Social services are responsible for providing preschool child care, relief care, advice about benefits and assessment for services needed on leaving school. Child protection concerns also fall into their area.

Voluntary organizations Voluntary organizations provide support and information for families, run play facilities, provide educational opportunities and sitting services. Some are large national agencies with numerous local branches, others are smaller groups concerned with a local issue or a single diagnosis.

Education

The Statement of Special Educational Needs

As a result of the 1981 Education Act, the education authority is obliged to assess children who are likely to need additional educational provision because of severe or complex difficulties. Following this assessment a legally binding document is produced known as the Statement of Special Educational Needs.

The statement is drawn up on the basis of a formal assessment by an educational psychologist, a medical report and reports from any other involved professionals such as thera-

pists and the child's nursery or school. The child's educational needs and the provision which must be made to meet them is clearly outlined. The statement is reviewed on an annual basis.

Mainstream and special schools

Where possible, children with special needs are educated in mainstream schools, with extra help provided in the classroom as needed. This often involves the employment of a special needs assistant for the child, along with physiotherapy, occupational therapy and speech and language therapy support as specified. Mainstream placement has the advantage of integrating children with special needs into a normal peer group in their own locality, and encouraging their adaptation to normal society at an early age. It is also advantageous for other children to learn to live alongside children with disabilities. However, there may be disadvantages as mainstream schools usually suffer from comparatively large classes, may have inadequate support and the buildings may be poorly adapted for the child with physical difficulties.

Special schools, on the other hand, provide expert teaching in small classes, by staff who have an understanding of handicapping conditions. Transport and health service support is also provided. However, the disadvantage lies in the child's limited exposure to 'normal life'. Often, a satisfactory compromise between mainstream and special schools is the establishment of special units for children with disabilities in the mainstream setting.

Support

Having a child with a disability places extra pressures and stresses on every such family. It is important therefore to determine how much support is available. Informal support in terms of family and friends is variable, and additional support is often appreciated. This may take a number of forms. Voluntary organizations and parent support groups give families the opportunity to meet others in similar circumstances and so can reduce the sense of isolation. Sitting services and respite care give parents a break from the burden of constantly caring for the child, and help in the home can also be provided. As regards financial benefits, a child with disabilities is entitled to receive the Disability Living Allowance, with a mobility component from the age of 5 years, and the parents may receive the Invalid Care Allowance provided they are not in full-time work.

Issues for the family

Families differ greatly in their reaction to having a child with a disability. However, on first receiving the news, they all tend to pass through similar emotional stages to those experienced in coping with bereavement. The first reaction is one of shock, when often only a small proportion of what is said is taken in. Negative feelings of fear and loss, anger and guilt then ensue. Gradually adaptation follows and leads to the final stage of acceptance. Some parents have difficulty in reaching this last stage, in which case supportive counselling by a psychologist may be necessary.

The family needs to adapt again at each stage of the child's development. Independence becomes an issue at each step, but particularly so at adolescence. An important part of the child's education is to foster independence, and this is usually addressed well at special schools. Young adult disability teams provide a service to advise about options beyond secondary school.

The impact of having a disability for the child and the family is similar in many ways to that of having a chronic illness. This is discussed in some detail in Chapter 10 (see p. 315)

Issues for the school

When a child with a disability is accepted at a mainstream school, the school needs to be prepared and informed about any anticipated difficulties. If the child needs occupational therapy, physiotherapy or speech and language therapy, the

---

Principles of management
The child with a disability

- A detailed assessment of the child's difficulties and abilities

- Explanation of the nature and possible causes of the child's disability

- Devising a programme to cover the child's and family's needs

- Helping the family cope practically and emotionally

- Advising on educational needs and schooling

THE CHILD WITH A DISABILITY AT A GLANCE

Epidemiology

10–20 per 1000

Presentation and how the diagnosis is made

Antenatally or at birth if anomalies are present
In the first year for motor handicaps and severe learning disabilities
In the second or third year for moderate learning disabilities, language disorder and autism
After cranial insults

Assessment of the disability

- Detailed assessment of the child's abilities
- Recognition of the child's underlying medical problem
- Assessment of the likely long-term effects
- When difficulties are complex a multi-disciplinary approach is needed. This involves the **child development team**: paediatrician, physiotherapist, occupational therapist, speech and language therapist, psychologist, teacher, social worker, health visitor

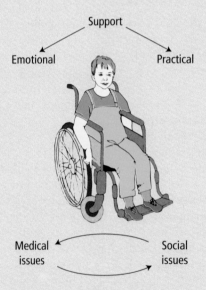

Support
Emotional   Practical

Medical   Social
issues   issues

Issues for the family

The initial impact is similar to bereavement
The impact of disability is similar to that of chronic illness (see p. 315)

Issues for the school

School needs information and guidance, and may need to make adaptations

Practical aspects of management

Breaking the news
This must be done by an experienced senior professional

Medical management
Usual paediatric care
If therapeutic input is needed it should be provided initially at home, and then in nursery and school

Genetic counselling
Required for many families even if no genetic cause is identified

Provision of services
Additional services are provided by education, social services and voluntary agencies

Education
The Statement of Special Educational Needs describes the provision that must be made for children with disabilities.
Mainstream versus special schools: where possible children with disabilities should be integrated into mainstream school

Support
This includes informal support, voluntary organizations, sitting services, respite care, home help, and social service allowances

staff will need to work with the therapists in order to implement their recommendations. In some circumstances the school may need to make alterations to accommodate physical disabilities. Special guidance or counselling may be required and help may be needed to integrate the child into the classroom.

CEREBRAL PALSY

Cerebral palsy is a disorder of movement and posture caused by an early permanent and non-progressive cerebral lesion. It is often associated with epilepsy, hearing and vision problems and learning and feeding difficulties.

Prevalence

Cerebral palsy affects two to three per 1000 children and is the commonest cause of physical disability in childhood.

Aetiology/pathology (Table 7.9)

Although the brain lesion itself in cerebral palsy is non-progressive, the clinical picture changes as the child grows and develops. The underlying brain lesion may result from different insults occurring at various times in the developing brain. The clinical picture resulting from these insults varies depending on the area of the brain involved.

Table 7.9 Causes of cerebral palsy

Prenatal
Cerebral malformations
Congenital infection (p. 243)
Metabolic defects
Perinatal
Complications of prematurity
Intrapartum trauma
Hypoxic–ischaemic insult* (p. 234)
Postnatal (if incurred before 2 years of age)
Non-accidental injury
Head trauma
Meningitis/encephalitis
Cardiopulmonary arrest

* In term babies this is an uncommon cause. Cerebral palsy should not be attributed to these insults unless they were severe and followed by neurological problems in the neonatal period.

Spastic cerebral palsy (85%) This is the commonest form and results from damage to the cerebral motor cortex or its connections.

Dystonic (athetoid) cerebral palsy This results from damage to the basal ganglia and is characterized by irregular and involuntary movements which may be continuous or occur on voluntary movement.

Ataxic cerebral palsy This is rare and results from damage to the cerebellum and is characterized by hypotonia, incoordination and intention tremor.

Clinical features of spastic cerebral palsy

Spastic cerebral palsy is classified according to the extremities affected (Fig. 7.3). Clasp knife hypertonia, brisk deep tendon reflexes, ankle clonus, and a Babinski response (extensor plantar) are demonstrable in the affected limbs.

Spastic hemiplegia (Fig. 7.3a)
In spastic hemiplegia paresis affects one side of the body only and the arm is often more involved than the leg. During

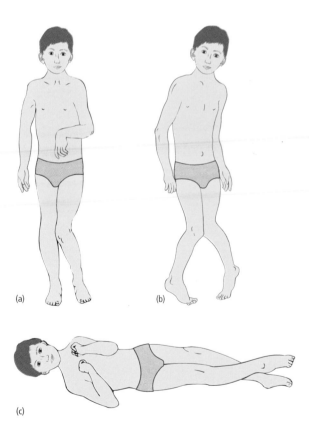

(a)   (b)

(c)

Fig. 7.3 Types of cerebral palsy: (a) spastic hemiplegia; (b) spastic diplegia and (c) spastic quadriplegia.

infancy decreased spontaneous movements are seen on the affected side. Walking is usually delayed until 18–24 months and when it develops has a characteristic gait. The child often walks on tiptoe because of the increased tone, and the affected arm is held in a dystonic posture when running.

Spastic diplegia (Fig. 7.3b)
In spastic diplegia both legs are predominantly involved and the arms are less affected, if at all. The first indication of a problem often occurs when the baby starts to crawl and the legs tend to drag behind. There is excessive adduction of the hips and the parents may find difficulty in putting on a nappy. When the baby is suspended by the axillae the legs take up a scissoring posture. Walking is delayed, and the gait characteristic. The feet are held in the equinovarus position and the child walks on tiptoes.

Spastic quadriplegia (Fig. 7.3c)
Spastic quadriplegia is the most severe form of cerebral palsy because of marked motor impairment of all extremities and the high association with severe learning disabilities and fits. Swallowing difficulties and gastro-oesophageal reflux are also common and often lead to aspiration pneumonia. Microcephaly is common and flexion contractures of the knees and elbows are often present by late childhood. Associated disabilities, especially speech and visual problems are particularly prevalent.

Associated problems

Children with cerebral palsy commonly have additional problems, especially if they have the quadriplegic or severe hemiplegic form of the condition. These problems include the following:
• learning difficulties;
• epilepsy;
• visual impairment;
• squint;
• hearing loss;
• speech disorders;
• behaviour disorders;
• feeding difficulties;
• undernutrition and poor growth;
• respiratory problems.

Presentation and how the diagnosis is made

Surveillance of babies who have suffered a cerebral insult is the commonest way in which cerebral palsy is diagnosed, others may be detected in the course of child health surveillance. In the neonatal period the diagnosis may be suspected if a baby has difficulty sucking, irritability, convulsions or an abnormal neurolgical examination. However, many of these infants subsequently develop normally, so it is important that cerebral palsy is not mistakenly diagnosed too early.

The diagnosis is usually made later in the first year of life when the following features emerge.
• *Abnormalities of tone.* Initially the tone may be quite reduced but eventually spasticity develops.
• *Delays in motor development.* Marked head lag and delays in sitting and rolling over are usually found.
• *Abnormal patterns of development.* Movements are not only delayed but also abnormal in quality.
• *Persistence of primitive reflexes.* Primitive reflexes such as the Moro, grasp and asymmetric tonic neck reflex (see p. 26) persist beyond the age when they normally disappear.

The diagnosis is made on clinical grounds. As the clinical picture takes time to evolve, repeated examinations are often required to establish the diagnosis. Once made, a multidisciplinary assessment is needed to define the extent of the difficulties.

Investigations

The aetiology of the cerebral palsy is often evident from the history. Rarely, further investigation is required to rule out progressive disorders. Computed tomography (CT) or magnetic resonance imaging (MRI) scans may be useful in demonstrating cerebral malformations, delineating the extent of structural lesions and ruling out very rare progressive or treatable causes such as tumours.

Principles of management

The goals of management fall into two categories: those specific to cerebral palsy, and those related to any child with a disability. As regards cerebral palsy itself, the effects of spasticity and the development of contractures must be minimized by regular physiotherapy and the child provided with aids to allow for independent mobility. The associated problems that commonly occur in cerebral palsy must be actively sought and management provided.

As for any child with a disability, appropriate schooling and educational resources must be provided to meet any special educational needs. One must ensure that the family are provided with adequate financial, practical and emotional support, and the child must be helped to integrate as much as possible into society.

Practical aspects of management

Most children with cerebral palsy have multiple difficulties and require a multidisciplinary input. This is best provided by a child development team, in order to ensure good

Principles of management
Cerebral palsy

- To minimize the effects of spasticity and development of contractures

- To identify and manage associated problems

- To ensure the child is provided with appropriate support for their special educational needs

- To ensure the family has adequate support: financial, practical and emotional

- To maximize the child's integration into society

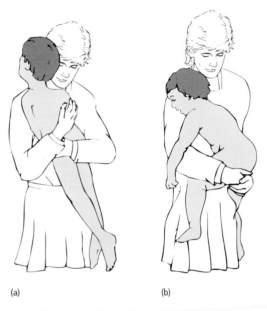

(a)   (b)

Fig. 7.4 Holding a child with cerebral palsy. (a) Incorrect. (b) Correct.

liaison between professionals and parents, and to structure a coordinated programme of treatment to meet all the child's needs.

Therapy

Physiotherapy

The role of the physiotherapist is crucial in the management of the child with cerebral palsy. It is the physiotherapist who advises on handling and mobilization (Fig. 7.4). The family must be taught how to handle the child in daily activities such as feeding, carrying, dressing and bathing in ways that will limit the effects of abnormal muscle tone. They are also taught a series of exercises designed to prevent the develop-

ment of deforming contractures. The physiotherapist may also provide a variety of aids, such as firm boots, lightweight splints and walking frames for the child who is beginning to walk.

Occupational therapy

The role of the occupational therapist overlaps with that of the physiotherapist. The occupational therapist is trained to advise on special equipment such as wheelchairs and seating, and also on play materials and activities that best encourage the child's hand function.

Speech therapy

The speech and language therapist is involved in advising on feeding and language. In the early months advice may be required for feeding and swallowing difficulties. Later, a thorough assessment of the child's developing speech and language is often required and help given on all aspects of communication including non-verbal systems when necessary.

Medication

Drugs, other than anticonvulsants for epilepsy, have a limited role in cerebral palsy. If spasticity is severe and causing pain, a drug to reduce muscle spasm is sometimes prescribed.

Orthopaedic surgery

Even with adequate physiotherapy, orthopaedic deformities may develop as a result of long-standing muscle weakness or spasticity. Dislocation of the hips may occur as a result of spasticity in the thigh adductors and fixed equinus deformity of the ankle as a result of calf muscle spasticity. Both of these may require orthopaedic surgery.

Nutrition

Undernutrition commonly occurs in children with cerebral palsy, and can reduce the child's chances of achieving his or her physical and intellectual potential. Food must be given in a form appropriate to the child's ability to chew and swallow. Energy-rich supplements and medical treatment for reflux, if present, may be required. If the child is unable to eat adequate amounts a gastrostomy may need to be placed.

Routine review of the child with cerebral palsy

The child with cerebral palsy requires regular review by the child development team to ensure that needs are being met, and that new needs are recognized. The role of the doctor in

school various facilities should be available for the young adult with learning disabilities, including an adult training centre, special hostels, communities and vocational training schemes.

THE DEAF CHILD

Prevalence

About 4% of school children have a hearing loss. Most of these are mild, usually resulting from secretory otitis media (p. 105). Two per 1000 children have moderate deafness and require a hearing aid, and a further one per 1000 is severely deaf requiring special education. Some children are at a higher risk for hearing impairment, as shown in Table 7.11.

Aetiology/pathophysiology (Table 7.12)

Conductive deafness is an extremely common problem in childhood. It results from persistent effusions in the middle ear, a complication of otitis media (see p. 105), and is known as chronic secretory otitis media or glue ear. Sensorineural deafness occurs as a result of damage to the cochlear or auditory nerve. It is rarer, but a cause of more significant disability.

Presentation/diagnosis

Children may present either when parents become concerned that their child is not responding to sound, or if the child's speech and language development is delayed. Children may also be identified if they fail to respond to the routine hearing test which is carried out at the age of 7 months. If the hearing loss is secondary to secretory otitis media, the tympanic membranes look dull and may be retracted.

The hearing deficit is confirmed by audiological testing (see p. 285). If a child is unable to cooperate, or if an objective test is required, brain stem evoked responses (BSER), an electrophysiological measure, is carried out.

Clinical features

The clinical features vary with the severity of the hearing deficit and the age at which it presents. If it is congenital, the child will be delayed in talking. If the onset is later, the child may present with behavioural difficulties which may not be immediately identified as a result of lack of hearing. Deafness is particularly common in certain medical conditions such as cerebral palsy.

Chronic secretory otitis media may be characterized by fluctuating hearing loss as the middle ear fluid may resolve only to return with each upper respiratory tract infection (URTI).

Associated problems

Hearing deficits frequently occur in association with learning disabilities, visual deficits and neurological disorders.

Principles of management

If the hearing deficit is secondary to secretory otitis media, the management is surgical (see below). Neurosensory loss is only rarely correctable surgically and the most important aspect of management therefore is to promote the child's ability to communicate from an early age. If the hearing deficit is significant this will usually require sign language, which is used in conjunction with oral speech.

Deafness is an enormous social barrier, and an important part of management must be to encourage the child to participate fully in school and society at large.

Table 7.11 Children at risk for hearing impairment

History of meningitis
History of recurrent otitis media
Significantly delayed or unclear speech
Family history of deafness
Parental suspicion of deafness
Children with cerebral palsy
Children with cleft palate
Children with absent or deformed ears

Table 7.12 Causes of deafness in school children

Conductive deafness
Almost all cases due to glue ear following otitis media
Sensorineural deafness
Damage to the cochlear or auditory nerve
Genetic
Various types 50%
Intrauterine
Congenital infection e.g. rubella, cytomegalovirus (CMV)
Perinatal (12%)
Birth asphyxia
Severe hyperbilirubinaemia
Postnatal (30%)
Meningitis
Encephalitis
Head Injury

Practical aspects of management

Conductive hearing loss

Medical treatment in the form of decongestants and anti-histamines are ineffectual in the management of middle ear effusion. If the effusion is causing persistent hearing loss surgical intervention is required. Tiny plastic tubes (grommets) are inserted into the tympanic membrane to aerate the middle ear and drain the fluid. Adenoidectomy may be performed at the same time. When grommets are in place the child must take care not to allow water to enter the ear canal at bath time or when swimming. The grommets usually eventually fall out spontaneously. They may not need to be replaced as the condition resolves as the child grows.

Sensorineural deafness

Hearing aids
A hearing aid is a device which amplifies sound. It may be

Principles of management
Hearing loss

Conductive hearing loss
- Correct by placement of grommets

Sensorineural hearing loss
- Ensure the child has a means of communication

- This may involve sign language

- Maximize hearing by use of a hearing aid

- Ensure schooling is appropriate and that support is provided

---

worn behind the ear or in a pocket or harness. Some aids have special features such as amplification of low or high frequencies and circuits to reduce intense peaks of noise. Most aids can be used with the 'loop' wiring system which transmits the teacher's voice, bypassing background noise. Selection of the most suitable aid is made by a

---

HEARING LOSS AT A GLANCE

Prevalence

4% of children have hearing deficits
3 per 1000 are moderately or severely impaired

Aetiology/pathophysiology

Most mild to moderate hearing loss is conductive and a result of secretory otitis media
Sensorineural deafness may be genetic, a result of pre or perinatal problems or follow a cerebral insult later in life

Clinical features

Lack of response to speech
Delayed speech
Behavioural problems

Associated problems

Learning difficulties
Neurological disorders
Visual deficits

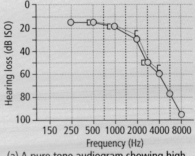

(a) A pure tone audiogram showing high frequency sensorineural deafness

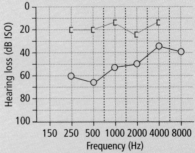

(b) A pure tone audiogram showing conductive deafness. The bone conduction is normal but the air conductive curve is impaired. There is 20–30 dB hearing loss

Presentation and how the diagnosis is made

Child health surveillance
Parental concern

Practical aspects of management

Grommets for conductive hearing loss
Hearing aids
Communication
Education

Issues for the family

Communication with child may involve learning sign language
Genetic counselling

Issues for the school

Moderately deaf children can attend a normal school
The severely deaf require specialist education at a school for the deaf or a partially hearing unit attached to a normal school

paediatric audiologist, who also teaches the family about its management and maintenance.

Communication

In the past there has been some controversy over teaching sign language on the basis that children must learn to live in a hearing world. However, it is now generally accepted that providing an alternative non-verbal means of communication increases a child's ability to relate to others, reduces the isolation and frustration of being unable to hear, and even encourages language development. Sign language is taught in conjunction with oral speech. Lip-reading is also valuable, and electronic analysers are a new development which can help the child to speak more clearly by converting voice patterns to visual displays.

Education

The peripatetic teacher of the deaf, who is employed by the local education authority is responsible for the child's early education and management, and later in advising on school placement.

Issues for the family

If the hearing deficit is sensorineural, the parents need to learn how to communicate with their deaf child and promote the child's communication skills. Some causes of deafness are genetic and in these circumstances genetic counselling is required.

Issues for the school

Many moderately deaf children can attend a normal school. The child is helped by sitting near to the teacher in order to maximize concentration. The 'loop' wiring system is a valuable development. More severely affected children require specialist education either at a school for the deaf or at a partially hearing unit attached to a mainstream school.

THE BLIND OR PARTIALLY SIGHTED CHILD

Blindness and partial sight are best defined functionally rather than by the degree of visual acuity. A child is defined as blind if he or she requires education by methods which cannot involve sight. If the child is of adequate intelligence this will include Braille. A child is defined as partially sighted if he or she requires special education but can use methods which depend on sight, such as large print books. In practice, most blind children have some vision even if it is only recognition of light and dark.

Prevalence

One in 2500 children is registered blind or partially sighted. Fifty per cent have additional handicaps.

Aetiology/pathophysiology

The commonest causes of blindness are optic atrophy, congenital cataracts, and choroidoretinal degeneration. In almost half of cases the cause is genetically determined, and in one third it is related to perinatal problems such as retinopathy of prematurity (see p. 246).

Clinical features

The eyes may be obviously abnormal in appearance, and nystagmus or roving, purposeless eye movements may be present. Babies who have a visual deficit from birth follow an altered pattern of development. Smiling tends to occur at the usual age, but is less consistent and reliable and, as the baby develops, his or her response to sound is unaccompanied by turning towards the source. Motor skills, both gross and fine are likely to be delayed. Hand regard is poor and reaching for objects and the development of a fine pincer grip is slow. Early language development may be normal, but the acquisition of vocabulary and more complex language may be delayed.

The child with visual deficits frequently develops mannerisms such as eye poking, eye rubbing and rocking. These are known as blindisms and probably occur as they induce pleasurable visual gratification of retinal origin. Neither these mannerisms, nor the delayed development should be regarded as evidence in themselves of significant learning difficulties.

Associated problems

Intelligence has an important influence on the child's ability to cope with visual difficulties. However, 50% of children with visual deficits have additional disabilities such as hearing deficits or severe learning difficulties and do less well.

Presentation and how the diagnosis is made

Babies may be identified in the neonatal period if for example cataracts are found (p. 235), or nystagmus or roving, purposeless eye movements are present. If, however, the eyes appear normal, it is frequently the mother who first suspects a problem when she fails to elicit eye contact. Children may also be identified in the course of child health surveillance (see p. 47). It must be emphasized that if a parent raises concern about poor vision this should be taken seriously.

VISUAL IMPAIRMENT AT A GLANCE

Definition

A child is defined as blind if education can only be provided by methods not involving sight e.g. Braille
A child is partially sighted if educational methods, such as large print books, can be used

Epidemiology

1 in 2500 children are registered blind or partially sighted
50% have additional handicaps

Aetiology/pathophysiology

Commonest causes are
Optic atrophy (**a**)
Congenital cataracts (**b**)
Choroidoretinal degeneration (**c**)

Clinical features

- The eyes may look abnormal or have unusual movements
- If the deficit is congenital, early smiling is inconsistent and there is no turning towards sound
- Reaching for objects and the pincer grip is delayed
- Early language may be normal, but complex language may be delayed
- 'Blindism' (eye poking, eye rubbing and rocking) may occur

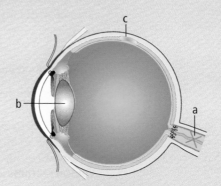

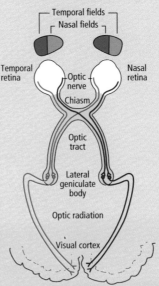

Associated problems

Hearing deficit or severe learning difficulties are common

Presentation and how the diagnosis is made

Malformations at birth, or later when developmental delay is evident

Practical aspects of management

Early intervention to improve developmental progress, reduce blindisms and increase parental confidence
Preschool: a peripatetic teacher from the Royal National Institute for the Blind
Advice on appropriate schooling
Mobility training
Supportive services

Issues for the family

Advice on non-visual stimulation and child-rearing
Adaptation of the home

Issues for the school

Mainstream nursery and nursery school with supportive services are often appropriate
Beyond this, mainstream school, a partially sighted unit, or a school for the blind (depending on learning abilities)

If a visual defect is suspected examination by an ophthalmologist is indicated. In the young child visual evoked response (VER) testing is often required. The VER is an electrophysiological method of evaluating the response to light and special visual stimuli.

Principles of management

Management is directed towards providing early intervention in order to promote developmental progress, reduce blindisms and to increase parental confidence. The family needs supportive services and the child requires appropriate educational resources.

Practical aspects of management

A peripatetic teacher is provided either by the local authority or the Royal National Institute for the Blind to advise parents in the preschool years.

At school level, improvements in equipment have occurred in recent years so that the child with partial sight may now be able to cope in a mainstream school. These improvements include better optical aids, good illumination, and reading material in very large type. Braille remains the essential method of reading for the child with a severe visual deficit, providing learning disabilities are not present.

Principles of management
Visual impairment

- To provide early intervention in order to improve developmental progress

- To support the family and increase parental confidence

- To provide appropriate educational resources

Mobility training is an essential part of education. As the child matures, instruction must be given in travel outside of school, initially under supervision and then independently.

Issues for the family

Parents of a blind child need help at a very early stage. They must be taught to stimulate their infant using non-visual means, such as touch and speech, and must continue to provide stimulation through the early years with appropriate play materials. The home is likely to require adaptation so that the child can explore this environment safely.

Issues for the school

Mainstream nursery and nursery school are often appropriate for the child with a visual handicap, provided support from the peripatetic teacher is available. Beyond this, factors such as the child's intellect and ability to make use of residual vision, the wishes of the family and the long-term prognosis determine whether placement should be in a mainstream school, partially sighted unit or a school for the blind.

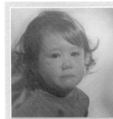

8 Emotional and Behavioural Problems

Introduction, 289
Approach to the child with emotional, behavioural and school problems, 289
Common behavioural and emotional problems in childhood, 291

Sleeping problems, 291
Eating difficulties, 292
Unwanted habits, 292
Psychosomatic symptoms, 293

Difficult and disobedient behaviour, 293
School-based problems, 294
Causes of failure at school, 295

She was not really bad at heart,
But only rather rude and wild;
She was an aggravating child.

Rebecca, Who Slammed Doors for Fun
Hilaire Belloc

Introduction

This chapter covers some common problems (Table 8.1) that are rather different from other conditions presenting to a doctor during childhood, as in the main they do not require a differential diagnosis. On the surface they may seem to lie more in the province of a psychologist, but parents very commonly turn to their doctor for advice about these problems and it is very important that the doctor learns to feel comfortable in addressing them.

Many of these emotional and behavioural problems occur to some degree in all children, but can become exaggerated for a variety of reasons, either related to the child, or as a result of the way they are handled. Other difficulties arise as a result of stresses in the family, such as death or divorce, or are caused by problems at school.

Some childhood behaviours, notably deliberate destructive conduct and self harm, running away, encopresis and age inappropriate sexual behaviour are indicative of serious disturbance (Table 8.2).

Factors that contribute to emotional and behavioural problems, and those that protect against their development are shown in Tables 8.3 and 8.4.

Approach to the child with emotional, behavioural and school problems

In addressing emotional and behavioural problems, more than any other problems in childhood, it is essential that the focus does not rest on the child alone. An understanding of the difficulties must be seen in the context of the family and the child's environment. Even if these factors are not directly responsible for the problem (and they often are), it is impossible to address the issue without a good understanding of the broader picture. It is also important to remember that handling these problems well takes both time and empathy.

History

• *The problem.* A full picture of the problem or difficulty must be obtained, with parents' perceptions of the cause, and how the situation is handled. Where the child is old enough, it is worthwhile to include him or her in this process.
• *The child.* It is important to gain an understanding of the child's temperament and personality, an idea of how the child is viewed by the parents, and how he or she relates to friends and family.
• *Recent events.* Childhood disturbances often occur as a reaction to events in the family. Common triggers include the birth of a sibling, the death of a grandparent or a move to a new house or school.
• *The family.* An understanding of family circumstances is essential. Marital friction is a common source of childhood emotional and behavioural problems, and single parents are likely to have more difficulties in disciplining and coping with their children single handed. Isolation compounds any problem, and the level of support in terms of relatives and friends is important to assess.
• *School or nursery.* School life brings its own problems and also affects how the child adjusts to difficulties at home. Peer and teacher relationships are as important to assess as the level of academic achievement.

Management

While emotional and behavioural problems differ from one another and from family to family, there is a commonality to approaching their management. Perhaps the most important aspect is to listen well, hearing a full account of the problem. This in itself can be therapeutic, and can lead the family to find solutions themselves. The process of listening cannot be rushed: adequate time must be given.

Table 8.1 Common emotional and behavioural problems in childhood

Sleeping difficulties
Eating problems
Unwanted habits
Difficult and disobedient behaviour
School-based problems
Psychosomatic symptoms
Enuresis

Table 8.2 Behaviour indicative of serious disturbance

Behaviour	Disturbance
Deliberately destructive	Low self esteem, hostile relationships
Deliberate self harm	Severe distress, low self esteem
Running away	Lack of affection, severe distress
Encopresis	Lack of self worth, inadequate care
Age inappropriate sexual behaviour	Sexual abuse

Table 8.3 Factors contributing to emotional and behavioural problems

In the child
Difficult temperament
Developmental delay
Poor self image
School failure
Abuse
In the family
Marital problems
Death of a relative, friend or pet
Poor discipline
Poverty
In school
Change of school
Bullying
Poor peer relationships

Table 8.4 Protective factors against emotional/behavioural problems

Consistent loving relationships
Adequate income
Stable family relationships
Support outside the family

Focal points
Evaluating the child with emotional and behavioural problems

- Allow adequate time to make a full assessment

- If the child is old enough to cooperate, obtain his or her account too

- Ensure that you obtain a full picture of the problem, the child, the family and the environment

- Where relevant, confer with other adults involved such as grandparents, teachers, childminders, etc.

Guidelines for parents in preventing and managing difficult behaviour

- Provide structure and routine in everyday life

- Set clear limits of acceptable behaviour

- Be consistent

- 'Catch your child being good' and reward positive rather than punish negative behaviour

- Enforce the above with love and affection

Many parental concerns relate to normal behaviour, for example food fads in toddlers or nightwaking in infants and it may be adequate simply to provide reassurance. Other concerns relate to difficult behaviour, and guidance regarding effective discipline is required.

The general principles of effective discipline include providing structure and routine in everyday life, setting clear limits of acceptable behaviour, rewarding good behaviour, and being consistent with punishments. Punitive anger is often ineffective and does not encourage the child to learn to control their actions and emotions. It is helpful to remind parents that positive results can be obtained by simply 'catching their child being good', rather than always looking to punish negative behaviour.

Star charts
A useful strategy in overcoming difficult behaviour is using a star chart, which can be adapted to improve and motivate a variety of behaviours, from enuresis to temper tantrums and disruptive behaviour at school. A calendar is drawn up and each day the child has behaved as required, a star or smiley face is awarded. When a certain number of stars have been earned the child is rewarded with a prize. This method can be very effective in reinforcing desirable behaviour, while alleviating focus on the negative.

Guidelines for managing emotional and behavioural problems

- Family and school issues must be addressed as well as the child's problems

- Parents need to be provided with guidelines for effective discipline, to be enforced with love and affection

- Star charts and time out are useful strategies

- Do not wait for a child to grow out of a problem. Even if the problem resolves the child may remain psychologically damaged

- Medication has a very limited role and should only be prescribed by specialists

Guidelines for preventing and managing sleeping problems

- Set a bedtime

- Have a relaxing bedtime routine

- Say goodnight

- If the child cries, ignore or at least give no positive attention

- If the child gets out of bed return him or her promptly and firmly

- Give positive reinforcement following good nights

Time out

Time out is a strategy used during an episode of difficult behaviour. The child is required to stay in a quiet spot for a fixed short period of time. One minute per year of age is a good guide, and a kitchen timer a useful way of enforcing the time. This method allows the child (and the parent) time to cool off, and also gives the parent a clear but limited non-violent means of discipline.

An important aspect of good management is to arrange a follow-up appointment for the parents. Other professionals may also provide support and help for the child. The health visitor is a particular asset for the preschool child, and the teacher for the child at school. More intransigent cases may require referral to a child psychologist or psychiatrist.

COMMON BEHAVIOURAL AND EMOTIONAL PROBLEMS IN CHILDHOOD

Sleeping problems

Difficulties in settling to sleep and waking through the night

Babies and children differ in their requirements for sleep, and parents vary in their ability to tolerate their child waking in the night. A substantial number of children have struggles around bedtime, and reports indicate that as many as one third of preschool children have disturbed sleep.

In most babies sleeping 'difficulties' are simply habit. They result from a lack of early establishment of routine, and develop so that toddlers readily realize that by playing up at bedtime they can control their parents. Sleep difficulties can also occur as a result of conflict in the family, or anxieties, such as starting school or fear of dying.

Clinical features Sleeping problems include a refusal to settle at night and waking through the night. Difficulties in settling commonly develop if babies are only put to bed once they are already asleep, and may also persist after a child wakes at night as a result of having been unwell. A common mistake is for parents to take the child into their bed or to sleep with the child for comfort. Once this pattern is established, it is difficult to break.

Management Parents may be resigned to sleepless nights and may not be aware that they are capable of controlling the situation. The problem can only be overcome if they are determined to tackle it. This is most easily achieved at an age when the child cannot climb out of bed. Night sedation is best avoided and should only be used as a last resort.

Successful management involves the following principles. A regular routine should be firmly established with parents adopting a calm, understanding but determined attitude, while avoiding angry threats and punishments. Bedtime should be set at a regular time, with time for a quiet, restful prebedtime routine, which might include a warm bath, light snack and reading a story. At the set time the child should resolutely be put to bed. If the child cries then, or later through the night, the crying should be ignored, or if that proves to be too stressful for the parent, the child may be checked but no positive attention given. On no account should the child be taken to the parental bed. If the parents are resolute, the sleeping problem resolves within a short period. However, it is usually a stressful undertaking and plenty of support, reassurance and encouragement are required.

Nightmares and night terrors

Nightmares

In a nightmare the child wakes as a result of a bad dream, becomes lucid quickly and usually remembers the dream's content. The child can often simply be reassured and returned to sleep. Nightmares may occur as a result of stresses and if persistent may need psychological help.

Night terrors

Night terrors (see p. 180) are a sleep problem of the preschool years. By contrast with a nightmare the child wakes confused, disorientated and frightened, and fails to recognize the parent. Minutes pass before orientation occurs and the dream cannot usually be recalled. Night terrors should not be confused with epilepsy. They are shortlived and reassurance alone is required.

Eating difficulties

Most children at some stage or another develop food fads. Difficulties frequently result if there is excessive parental insistence on eating and subsequent anxiety when the child refuses to do so. In fact, most of the worry about children's eating is unnecessary, and the majority of children come through this phase thriving and unscathed. Mismanagement by the parent can result in a great deal of conflict and stress at mealtimes, which is particularly distressing as it challenges the parents' basic need to nurture. The problems are compounded if the eating problems are associated with failure to thrive (see p. 61).

Occasionally, severe eating problems are caused by emotional stress and can be associated with problems in the parent–child relationship. Eating difficulties in adolescence are discussed in Chapter 11.

Clinical features Eating difficulties may present early in infancy, or more commonly develop during weaning. They may follow a minor illness, where appetite is naturally reduced, and negative reactions to food are set up as a result of parental insistence to eat. The child then develops adversive behaviour such as refusing to eat, spitting out or throwing food, or even vomiting. Parents may respond by force feeding, playing games, preparing alternative meals or persisting with lengthy mealtimes in order to get just another mouthful in.

Management Eating difficulties can be hard to tackle. It is important to reduce the parents' anxiety, and it is often helpful to demonstrate that the child is growing normally according to a growth chart. Battles over food are always best avoided and relaxed, social family meals should be encouraged. A high chair is invaluable for the toddler at meal times, both for comfort and restraint. The child's

Guidelines for preventing and managing eating difficulties

- Be guided by the child's appetite
- Mealtimes should be relaxed social events
- Do not resort to bribery, games or force
- End the meal at first sign of adverse behaviour
- Do not provide alternatives if a meal is refused

appetite should be respected and no attempts made to make the child eat by bribery, games or force. With reduction in anxiety and pressure the problem usually resolves.

Although the diet often lacks variety it is usually nutritionally adequate and prescription of vitamins is not necessary.

Unwanted habits

Children not infrequently indulge in habits that concern their parents. These include thumb-sucking, head-banging, body-rocking, nail-biting, hair-pulling, teeth-grinding and tics. The child may not be able to control these habits, which may be further reinforced by parents attempting to stop the child exhibiting them. As the child grows older he or she often learns to inhibit the habit, particularly in social situations.

Thumb-sucking

Thumb-sucking is normal in early infancy. However, beyond a certain age it makes the older child appear immature and may interfere with normal alignment of the teeth. It is a difficult habit to influence, and it is best to ignore it as it resolves over time. The child who actively tries to restrain thumb-sucking should be given praise and encouragement.

Nail-biting

Nail-biting is a difficult habit to break, and it is only possible to influence if the child is resolved to do so. Application of bitter tasting nail varnish can be helpful. In some children it is a sign of tension.

Masturbation

Masturbation is common in children, and this sometimes presents as a problem, particularly if it occurs publicly. It is more likely to appear when the child is bored, anxious or tired, and the child can often be distracted at these times. Dressing the child in clothes that makes access more difficult may help. Parents should be told to ignore the habit in younger children. The older child should not be reprimanded, but does need to be informed that it is not a social activity and should not be carried out publicly.

Enuresis

Failure to achieve toilet training or regression to wetting may be, and often is, a sign of stress. Common precipitating events include the birth of a sibling, death in the family, move to a new home and marital conflict. Enuresis may also result from inadequate or inappropriate toilet training. Enuresis is fully discussed in Chapter 5 (p. 186).

Encopresis

Encopresis, or the passage of faeces in inappropriate places, usually indicates a serious emotional disturbance. It needs to be distinguished from soiling, which results from leakage of liquid faeces around hard stool when a child is constipated. Encopresis and soiling are covered in Chapter 5 (p. 172).

Psychosomatic symptoms

Some children manifest emotional problems in the form of psychosomatic symptoms. The commonest of these symptoms are abdominal pain in the younger child and headaches in the older child. Once organic causes for these complaints have been excluded (see Chapter 5) the possibility of an underlying emotional cause must be explored.

Difficult and disobedient behaviour

Temper tantrums

Temper tantrums are a normal aspect of a child's development and peak at around the ages of 18 months to 3 years.

Clinical features Frustration, anger and tantrums are typical for toddlers, and may involve hitting, biting and other potentially harmful behaviour. Some babies and toddlers may resort to breath-holding (see p. 179) as part of the tantrum and this is often a frightening event to witness.

Management The parental response to tantrums is very important. Caregivers who respond to toddler defiance with

---

Guidelines for preventing and managing temper tantrums

- Prevent tantrums by avoiding high-risk situations such as hunger and tiredness
- Attempt to divert the tantrum if possible
- Teach control by example
- Reward good behaviour
- Ignore the behaviour and leave the child until calm
- Use time out as a strategy

---

punitive anger run the risk of reinforcing defiance, and teach the child that out of control emotions are a reasonable response to frustration. Temper tantrums need firm handling, without anger and aggression. They can often be averted by avoiding high-risk situations like hunger and tiredness, and the episode diverted by providing distraction or allowing the child to have simple choices of activities. Once the tantrum is in full cry, it is best to ignore it until the child has calmed down. Time out is an excellent strategy for managing the tantrum after the event.

Aggressive behaviour

Young children often have aggressive outbursts ranging from temper tantrums, hurting others or destroying toys or furniture. This behaviour usually results from frustration and the child's inability to deal with it. Most children learn to control their aggression, but some fail to do so, and it escalates as a problem, leading to bullying in primary school and delinquency beyond. If the behaviour is extreme, the psychiatric term conduct disorder is applied.

Clinical features Several factors contribute to aggression. Boys more than girls, large, active children and children from larger families tend to show more aggressive behaviour. Marital discord and aggression within the home contribute to its expression, and exposure to aggression on television may also have an effect. There is a relationship between aggression and emotional disturbance, school failure, brain damage and overactivity.

Management Parents need to be consistent in their management of the child exhibiting aggressive behaviour, and, difficult though it may be, must resist from counteracting aggression with more aggression. Both time out and star charts are positive methods for managing the child. It is important for the doctor to explore whether frustration, disturbance and tensions in the home can be reduced.

For the school-age child, management must involve the staff at school in order to address any academic or social problems, and to gain cooperation in instituting behaviour modification. If aggression and bullying (see below) are general problems for the school, instituting school based intervention can be effective.

Hyperactivity (see Attention deficit disorder, p. 295)

Hyperactivity is characterized by poor ability to attend to a task, motor overactivity and impulsivity. In the preschool years, children are naturally active and tend to have a short attention span for activities. How this is viewed often depends on parental perceptions, and a child with high spirits in one family may be perceived to be hyperactive in another.

Boys tend to suffer from hyperactivity more than girls, and there is often a family history. Babies who have been temperamentally difficult are more likely to develop into hyperactive children, and it is more common in children with delay of developmental milestones. Hyperactivity is also seen in children who have never been given limits or taught to develop self control, and it occurs as a reaction to tensions and problems in the home.

Clinical features It is important to be aware that the hyperactive child may not demonstrate the extent of his or her hyperactivity in the visit to the doctor, and the history is therefore more important than observation in the clinical setting. The hyperactive child is restless, impulsive and excitable, and fails to focus on any activity for long. The child tends to have little sense of danger, and requires great vigilance. As such children are unable to concentrate for long on any quiet activity, they often have difficulties on starting school.

Management The hyperactive child benefits from routine and regularity in everyday life. He or she needs to have firm boundaries set for his or her behaviour and consistency in discipline. On starting school, the support of the teacher is essential in helping with adjustment. Medical management is discussed on p. 295.

School-based problems

Teasing and bullying

Bullying is a major problem for many children. Overall, about 10% of children report being bullied once per week and 7% of children are identified as bullies. It is important to remember that victims may be bullies themselves and that most bullying goes undetected by parents and teachers. Bullying tends to be more common in primary schools, and varies from school to school according to the ethos.

Clinical features A child may or may not admit to being a victim of bullying, and it should therefore be considered as a possible cause of distress whenever a school child is disturbed. The child may react to bullying by becoming withdrawn, aggressive or develop psychosomatic symptoms. It is a common cause for school refusal.

Management In schools where bullying is a problem, a whole school approach is most effective so that the ethos of bullying becomes unacceptable, and both the victims and the bullies are helped. The individual child needs help in handling the situation and increasing self esteem. Any school refusal must be addressed instantly (see p. 295).

Non-attendance at school

Most absences from school (Table 8.5) occur as a result of illnesses, which are usually minor. These absences may be prolonged through parental anxiety, particularly if the child has a chronic illness (see p. 315). In some circumstances, parents may keep their child at home to help care for younger siblings or elderly relatives or even to help out at work. The two situations where the doctor may become involved are school refusal and truancy.

Clinical features The main distinction between school refusal and truancy is that in the former everyone knows where the child is, but in the latter the child's whereabouts are unknown during school hours.

School refusal may result from either separation anxiety or school phobia. Anxiety on separating from parents is common on first starting school, and also may be precipitated by a traumatic event, such as a family death. School phobia is usually triggered by distressing events at school,

Table 8.5 Reasons for school absence

Illness
Kept at home by parent
School refusal
Truancy

such as problems with peers or teachers. In both types of school refusal the child is usually well behaved with no academic problems, although there may be associated neurotic behaviour.

Truancy is commonest in secondary school particularly in the last years, and is probably universal to a degree. Persistent truancy is associated with generally antisocial behaviour, poor academic achievement and unsettled family background.

Management Management of school absenteeism must involve close collaboration between the parents and the teachers. In most cases of school refusal the child should be returned to school as quickly as possible, while addressing underlying problems. Delaying the return only exacerbates the problem. Truancy is harder to tackle and requires a total treatment package. The needs of the child must be met, including any learning problems. The education welfare officer should become involved if the truancy is persistent.

School failure

Failure at school has profound effects for the individual not only in terms of his or her achievements in adult life and chances of employment, but also in terms of quality of life in the school years. School failure is associated with low self esteem, behavioural difficulties and psychosomatic disorders. Children may fail at school for a number of reasons, both educational and social, that may compound each other (Table 8.6). From the educational point of view it is particularly important to address causes such as dyslexia, attention deficits and visual or hearing impairments that reduce the child's potential to learn, and can lead to frustration and other negative psychological reactions.

Table 8.6 Causes for failing at school

Educational
Limited intellect
Attention deficit disorder
Hearing or visual deficit
Dyslexia
Dyspraxia
Social
Problems at home
Peer problems
Absence from school

Causes of failure at school

Dyslexia

Dyslexia is the commonest type of specific learning difficulty. The dyslexic child is unable to process effectively the information required in order to read. The result is a reading ability below that expected for the child's general level of intelligence. Dyslexia must be differentiated from slow reading as a result of limited intellect or inadequate teaching. It is much more common in boys and there is often a family history.

Clinical features The child often has a history of delay in learning to talk. There may be difficulties other than reading, and spelling is affected more than reading. If not recognized, the child is likely to fail at school and commonly responds by withdrawing or exhibiting disruptive behaviour.

Management If suspected the diagnosis must be confirmed on testing by an educational psychologist. The child needs individual help in overcoming the difficulty, and may need statementing (see Chapter 7, p. 275).

Attention deficit disorder

Attention deficit disorder refers to a difficulty in generally focusing on tasks or activities. It may or may not occur with hyperactivity (see p. 294) and is far commoner in boys than girls. These children often have a history of being colicky, temperamentally difficult babies.

Clinical features The child is fidgety, has a difficult time remaining in his or her seat at school, is easily distracted and impulsive, has difficulty following instructions, talks excessively and flits from one activity to another. Daydreaming is more obvious if hyperactivity is not a feature.

Management The child benefits from a regular daily routine with simple clear rules, and firm limits enforced fairly and sympathetically. Overstimulation and overfatigue should be avoided. In school a structured programme is required with good home communication to ensure consistency.

Attention deficit problems, particularly if associated with hyperactivity, can be very stressful to the family and counselling may be needed. Central nervous system stimulants such as methylphenidate, prescribed during school hours, have been shown to be helpful in selected cases. Therapies such as megavitamins and low sugar diets have not been proved to be effective. Diets with no artificial colourings or flavourings remain controversial, but in general do not help the majority of these children.

Prognosis Both the hyperactivity and attention difficulties tend to improve through adolescence, but the educational deficit may persist as a handicap later in life.

Dyspraxia

Clumsiness, or dyspraxia, can cause problems at home and at school. Fine motor incoordination leads to untidy writing, and gross motor incoordination leads to difficulty with sports. The academic and social difficulties that ensue can cause the child considerable unhappiness and lead to behavioural problems if they are not recognized and dealt with helpfully. An occupational therapist can assist the school in devising a programme which will help overcome the difficulties and build self confidence.

9 Emergency Paediatrics

Introduction, 297
The child presenting as an emergency, 297
Cardiorespiratory arrest, 299
Respiratory failure, 300
Upper airway obstruction, 300

Shock, 303
Causes of shock, 304
Coma, 306
Poisoning, 309

Types of poison ingestion, 310
Accidents and burns, 310
Acute life-threatening events and sudden
  infant death syndrome, 312

Elisha came into the house and behold!—the boy was dead, laid out on his bed. He entered and shut the door behind them both. Then he went up ... and placed his mouth upon his mouth ... and he warmed the flesh of the boy ... the boy sneezed seven times, and the boy opened his eyes.

Kings 2. Ch 4, 32–34

Introduction

This chapter discusses the presentation and treatment of children with acute life-threatening disorders. Children may become critically ill very rapidly and survival depends on rapid recognition of the ill child, appropriate first aid, rapid transfer to hospital and appropriate use of therapies. This chapter deals with the important basics of each of these aspects of the problem.

THE CHILD PRESENTING AS AN EMERGENCY

Pathophysiology

The homeostatic physiological milieu is relatively fragile in children and particularly so in infancy. The child has an ability to preserve intravascular volume against abnormal fluid losses as occurs in diarrhoea or excessive vomiting, but once these physiological mechanisms have been fully deployed, collapse with shock can rapidly occur.

Although life-threatening disorders often start insidiously it is important to remember that progression from minor symptoms to moribund state may occur very rapidly. This is particularly likely if the child has an underlying predisposition to severe illness (Table 9.1).

The major presenting features of children with severe illness are listed in Table 9.2. Many of these conditions are described elsewhere in this book.

Approach to the child presenting as an emergency

Initial assessment

Unlike any other aspect of paediatrics, management must precede history and examination. After very rapid assessment, the critically ill child must be resuscitated, the airway secured and the child's condition stabilized. The initial management of the critically ill child is discussed below, but the difference between life and death may depend on the management in the first hour after the collapse.

Once the initial resuscitation has taken place, the child must be carefully assessed for evidence of disease in other systems which may have caused the initial collapse, although the underlying disease may be obvious as in trauma or asthma.

History

• *Description of the events leading up to the collapse.* A detailed history from a witness of the collapse may be very helpful. This may be a teacher or a playmate if the child collapsed away from home. Establish whether the child was well immediately before the collapse or whether there was a rapidly progressive illness.

• *Previous medical history.* Knowledge of previous medical history is very important to establish whether the child has an underlying illness predisposing to collapse, such as diabetes or asthma. Has the child been on prescription drugs and could he or she have been indulging in substance abuse? In infants a recent minor illness may be significant and the severity of diarrhoea and vomiting may have been underestimated by the parents.

Physical examination

After the initial emergency assessment of the child a more careful physical examination must be carried out. Important clues as to the cause of the collapse may be obtained from the physical examination and Table 9.3 lists the important features to assess.

Table 9.1 Predisposing causes of severe illness in children

The very young
Poor nutritional state
Immunodeficiency
cancer
steroid treatment
Chronic disease

Table 9.2 The major presenting features of severe illness in children

Cardiorespiratory collapse
Respiratory failure
Upper airway obstruction
Shock
Coma
Poisoning or drug abuse
Infection (p. 103)
Dehydration (p. 116)
Metabolic disease (diabetic ketoacidosis, p. 328)
Trauma and burns

Table 9.3 Specific abormalities on clinical examination which may help in diagnosis of the underlying cause of severe illness

Rashes, particularly petechial or purpuric (see p. 198)
Depth of coma (Table 9.12)
State of hydration (p. 117)
Vital signs (blood pressure, pulse, respiratory rate, temperature)
Signs of respiratory distress
Stridor
Signs of injury
Surface area of burns

Investigations

Investigations are directed towards:
• *Diagnosis.* The appropriate investigations are discussed below in the relevant sections on causes of collapse.
• *A guide to appropriate management.* If the child requires respiratory support, a chest X-ray and regular blood gases are essential to guide management.

Management

Emergency treatment should occur where the child presents. This in practice is in an Accident and Emergency room. As soon as the child is stable he or she should be moved to an Intensive Care Unit for further monitoring and management.

Focal points
Evaluating the child presenting as an emergency

• Rapidly assess the state of the child

• Stabilize the condition

• Only then take a full history and carry out a physical examination

• Assess the child for evidence of disease in other systems which may have precipitated the emergency

---

Principles of management
The child presenting as an emergency

Assessment
This must be conducted rapidly
Is the airway clear?
Is the child breathing?
Is there adequate blood pressure?
Are there obvious injuries?
• fractures
• lacerations
• burns
What is the level of consciousness?

Resuscitation
Clear the airway
Intubate if not breathing
Cardiopulmonary resuscitation if poor cardiac output
Establish intravenous access
Pressure to stop bleeding
Immobilize fractured limbs, and neck if trauma suspected

Problem directed management
Blood gases
Treat shock with fluids (p. 304)
Investigate cause of illness
Investigate function of other organs
Ensure adequate hydration
Specific drugs once a diagnosis is made

Management of the pulse-less or moribund child must be prioritized into these four areas in sequence.

A	Airway	PLUS	D	Don't
B	Breathing		E	Ever
C	Circulation		F	Forget
D	Drugs		G	Glucose

Management of shock is discussed on p. 303. Management of the traumatized child is beyond this book's scope.

Support for relatives

During resuscitation, relatives must be kept closely informed. This is best done by taking them to a separate room out of sight and hearing of the resuscitation. A member of the resuscitation team—usually a nurse—should stay with the relatives and keep them informed of progress and give emotional support. It is best if only one person is involved in talking to the relatives during the process of resuscitation. Once the child is stabilized the most senior member of the team should inform the parents of the situation and answer their questions as honestly as possible.

CARDIORESPIRATORY ARREST

Cardiac arrest occurs as the end result of a large number of conditions affecting infants and children. The commoner causes are listed in Table 9.4.

There must be a well-rehearsed protocol for cardiac arrest that occurs in hospital. All medical staff involved in resuscitation should be appropriately trained. It is beyond the scope of this book to describe the detailed approach to the management of cardiac arrest, but the following are important principles.

Management

The process of resuscitation is a team effort and requires an experienced paediatrician and anaesthetist together with

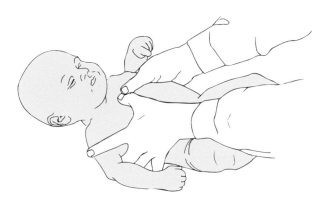

Fig. 9.1 External cardiac massage in an infant. The compression rate should be 120 per minute with six compressions to each ventilatory breath.

nursing support. The most senior doctor on the team should take charge of the resuscitation and if necessary be the person who decides how long resuscitation should continue if there is no response.

The principles of managing the child with cardiac arrest is the same for any critically ill child. Proceed in the sequence:
- Clear the airway by suction under direct vision if necessary.
- Establish ventilation through an endotracheal tube.
- Give external cardiac massage (Fig. 9.1).
- Give cardiac stimulant drugs.

Once the initial resuscitation has been established, then con-

Table 9.4 Commoner causes of cardiorespiratory arrest

Severe respiratory disease
Upper airway obstruction
Cardiac disease Arrhythmia Cardiac failure Myocarditis
Neurological disorder Birth asphyxia Cerebral oedema Coning Head injury
Drug ingestion
Severe hypoxic–ischaemic insult Suffocation Drowning
Drug or toxin

Principles of management
Cardiorespiratory arrest

Airway
Clear oropharynx
Intubate

Breathing
Ventilate with a self-expanding resuscitation bag
Mouth-to-mouth if nothing else available

Circulation
External cardiac massage
Alternate one lung inflation with six cardiac compressions
Display ECG trace and defibrillate if appropriate

Drugs
Establish vascular access for drug administration
Alternatively, some drugs can be given down the endotracheal tube or by
    direct intracardiac injection
Check blood sugar, give glucose if low

sideration should turn to the cause of the collapse and the child should be monitored very closely in an intensive care environment.

RESPIRATORY FAILURE

Respiratory failure is the end result of a large number of causes, but its definition is usually based on abnormal arterial blood gases with both severe hypoxia and hypercapnia (see p. 358).

A careful history and physical examination should elicit the underlying cause of the child's respiratory failure and a diagnosis is essential for specific management of the condition.

The causes of respiratory failure are listed in Table 9.5.

The approach to the child with respiratory failure

The clinical diagnosis of respiratory failure is obvious if the child is apnoeic or severely cyanosed, but impending respiratory failure may be more difficult to recognize.

History

Asthma is the commonest cause of respiratory failure in children over 1 year of age and a careful history of previous episodes should be taken (p. 123). Wheeze and night cough

Table 9.5 Causes of respiratory failure

Upper airway obstruction
Inhaled foreign body
Epiglottitis
Croup
Lower airway disease
Asthma
Bronchiolitis
Pneumonia
Cystic fibrosis
Neonatal lung disease
Neurological
Head injury
Meningitis
Raised intracranial pressure
Muscle disorder
Cardiac
Severe cardiac failure
Toxic
Drug ingestion

Table 9.6 Investigations and their relevance in a child with respiratory failure

Investigation	Relevance
Blood gases	Falling pH and increasing $Paco_2$ indicates respiratory failure with need for ventilation
	Low Pao_2 indicates need for additional oxygen
Oxygen saturation	Monitor progress of respiratory disease
Chest X-ray	Lobar or segmental collapse?
	Aspiration

are important features of this condition. A list of prescribed medication should be recorded and how much of each drug has been given in this episode ascertained.

In infants, infection, particularly bronchiolitis (p. 119), is the commonest cause and the history should focus on exposure to infectious agents, recent fever and a history of apnoea associated with the present illness.

Physical examination

Inability to speak because of breathlessness is a worrying sign that should be carefully assessed. Signs of respiratory distress include dyspnoea, recession, cyanosis and grunting in babies, but these may all be present in children who do not go on to develop respiratory failure.

Investigations

The relevant investigations and their significance are shown in Table 9.6.

Management

- Direct treatment at the underlying cause of the respiratory failure.
- Support the respiratory physiology. If the child is hypoxic (cyanosed), but the $Paco_2$ is normal he or she requires oxygen therapy and careful observation. A rising $Paco_2$ indicates the need for respiratory support with mechanical ventilation. This should take place only on an Intensive Care Unit. Oxygen saturation monitoring may be helpful in following progress of the illness.

Prognosis

This depends on the underlying cause and its severity.

UPPER AIRWAY OBSTRUCTION

Acute upper airway obstruction is an acute medical emer-

RESPIRATORY FAILURE AT A GLANCE

Aetiology

See Table 9.5

Clinical features

- Dyspnoea
- Tachypnoea
- Cyanosis
- Alar flaring
- Grunting in babies
- Intercostal, subcostal and suprasternal retractions
- Symptoms and signs of underlying disease
- In severe asthma, wheezing may not be heard because of poor air entry
- Restlessness, dizziness
- Impaired consciousness and confusion

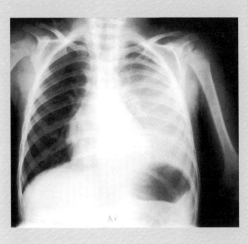

Investigations

Blood gases
Chest X-ray

Management

See Principles of Management Box, below

Principles of management
Respiratory failure

- Initial assessment of arterial blood gases with regular reassessments

- Continuous assessment with oxygen saturation monitor and if desaturated give oxygen

- Mechanically ventilate if increasing $Pa\text{co}_2$ (but the need for mechanical ventilation is based on whole clinical picture, not just blood gases)

- Investigate cause of respiratory failure

- Treat underlying cause:
    antibiotics for infection (p. 109)
    steroids and bronchodilators for asthma (p. 321)
    remove foreign body via bronchoscope

gency as death may occur rapidly if it is unrelieved. Obstruction may be intrinsic (e.g. epiglottitis) or extrinsic caused by a foreign body in the upper airway. The major symptom of upper airway obstruction is inspiratory stridor which is discussed fully on p. 126.

Acute upper airway obstruction is most likely to occur as the result of aspiration of a foreign body. This is particularly likely in toddlers who tend to put small objects into their mouths. Peanuts are a particularly common object to inhale. Larger objects are most likely to obstruct above the level of the carina and the symptoms are immediate and dramatic.

The approach to the child with upper airway obstruction

Presentation is acute with sudden onset of choking, coughing and cyanosis.

History

Specific questions to be asked include whether there is the possibility of aspiration of foreign body (has the child had access to beads, peanuts, etc.) and whether there has been a history of stridor and malaise suggestive of acute epiglottitis or croup (p. 126).

Physical examination

If obstruction is severe the child will be cyanosed and collapsed. Stridor may be present if the child is able to move enough air around the obstruction. Marked recession will be present. If epiglottitis is suspected the doctor must not examine the child's throat.

Investigations

All investigations must be delayed until a safe airway has been established. Undertaking any painful procedure such as blood tests or moving the child from the mother's arms to examine or take to an X-ray may precipitate complete airway obstruction.

Management

If an object is blocking the larynx or trachea it must be removed as rapidly as possible as death may occur within minutes. Every effort must be made to avoid pushing the object further down as this may cause complete airway obstruction.

Tracheostomy may be necessary as a life-saving procedure in hospital.

The Heimlich manoeuvre

This is a first aid measure to relieve acute upper airway obstruction such as that which occurs as the result of choking on a piece of food or partially aspirating a foreign body. The operator stands behind and embraces the child, with his or her hands grasping each other under the costal margin. The operator then vigorously squeezes the child's abdomen, increasing intra-abdominal pressure and forcing

---

Principles of management
Upper airway obstruction

• If a foreign body is suspected in the trachea perform the Heimlich manoeuvre

• If cardiorespiratory arrest occurs first establish the airway with a tracheostomy if intubation is impossible

• If intubation is required avoid distressing the child until an anaesthetist arrives

• Support the child with cardiopulmonary resuscitation if necessary

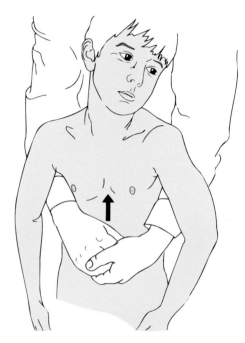

Fig. 9.2 The Heimlich manoeuvre.

UPPER AIRWAY OBSTRUCTION AT A GLANCE

Aetiology

Intrinsic: epiglottis, croup
Extrinsic: foreign body

Clinical features

• Choking, coughing
• Inspiratory stridor
• Decreased air movement
• Marked recession
• Cyanosis
• Collapse if complete obstruction occurs

Investigations

Delay until airway is established

Older children   Younger children

Heimlich manoeuvre

Management

See Principles of Management Box
p. 302

the air out of the lungs. This should also result in the foreign body being blown out.

SHOCK

Shock is the term used to describe a state where the cardiac output is insufficient to perfuse the tissues adequately. The best clinical measure of shock is the blood pressure. Hypotension will cause perfusion to fall in vital organs resulting in multiple organ failure of which the brain and kidneys are the most vulnerable. The body has a variety of physiological mechanisms to protect vital organs during periods of hypotension. These include redistribution of blood flow from the skin, muscles and bowel to the vital organs, brain, myocardium and kidneys. This is why children in shock are pale with poor skin perfusion. Uncorrected shock will lead to cardiac arrest.

The causes of shock are shown in Table 9.7.

Approach to a child in shock

History

A careful history must be taken to elucidate the cause of the shock concentrating on those listed in Table 9.7. Enquire into obvious sources of fluid loss (e.g. diarrhoea, vomiting, history of diabetes). Ask whether the child has had a cardiac problem and enquire about allergies (e.g. bee stings, peanuts, etc.). Enquire whether there was a close relationship between ingesting an unusual food and the onset of shock.

Physical examination

Two distinct assessments must be made on physical examination; the severity of the shock and its underlying cause.
- *Signs of shock.* It is important to recognize the signs of shock in its relatively early stages before the child collapses. Early symptoms include restlessness, tachycardia with a thready pulse and pallor with cold clammy extremities. At this stage the blood pressure may be normal. Poor skin perfusion can be assessed by blanching the skin by pressing on it with a finger and seeing how long it takes for the capillaries to refill. Oliguria is a common feature of the shocked child. Once hypotension occurs the child is extremely ill.
- *Signs of the underlying cause of the shock.* Signs include petechial or purpuric skin lesions in meningococcaemia, evidence of trauma and hepatomegaly in cardiac failure. The focus of a septicaemic illness may be otitis media (examine tympanic membranes), meningitis (assess for neck stiffness), osteomyelitis and septic arthritis (examine joints and limbs for sites of swelling and tenderness).

Investigations

The relevant investigations and their significance are shown in Table 9.8.
- Temperature. The failure of skin perfusion will result in the child having a widening difference between peripheral temperature and core (rectal) temperature.
- Blood gases. Metabolic acidosis occurs as the result of anaerobic tissue metabolism.
- Electrolytes and urea to assess dehydration.
- Blood glucose to exclude hypoglycaemia or diabetic ketoacidosis.
- ECG to evaluate cardiac function.
- A central venous pressure (CVP) line is helpful to assess the degree of fluid loss and to monitor replacement.

Table 9.7 Causes of shock

Hypovolaemic	Cardiogenic	Anaphylactic
Haemorrhage	Myocardial impairment	Allergic reaction
Infection (e.g. meningococcal)	Heart failure	
Loss of intravascular fluid (p. 117) (e.g. vomiting, diarrhoea)		
Diabetic ketoacidosis		
Trauma		
Burns		

Table 9.8 Investigations in shock and their relevance

Investigation	Relevance
Temperature difference between core and periphery	Wide difference (rectal/skin) suggests peripheral shut-down
Full blood count	Neutrophilia suggests infection
Blood cultures	Septicaemia
Blood pH	Metabolic acidosis suggests tissue hypoxaemia
Serum electrolytes and urea	High urea/creatinine indicates dehydration or renal impairment
Blood glucose	Hypoglycaemia Hyperglycaemia as a result of diabetic ketoacidosis
ECG	Cardiac function
Central venous pressure	Low in dehydration High in cardiac failure

Management A severe allergic reaction should be treated rapidly. If the airway is compromised, the child should be intubated. Drug treatment includes:

• *Adrenaline* given intravenously as an emergency.
• *Corticosteroids* (hydrocortisone intravenously). These may take several hours to have an effect.
• *Antihistamines.*
• *Aminophylline* if bronchospasm develops (p. 322).

In children who have had one episode of anaphylaxis, the parents should be given adrenaline to adminsiter subcutaneously and hydrocortisone to keep with them to treat the child following a subsequent inadvertent exposure to the allergen. In addition, they must be taught basic life support techniques.

COMA

Coma is a poorly understood condition and refers to a markedly reduced state of consciousness caused by a reduction in cerebral metabolic rate. Sometimes the term encephalopathy, which refers to altered state of consciousness, is used to describe a precomatose state. The causes of coma are listed in Table 9.9.

Approach to the comatose child

In any child presenting with coma the first task is to stabilize the child (see below) prior to further evaluation.

History

Once the child is stable a careful history should be taken. Particular attention should focus on whether there has been a prodromal illness, history of recent contacts with infectious diseases, possibility of drug ingestion (either deliberate or accidental in young children) or a recent head injury.

Enquiries should be made concerning the risk of non-accidental injury.

The duration of the convulsion must be ascertained and whether there have been previous convulsions. The neurodevelopmental state of the child prior to the status should be documented but is usually normal. Precipitating factors such as playing computer games or a history of diabetes must be clarified.

• *Past medical history.* Ascertain whether the child has suffered from convulsions and whether there is a history of diabetes.

Physical examination

A careful neurological examination must be carried out to establish the degree of coma.

• *Vital signs.* Bradycardia suggests raised intracranial pressure and fever with tachycardia suggest infection or dehydration. Cardiac arrythmia occurs in some types of drug overdose. Tachypnoea occurs in respiratory distress and deep sighing (Kussmaul) respirations are a feature of diabetic ketoacidosis.

• *Focus of infection.* The child should be examined for a focus of infection which might have precipitated coma. This includes signs of consolidation in the chest, meningeal irritation and otitis media.

• *Depth of coma.* This can be determined clinically by assessing the child's best response to commands (Fig. 9.3) The lighter the coma the more appropriate the response and the deeper the coma the less the response. In deep coma there is no response at all.

• *Papilloedema.* The fundus should be examined for papilloedema which is a sign of raised intracranial pressure and may be accompanied by a slow pulse and raised blood pressure.

• *Pupillary light reflex should be elicited.* A unilateral

Table 9.9 Causes of coma

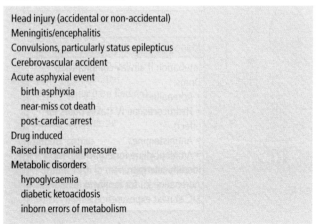

Head injury (accidental or non-accidental)
Meningitis/encephalitis
Convulsions, particularly status epilepticus
Cerebrovascular accident
Acute asphyxial event
  birth asphyxia
  near-miss cot death
  post-cardiac arrest
Drug induced
Raised intracranial pressure
Metabolic disorders
  hypoglycaemia
  diabetic ketoacidosis
  inborn errors of metabolism

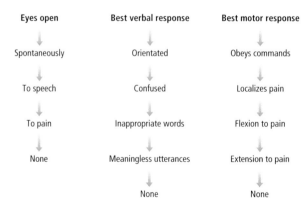

Fig. 9.3 Clinical assessment of depth of coma. The less the response, the deeper the coma.

Table 9.10 The relevance of various investigations in elucidating the cause of coma

Investigation	Relevance
Blood glucose	Hypoglycaemia: rapid coma Hyperglycaemia: ketoacidosis and slower onset of coma
Full blood count	Elevated WCC and shift to left in infection Decreased PCV and decreased Hb in acute haemorrhage
Blood and urine culture	Organisms identified if infection
Urea and electrolytes	Elevated urea if dehydrated
Blood gases	Indicates metabolic or respiratory acidosis (see p. 358 for interpretation)
Chest X-ray	Infection or cardiac failure
CT or MRI scan	Focal pathology (tumour, haemorrhage, abscess) Cerebral oedema
Lumbar puncture	Only if no cerebral oedema or raised ICP on imaging Positive in meningitis (see p. 361 for interpretation)

WCC, white cell count; PCV, packed cell volume; Hb, haemoglobin; CT, computed tomography; MRI, magnetic resonance imaging; ICP, intracranial pressure.

dilated pupil with impaired light reflex indicates a third nerve palsy caused by temporal lobe herniation.

Investigations

Investigations required and their relevance is shown in Table 9.10. The commonest and most treatable metabolic cause of coma is hypoglycaemia and all children with an altered level of consciousness should have an urgent finger prick stick test for blood glucose.

All unconscious children must have a brain scan before lumbar puncture to avoid the risk of coning (p. 110). Computed tomography (CT) or magnetic resonance imaging (MRI) scans will show focal pathology (tumour, haemorrhage, infarction) and will indicate whether severe oedema is present. If cerebral oedema is not present, lumbar puncture must be performed.

Management

Specific therapy for cerebral oedema include the use of osmotic agents (e.g. mannitol) and hyperventilation. Steroids are only used for focal oedema around a tumour. High dose barbiturates are commonly used to reduce cerebral metabolic rate.

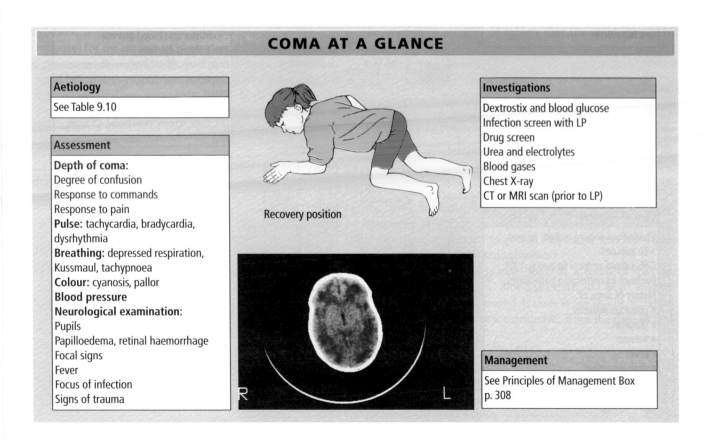

COMA AT A GLANCE

Aetiology
See Table 9.10

Assessment

Depth of coma:
Degree of confusion
Response to commands
Response to pain
Pulse: tachycardia, bradycardia, dysrhythmia
Breathing: depressed respiration, Kussmaul, tachypnoea
Colour: cyanosis, pallor
Blood pressure
Neurological examination:
Pupils
Papilloedema, retinal haemorrhage
Focal signs
Fever
Focus of infection
Signs of trauma

Recovery position

Investigations
Dextrostix and blood glucose
Infection screen with LP
Drug screen
Urea and electrolytes
Blood gases
Chest X-ray
CT or MRI scan (prior to LP)

Management
See Principles of Management Box
p. 308

Table 9.12 Common poisons ingested by children

Drugs	Household agents
Aspirin	Paraffin
Paracetamol	Turpentine
	Disinfectants
	Bleach
	Weedkillers

ties. If aspirin or paracetamol overdose is suspected then measurement of serum levels of these drugs should be performed.

Management

- Discuss with the National Poisons Unit.
- Removal of the poison. The child should be made to vomit by giving ipecacuanha syrup. There are three important exceptions to this rule:
  1 If the child is semiconscious or unconscious, as aspiration may occur if vomiting is induced.
  2 If caustic or corrosive substances have been ingested, vomiting may exacerbate the oesophageal injury.
  3 Paraffin, turpentine or petrol may be aspirated during vomiting and cause lipoid pneumonia.
- Activated charcoal, an absorbent, can reduce the absorption of many drugs including aspirin, paracetamol, barbiturates and tricyclic antidepressants. It must not be given until ipecacuanha has been effective.
- Specific antidotes or therapy for the poison should be instituted if appropriate (e.g. naloxone for opiate poisoning).
- Supportive management. Respiratory and/or cardiovascular failure are important and common complications of many forms of poisoning. If the child is comatose, hypotensive or unwell a drip should be inserted and the child nursed in an environment where he or she can be very closely observed and respiratory support can be instituted if necessary.
- Advice to parents concerning the prevention of further accidents or ingestions in the home.
- In a child who has attempted suicide or parasuicide appropriate psychiatric advice should be obtained.

Types of poison ingestion

Salicylate poisoning

Owing to its easy availability in many homes, aspirin is the most common drug to be ingested accidentally by children.

Salicylate poisoning causes initially a respiratory alkalosis caused by stimulation of the respiratory centre and later a metabolic acidosis as a result of the acid load of the drug. Gastric bleeding may occur as the result of its effects on the mucosa.

Clinical features The earliest sign is overbreathing, often associated with vomiting and diarrhoea. Sweating may be a feature. If the overdose has been large, metabolic acidosis occurs about 6–8 hours after ingestion with ketosis, hyperglycaemia and glycosuria. Eventually collapse may occur with loss of consciousness. The physical and laboratory findings show a considerable similarity with those found in diabetic ketoacidosis and blood sugar levels should be measured to exclude this possibility.

A serum salicylate level helps to establish the likely severity of the overdose.

Management Salicylates are retained in the stomach for a long time so that vomiting should be induced even if ingestion occurred some hours earlier. If the patient is acidotic give sodium bicarbonate which promotes renal excretion of salicylate. Renal dialysis or exchange transfusion should be used in massive overdoses to remove salicylate.

Paracetamol poisoning

Paracetamol ingestion is rarely severe enough to cause serious problems, but liver failure is the major risk if >150 mg/kg is ingested.

Clinical features Early symptoms include anorexia, nausea and vomiting. Signs of liver failure occurs on the second day with abdominal pain, liver tenderness and hepatic failure with jaundice after 2–3 days.

Initially liver function tests are normal. The prothrombin time and liver enzymes become abnormal 12–24 hours after ingestion. The decision to treat depends on a paracetamol serum level 4 hours after ingestion.

Management Successful treatment depends on early recognition and institution of adequate treatment. Vomiting should be induced in all cases. In patients at risk of liver damage, oral methionine or *N*-acetyl-cysteine reduces the severity of liver necrosis. The decision to use these agents depends on the serum level of paracetamol 4 hours after ingestion.

ACCIDENTS AND BURNS

Accidents and accident prevention have been discussed elsewhere in this book (p. 50). Accidents are the most important

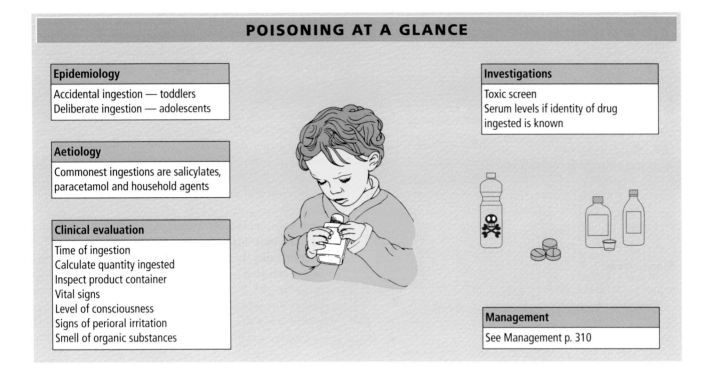

POISONING AT A GLANCE

Epidemiology

Accidental ingestion — toddlers
Deliberate ingestion — adolescents

Aetiology

Commonest ingestions are salicylates,
paracetamol and household agents

Clinical evaluation

Time of ingestion
Calculate quantity ingested
Inspect product container
Vital signs
Level of consciousness
Signs of perioral irritation
Smell of organic substances

Investigations

Toxic screen
Serum levels if identity of drug
ingested is known

Management

See Management p. 310

---

causes of death after 1 year of age and children may present to hospital critically ill as the result of trauma, burns or near-drowning.

It is beyond the scope of this book to discuss the medical approach to children who have been the victims of severe trauma. The principles of care are discussed under the heading of shock. Blood loss, either internal (e.g. ruptured spleen) or external (visible), must always be considered and rapidly treated.

Burns and scalds

Burns are the second commonest cause of accidental childhood death after road traffic accidents. One half of deaths are caused by smoke inhalation leading to respiratory failure (p. 300) and one half caused by thermal damage to the skin. Approximately one half of thermal injuries admitted to hospital are the result of scalds from hot water.

Thermal injuries cause death either as a result of massive fluid loss through the denuded skin or by infection. A second major problem in children who survive is scarring which may have major psychological consequences.

First aid

Scalds are first treated by removing the clothes over the affected area and the skin cooled under a cold tap. Children who are scalded or burnt should be wrapped in a clean towel or sheet and brought immediately to hospital.

Clinical assessment

The extent of the thermal injury must be assessed. This is done by estimating the surface area involved. This is illustrated in Fig. 9.4. The percentage body area affected is calculated.

If the child has suffered smoke inhalation respiratory failure with wheeze, cyanosis and dyspnoea may occur rapidly.

Management

• If there are burns to more than 10% of the surface area, insert an intravenous cannula to gain vascular access and give fluids in the form of colloid to prevent or treat shock caused by fluid loss. Details of the fluid management are beyond the scope of this book.
• Analgesia. Give morphine to control pain.
• Assess airway and respiratory function. Arterial blood gases may be necessary to decide whether mechanical ventilation is required (p. 358). Thermal injury to the airway may necessitate a rapid tracheostomy before severe oedema causes obstruction.
• Skin grafting. This is required for full-thickness burns. This can be assessed after a few days by testing for pain sensation. If a pinprick is not felt then the burn is full thickness.

Principles of management
Burns

- Give intravenous fluids to prevent severe fluid loss through burnt skin

- Analgesia to control pain

- If thermal injury to mouth or airway, assess the need for tracheostomy

- Skin grafting for full-thickness burn

- Psychological support for child and family

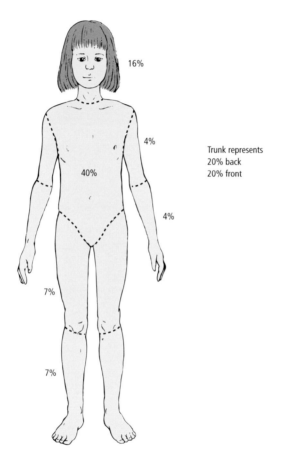

16%

4%

Trunk represents
20% back
20% front

40%

4%

7%

7%

Fig. 9.4 Estimating the surface area of burns in children.

- Psychological support for the child and his or her family.

Drowning

Most drowning incidents in Britain occur in fresh water (bath, river, swimming pool). The outcome following near-drowning in cold water (<10°C) is significantly better than in warm water. This is probably a result of the hypothermia that cold water induces.

First aid

The child must be resuscitated at the site of the drowning incident with mouth-to-mouth resuscitation and rapidly transferred to hospital.

Management

- Clear airway and institute mechanical ventilation. Assess circulation and treat if shock is present.
- If hypothermic, slowly warm over a number of hours.
- Secondary drowning is rare and refers to secondary respiratory failure 24 hours after the drowning incident. It is probably a result of surfactant deficiency.

Prognosis

It is well known that children can recover fully despite a very prolonged period of cardiac arrest following a drowning incident, particularly if the child was rescued from cold water. Prolonged resuscitation efforts are therefore necessary until the child is rewarmed.

Hypoxic brain damage rarely occurs after near-drowning and full recovery is the rule if the child can be resuscitated.

ACUTE LIFE-THREATENING EVENTS AND SUDDEN INFANT DEATH SYNDROME

The definition of sudden infant death syndrome (SIDS) is 'the sudden death of any infant or young child, which is unexpected by history, and in which a thorough postmortem examination fails to demonstrate an adequate cause for the death.' Some children are found in a collapsed apnoeic state looking grey and mottled, but can be resuscitated. This is referred to as an acute life-threatening event (ALTE) or a near-miss cot death.

Sudden infant death syndrome affects infants below the age of 1 year with the peak rate at 2–4 months. It is the commonest cause of death in infancy after the first week of life. In Britain the incidence of SIDS has fallen by over 50% in the last few years probably as a result of new advice on the sleeping position of babies (see below).

Pathogenesis

The cause of SIDS is unknown. There is no single cause and many factors are involved including infection, cardiac dysrhythmia and accidental suffocation. It is thought by many to be caused by an environmental factor on a susceptible infant. Recently most attention has been placed on sleeping position, the infant's temperature and exposure to tobacco smoke in the home.

It is thought that the baby's body temperature is related to sleeping position and overheating is an important factor in the control of respiration. Babies who are nursed prone in their cots have less skin surface area exposed for heat loss. Recently the Department of Health has issued advice to parents of young babies in the Back to Sleep health education campaign (p. 314). This advice appears to be the major cause of the reduction in the number of cot deaths.

Approach to the child presenting with acute life-threatening events or sudden infant death syndrome

In babies who die of SIDS there is often a preceding history of minor illness such as a cold or a cough but not severe enough to cause concern that the baby is seriously ill. The baby usually dies at home in his or her cot between the hours of 04:00 and 12:00. Death appears to have occurred rapidly and without warning. It is not uncommon for the child to be cold by the time he or she is found and postmortem lividity is seen. Rarely the baby may be found to have a major pathology at postmortem such as pneumonia or septicaemia, but this is uncommon and an obvious but unexpected cause for death is found in only 20% of cases.

Babies who have been found with an acute life-threatening episode are usually pale (indicating a poor circulation) and mottled in appearance. The pulse is usually slow and the blood pressure low. Only vigorous resuscitation will save the baby's life.

In those cases where the baby is found collapsed, but not dead in the cot, immediate first aid with mouth-to-mouth resuscitation and external cardiac massage may save the baby's life. Irreversible brain damage may occur as the result of prolonged hypoxia.

Investigations

In babies who have been successfully resuscitated from acute life-threatening episodes, investigation for an underlying cause is essential. The following should be undertaken:

ACUTE LIFE THREATENING EVENTS AND SUDDEN INFANT DEATH SYNDROME AT A GLANCE

Epidemiology

Commonest cause of infant death (past first week)
Affects babies under 12 months, peak age 2–4 months

Aetiology

Related to sleep position (a), temperature (b), smoking (c) and environment
In 20% a major unsuspected condition is found at autopsy

Prevention

'Back to sleep campaign' has halved deaths due to sudden infant death syndrome

History

Normally healthy baby
(Preceding minor illness)

Physical examination

Found collapsed
Pale and mottled
Slow pulse, low blood pressure

Investigations

Blood sugar
Infection screen
Chest X-ray and barium swallow
ECG monitoring
Screen for inborn errors of metabolism

Differential diagnosis

Sepsis
Gastro-oesophageal reflux
Neurological abnormality
Hypoglycaemia (rare)
Cardiac arrythmia (rare)
Inborn error of metabolism (rare)
Suffocation (rare)

Management

Immediate cardiopulmonary resuscitation
Admit for investigation and observation
Home apnoea monitoring not of proven benefit but relieves anxiety
Train caregivers in CPR

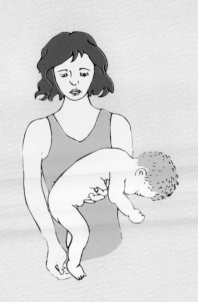

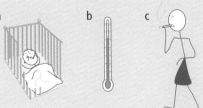

a   b   c

Back to Sleep campaign

Babies should be laid to sleep on their backs
If the side position is chosen, the lower arm should be well in front of the body to prevent the child from rolling into a prone position

Infants should not be exposed to cigarette smoke either before birth or afterwards

Avoid overheating the baby
Guidance to the parents includes:
• Sleeping room temperature 16–20°C
• Avoid excessive bedding for the temperature of the room
• Ensure bedding will not overlie the baby. Make it up so that the infant's feet come down to the end of the cot
• Avoid duvets in infants <1 year of age
• Do not increase the bedding when the child is unwell or feverish
• An infant >1 month does not require a hat for sleeping unless the room is very cold

• infection screen, particularly blood cultures, urine culture and consider lumbar puncture;
• investigations for gastro-oesophageal reflux (p. 158);

• continuous monitoring for episodes of apnoea;
• ECG monitoring for cardiac dysrhythmias;
• metabolic investigations including blood sugar (hypoglycaemia) and inborn errors of metabolism.

Management

The management is the same as for any baby with cardiopulmonary arrest and is described on p. 299.

Prevention

The family of a previously affected child The family of a SIDS victim will be extremely anxious about the outcome for subsequent siblings. Apnoea monitoring at home is usually offered although there is no evidence that this will prevent further deaths. If the new baby is unwell there should be early referral to the GP with admission to hospital for close monitoring if the doctor is concerned.

General prevention The advice given by the Department of Health should be given to all new parents. Additional advice includes the encouragement of breast-feeding, and warning about not overwrapping the baby if he or she develops a mild infection.

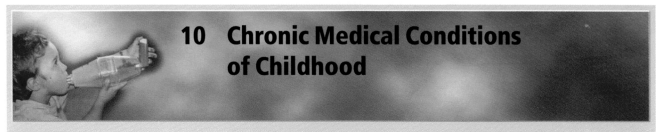

10 Chronic Medical Conditions of Childhood

Introduction, 315
Approach to the child with a chronic illness, 316
Asthma, 318
Management of asthma, 319

Diabetes mellitus, 325
Management of diabetes, 326
Epilepsy, 332
Management of epilepsy, 334
Congenital heart disease, 337

Management of congenital heart disease, 338
The child with cancer, 340
Management of the child with cancer, 341

Physicians of the utmost fame
Were called at once; but when they came
They answered, as they took their fees,
There is no cure for this disease.

Cautionary tales. Henry King
Hilaire Belloc, 1870–1953

Introduction

There is no universally accepted definition of childhood chronic conditions; however, the following definition is useful: *a chronic illness is a physical condition that lasts longer than 3 months, and is of sufficient severity to interfere with a child's ordinary activities to some degree.*

Some 10–20% of children will experience a chronic medical condition at some point in childhood, with 5–10% having a moderately to severely handicapping long-term illness or disability (Table 10.1).

Children with chronic disease have many needs in common with each other, irrespective of what disease they may have. Before tackling individual medical conditions (of which only a few are detailed in this chapter) it is important to take an overview and gain an understanding of the impact any chronic illness has on a child and the family, and the physical, emotional and social stresses which result. This is critical as psychosocial factors not only affect how the child functions in the family, with peers and at school, but also can affect the very course of the medical condition.

The effect of chronic illness on the child

In addressing chronic illness, it is important to understand the impact a chronic illness is likely to have on a child's development and functioning. This will vary depending on the age of the child and the age at which the condition developed.

Interestingly, factors other than the severity and prognosis of the condition affect the child's adjustment. In fact there appears to be little relationship between the severity of the condition and the degree of psychosocial difficulties encountered. Children with mild disabilities may suffer as much or more than those in whom the condition is severe. Factors which may influence a child's adjustment are shown in Table 10.2.

Common problems experienced

Given the impact that chronic illness has on a child it is perhaps not surprising that the child is two to three times more likely to experience emotional, behavioural and educational difficulties than their healthy peers. Low self esteem, impaired self image, behavioural problems, depression, anxiety and school dysfunction are all common observations. These problems may occur as a result of the child's own reaction to his or her chronic illness or the reaction of parents, peers, professionals and society as a whole.

The child and school

School is a central part of any child's life. The acquisition of academic and vocational skills, and the development of work-related habits are only one aspect. An equally important aspect is the development of social interactions with peers and adults outside the family.

The child's ability to perform at school can be affected, placing the child at risk for becoming an underachiever and failure in his or her own eyes and the eyes of his or her peers. Large amounts of school are often missed because of acute exacerbations, outpatient appointments and hospitalizations. If the child has adapted poorly, further days may be missed in addition.

Chronic illness affects the social aspects of school life too. Frequent illness episodes and restrictions can exclude the child from activities. Physical appearance, acute medical problems, taking medications at school and special diets all make the child different. As a result some children are made fun of by their healthy peers, and come to feel inferior to and isolated from their classmates.

In addition to contending with the special problems of his or her condition and the reaction of others, the child is also

Table 10.1 Prevalence of chronic conditions in childhood

Condition	Rates per 1000
Asthma (moderate and severe)	10.0
Epilepsy	8.0
Congenital heart disease	7.0–8.0
Dibetes mellitus	2.0
Arthritis	1.0
Cystic fibrosis	0.4
Chronic renal failure	0.1
Malignancy	0.1

Table 10.2 Factors affecting a child's adjustment to a chronic illness

The child
The age of the child
The age at which the illness developed. School entry and adolescence are particularly vulnerable periods
Low intelligence or unattractiveness increase the probability of maladjustment

The illness
Conditions with unpredictable flare-ups or recurrences are more stressful than stable conditions
'Invisible' conditions (e.g. diabetes) may be concealed and lead to a lack of acceptance

The family
The family's attitude and ability to function is the most critical factor in determining the child's adjustment

likely to be aggravated by concerns and difficulties that beset all children at school, such as peer acceptance, competition, anxiety about academic achievement and athletic prowess and concerns about physical appearance and sexual development.

The effect of chronic illness on the family

The development of a long-term medical condition in a child affects a family on a number of levels; practical, social and psychological. Altered daily routines, outpatient visits and hospitalizations, unexpected exacerbations and the administration of medications require organization, time and energy. Socially, the family may experience isolation from neighbours and friends, difficulty in finding babysitters, and may have to forgo activities and holidays and even change career plans.

The parents

There is usually a common response to learning that a child has a chronic illness, which is not dissimilar to that of bereavement. The initial reaction is one of shock or disbelief, which is followed by denial, anger and resentment. These feelings often induce a sense of guilt and then sadness. Acceptance should follow, although this may not occur if the parent gets stuck at an earlier stage.

It is not surprising that clinical anxiety, depression, guilt and grief are common problems particularly for mothers who often take the major role in caring for the child. It is also not surprising that marriages are more subject to dissatisfaction, differences and arguments, and that marital problems are often exacerbated.

Siblings

Although siblings often develop more kind and considerate relationships, they are also at higher risk. Parents are likely to be less available, and they may neglect, overindulge or develop unrealistic expectations for their healthy children. Anxiety, embarrassment, resentment and guilt are common, as are fears about their own well-being and the cause and nature of their sibling's health problems.

In discussing chronic illness in childhood the focus is often on psychopathology and psychosocial problems; however, it must be emphasized that the impact is not always negative. Some families seem to grow closer to each other and in working with families the question often arises, 'How do some families of chronically ill children survive so well?'

Approach to the child with a chronic illness

Time, rapport and skill must be invested in assessing the psychosocial consequences of a chronic illness on the family. It is important to allow adequate time for this, particularly at the onset of the condition, and when important changes occur, such as school entry and adolescence. If there are problems parents must be given the opportunity to express themselves without the child being present, and adolescents should always be seen alone. This is important, not only to allow the adolescent to talk about problems, but also as it transmits the message that they should begin to be responsible for their own health care.

In evaluating the child at an initial or follow-up visit a full picture of the child's physical, emotional and behavioural condition must be obtained

Management

Too often management of chronic illness by medical professionals focuses on the relatively simple clinical management alone. It cannot be emphasized enough that the child must be seen as a whole. If this is ignored the child's and family's needs are not met, so increasing their difficulties, which in itself is likely to affect adversely the course of the illness.

Counselling

In an age of technological medical advances there is still no substitute for the old-fashioned quality of caring for the child and the family. It is always remarkable how a thorough assessment in itself is a therapeutic intervention, and concern and empathy go a long way in assisting the family to make the best of the circumstances they face. It is important to note that it is rarely helpful to try to conceal chronic conditions where this is possible, as it encourages the child to believe that the illness is a secret and something of which to be ashamed.

Education

A vital aspect of management is education of the family about the condition. Gone are the days when doctors paternalistically 'protected' their patients from knowing about the condition and its prognosis. Including the parents increases their trust and also provides them with the skills to self-manage many aspects of the condition. This is particularly critical in conditions such as asthma and diabetes.

Coordination

Very often in chronic illness the child is looked after by a variety of health professionals: consultants, therapists and dietitians, not to mention teachers and social workers. Liaison and coordination is very important as differing opinions and advice can be very confusing for the family. The development of specialist clinics for the more common medical conditions has improved this problem, especially as clinics usually include specialist nurses whose role is one of support, education and liaison.

Genetic issues

Most parents have questions regarding genetic implications for subsequent children and the affected child's own chances of fertility. It is important that these are addressed, and where necessary referred to a geneticist.

Support

An assessment of support available to the family must be made. Chronic illness can be an isolating experience and many families do not have the support of the extended family and friends. Referrals to a social worker may be needed in order to advise on benefits and services offered by social services (see p. 275). If the child has emotional and behavioural difficulties, referral for counselling may be required. Self-help and voluntary organizations such as the British Diabetes or Epilepsy Association can be helpful and often run support groups and activities allowing families with similar problems to meet.

School

Involvement of the child's school is essential for a number of reasons.
- *Medical.* The staff need to understand the child's condition well in order for them to cope competently with problems arising. The greatest concern is usually the handling of acute exacerbations, but other requirements such as dispensing medication and dietary restrictions must be discussed. Asking teachers to report untoward events such as symptoms or drug side-effects can be helpful.
- *Educational.* These children are at risk for underachieving for the reasons explained above. This can be minimized with appropriate support, such as help in making up with school work lost through illness or hospital visits or providing preferential seating in class. The child may need extra encouragement, but care must be taken that this does not result in preferential treatment which may have social repercussions. Some children may have special educational requirements that need to be met (see p. 275).
- *Social.* Teachers can be instrumental in helping the child

---

CHRONIC ILLNESS AT A GLANCE

Epidemiology

10–20% of children have a chronic medical problem at some time in childhood, 5–10% have a severe or moderate condition

Effect on the child

Chronic illness:
- Impacts on the child psychologically
- Increases the risk of emotional, behavioural and educational difficulties
- Is associated with dysfunction at school

Effect on the family

The initial parental response is akin to bereavement
Parents must cope with:
- demands of appointments
- drug administration
- unexpected exacerbations
- social difficulties
Siblings may suffer from altered attention and expectations, and experience more emotional and behavioural problems

Effect on the child at school

Academic performance, achievements and social life may be affected
Concerns and difficulties experienced by any child are likely to be aggravated

Approach to the child

Time, rapport and skill required
A holistic approach is essential

Management

Management must extend beyond the medical to:
- counselling and support
- education
- coordination and liaison between professionals
- genetic issues
- medical, educational and social issues at school

---

cope and integrate socially into school life. Emotional and behavioural difficulties are likely to be expressed at school, and the teachers need to be sensitive to this. For the child where the family is failing to cope effectively, the school has a particularly important role.

ASTHMA

Prevalence

Asthma is the commonest chronic condition of childhood and its incidence is rising. It affects some 10% of children at some point in childhood. The increase in numbers may be related to pollution and there is clustering of cases in children living near motorways.

Aetiology and pathophysiology

The symptoms of asthma, cough and wheeze are caused by narrowing of the bronchi and bronchioles as a result of bronchoconstriction, mucosal swelling and viscid secretion obstructing the lumen (p. 120). Various allergic and non-specific stimuli may initiate this process in the susceptible individual by triggering the release of histamine and other mediators. These stimuli include dust mites, air pollutants, cigarette smoke, cold air, viral infections, stress and exercise.

Initial presentation of asthma

Most children with asthma become symptomatic in infancy or the preschool years. The diagnosis is made clinically on the basis of a persistent or recurrent cough or wheeze, which is responsive to medication. A family or past medical history of atopy contributes to the diagnosis.

Diagnosis in infancy

Many babies have episodes of wheezing, in part as a result of their relatively narrow airways which become readily obstructed. These episodes may be related to infection by the respiratory syncytial virus (RSV). The majority of wheezing babies do not persist in having troublesome symptoms, and there is therefore no advantage to labelling them as having a chronic medical condition, particularly as the treatment of the wheezy baby is the same whether he or she has a diagnosis of asthma or not (see p. 122). However, if the baby has another atopic condition or there is a family history of atopy and asthma, the wheezing is more likely to be a manifestation of asthma. In infancy, as the airways are so narrow, the contribution of secretions and mucosal oedema to the obstruction is greater, and there is often a poor response to bronchodilator treatment.

Diagnosis in childhood

Recurrent episodes of coughing and wheezing especially if aggravated or triggered by exercise, viral infection or inhaled antigens are highly suggestive of asthma. The diagnosis is made on the basis of the response to bronchodilator treatment. In the younger child this response is judged clinically by the reduction in respiratory distress and wheeze. In the older child reversibility of airway obstruction can be demonstrated by peak flow measurements. Although X-rays are not often indicated in the child with asthma, a chest X-ray should be obtained at the first episode to exclude a foreign body in the lung or oesophagus.

Allergy testing

Allergy tests are not usually carried out unless the diagnosis is in doubt. Skin testing is not usually helpful, as false positives and negatives are common and a skin response may not reflect airway hypersensitivity. Radioallergosorbent tests (RAST) may identify allergens to be avoided.

Management of asthma

Goals of management

The goals of management include those for any chronic condition of childhood (see p. 317). The principal goal is the prevention and relief of symptoms of wheeze and cough, both night and day. The child and the parents must be educated so that they can manage a large part of the disease themselves. Good management should promote normal growth and development and allow the child to become involved and participate in all types of exercise and sport.

Practical management

Medication

The drugs used for treating asthma may be classified into 'relievers' and 'preventers'.

• *Relievers.* All children require 'relievers' which are usually beta-agonists such as salbutamol or terbutaline, although the antimuscarinic ipratropium bromide is sometimes used.

• *Preventers.* If the child needs to use 'reliever' treatment frequently (more than 2–3 times a week) the condition warrants prophylactic management with 'preventer' medication. Sodium cromoglycate, which stabilizes mast cells, is the initial drug of choice, but if this fails to prevent symptoms inhaled steroids are required.

All medications should be delivered by inhalation, where possible, as this ensures delivery of the drug direct to the target organ, the bronchioles, causing a more immediate effect and at a lower dose than if the drug is taken orally.

**Goals of management
Asthma**

• Rapid relief of symptoms

• Prevention of symptoms both night and day

• Normal levels of activity, including sport

• Normal growth and development

• Self-management

The following step-by-step plan to control symptoms is recommended for management of the asthmatic child.
• *Step 1.* Inhaled beta$_2$-agonists as required for symptom relief, but no more than three times a week. If symptoms persist check that the child is having the treatment, the delivery system is appropriate and that the technique good.
• *Step 2.* Trial of sodium cromoglycate for at least 6 weeks to determine whether there is a prophylactic response. Continue inhaled beta$_2$-agonist as required.
• *Step 3.* If the trial of cromoglycate is unsuccessful, replace with inhaled steroids. Continue beta$_2$-agonists as required.
• *Step 4.* Increase dose of inhaled steroids. Consider introducing long-acting beta$_2$-agonists or slow-release xanthines (given orally) or ipratropium bromide.
• *Step 5.* When the maximum dose of inhaled steroids is reached, low dose, alternate-day oral steroids should be considered.

Route of administration

Medications need to be inhaled to be most effective. The delivery system chosen must be appropriate for the capability of the child, who will be affected by the severity of the attack. Table 10.3 summarizes the medical treatment of asthma at various ages.

Nebulizer
For infants, children who cannot cooperate and in severe asthma attacks, a mains pump and nebulizer are needed to provide an aerosol which is then delivered by a face mask held close to the child's face (Fig. 10.1).

Spacer device
Toddlers can usually cooperate by using a spacer device with a valve system (Fig. 10.2). A metered dose inhaler dispenses the dose into the chamber and the child inhales the medication over a number of inhalations. The device ensures that the medication reaches the lungs rather than landing in the mouth or throat. Even young infants can use a spacer device if a closely fitting mask is attached, and it can be effective

Age (years)	Delivery system	Reliever	Preventer
<2	Nebulizer Valved spacer and face mask	Salbutamol Terbutaline Ipratropium bromide	Sodium cromoglycate Inhaled steroids: beclomethasone, budesonide
2–4	Metered dose inhaler and valved spacer Nebulizer for acute episodes	As above	As above

5–8	Powder inhalers: MDI with
	    valved spacer for acute
	    attacks
		As above	As above

>8	Powder inhalers Metered dose inhaler with training	As above	As above

Table 10.3 The medical treatment of asthma for children of different ages

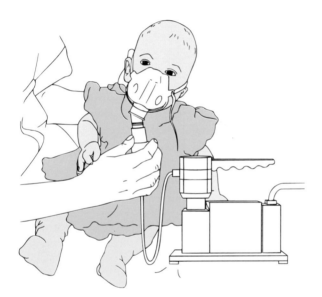

Fig. 10.1 Child using a nebulizer.

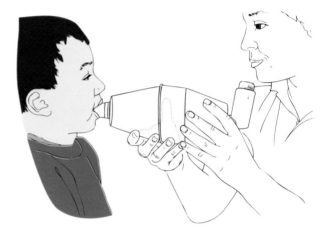

Fig. 10.2 Toddler using a spacer device.

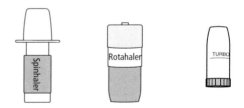

Fig. 10.3 Examples of dry powder systems.

even if a child is crying. It is useful for the older child too in an acute attack when he or she may not be able to use a dry powder system or metered dose inhaler directly. In this circumstance up to 20 puffs can be delivered into the chamber to provide a therapeutic effect.

Dry powder systems (Fig. 10.3)
These are suitable for the school-age child. A good inspiratory effort is needed to trigger the system and so in a severe attack the child may need to resort to a spacer device.

Metered dose inhaler (Fig. 10.4)
This device requires a good degree of coordination and it has been shown that many adults do not use it effectively. It should only be prescribed in children over the age of 8–10

years and only after thorough instruction and checking of technique.

Environmental control

Good environmental control, by reducing exposure to allergens and irritants, can effectively reduce symptoms and drug requirements. It is critical that the child is protected from exposure to cigarette smoke, and smoking in the home, at

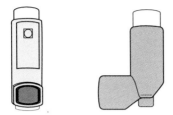

Fig. 10.4 Metered dose inhaler.

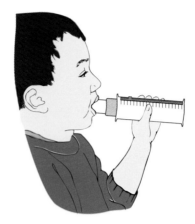

Fig. 10.5 A child using a simple meter to measure peak flow rate.

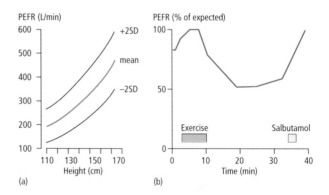

Fig. 10.6 Peak flow chart: how exercise can affect peak flow. (a) The peak flow rate must be related to the child's height to interpret whether it is low. (b) Fall in peak flow rate with exercise in an asthmatic child. Peak flow rate recovers on administration of salbutamol.

least in the child's presence or bedroom, must be avoided. The teenager must be warned of the undesirability of smoking.

House dust, house-dust mites, grass pollens and pets are the commonest allergens. Complete avoidance of house dust is impossible, but feather pillows, duvets and fitted carpets can be avoided. Mattresses should be covered with plastic and the child's room cleaned regularly. Pets, especially cats, may present a problem and while it is undesirable to remove the family pet, acquisition of new pets can be discouraged.

It is a common belief that certain foods can cause asthma. Exclusion diets are not generally indicated, but occasionally certain foods or fizzy drinks are identified as causing attacks. It seems reasonable to avoid these foods, although care must be taken to ensure the diet remains balanced.

Monitoring the condition

Asthma is monitored by keeping a diary of symptoms, where wheezing, cough and activity levels are recorded along with medications given. In the child old enough to cooperate, peak flow monitoring forms part of the record.

Peak flow monitoring (Fig. 10.5)
The majority of children do not need sophisticated lung function tests; however, the peak flow rate is a useful measure of asthmatic control. In the surgery or hospital, a Wright's peak flow meter is used, though it is also useful for the family to have a simple meter for home use.

Peak flow rate (PFR) measures the volume of air moved in a forced expiration. The child is instructed to inhale, place the mouth piece in his or her mouth and to blow out as hard as he or she can. The needle records the peak flow of that exhalation. The procedure should be repeated three times, and the highest reading recorded. Measurements can be taken before and after treating an attack, and in children on preventive medication measurements should be recorded daily, before morning and evening medications.

Peak flow rate is measured in litres/minute. Values must be related to the size of the child. The standardized chart is shown in Fig. 10.6, with an example of how PFR changes with exercise in an asthmatic child.

The diary
An example is shown in Fig. 10.7. The diary serves two functions. It allows the physician to review the child's course and in conjunction with regular clinical reviews to advise on changes in medication requirements. It also may alert him or her to other factors affecting the child such as stress, compliance or environmental triggers. The diary's second function is to help the family follow the course of the condition, make sensible decisions about the need for medication and alert them when to obtain medical advice.

Management of acute problems

If an acute asthmatic attack does not respond quickly to a child's usual treatment at home he or she will need urgent treatment by nebulizer attached to an air compressor or compressed oxygen supply. This may be administered by the

Date this card was started			1	2	3	4	5	6	7	8	9	10
1. WHEEZE LAST NIGHT	Good night .... 0 Slept well but slightly wheezy .... 1 Woke x 2–3 because of wheeze .... 2 Bad night, awake most of time 3		0	0	1	0	0	3	2	1	0	0
2. COUGH LAST NIGHT	None .... 0 Little .... 1 Moderately bad .... 2 Severe 3		0	0	0	0	1	2	2	0	0	0
3. WHEEZE TODAY	None .... 0 Little .... 1 Moderately bad .... 2 Severe 3		0	0	0	1	2	2	2	1	0	0
4. ACTIVITY TODAY	Quite normal...................... 0 Can only run short distance .... 1 Limited to walking because of chest .... 2 Too breathless to walk 3		0	0	0	1	1	2	2	1	0	0
5. NASAL SYMPTOMS	None .... 0 Mild .... 1 Moderate .... 2 Severe 3		0	0	0	0	0	0	0	0	0	0
6. METER (Best of 3 blows)	Before breakfast medicines		200	200	200	150	150	150	100	200	200	200
	Before bedtime medicines		200	200	200	125	125	100	150	200	200	200
7. DRUGS (Number of doses actually taken during the past 24 hours)	Name of drug Salbutamol	Dose prescribed 2 puff prn	–	–	–	1	2	4	4	2	–	–
8. COMMENTS	Note if you see a doctor (D) or stay away from school (S) or work (W) because of your chest and anything else important such as an infection (I)											

Fig. 10.7 Diary in asthma.

GP, but if a doctor is not immediately available the child must be taken to hospital for treatment. If there is a good response, the child may be sent home after a period of observation. If the episode is severe or recurrent a short course of oral steroids may be required. Prednisone given for only 3–4 days does not require tapering off, and will not cause adrenal suppression or affect growth.

If there is inadequate improvement to the nebulized beta-agonist, the child must be admitted for intravenous therapy of a beta-agonist, steroid and possibly aminophylline treatment. Most severe attacks respond rapidly to this treatment, but occasionally intubation and ventilation is required. The treatment of a severe asthma attack is covered in more detail in Chapter 4.

In general, children with asthma are often subjected to a large number of unnecessary chest X-rays. Beyond the initial episode at diagnosis X-rays are only indicated if another problem such as pneumonia, pneumothorax or foreign body is suspected. This is best assessed after the bronchospasm has been relieved.

Routine follow-up of the child with asthma

Regular follow-up is required for all children with asthma, the frequency depending on the severity of the condition and the capabilities of the family in making management decisions.

History

If a diary has been diligently kept, most of the information will be recorded. If this is not available it is important to determine the frequency of symptoms of cough and wheeze and the degree to which it is affecting activity. It is also important to ascertain whether there have been any severe attacks in the interim or absences from school, and whether there are any psychosocial difficulties related to asthma.

Physical examination

At routine appointments, more often than not there is no

Principles of therapeutics
Asthma

- Medications must be delivered by inhalation whenever possible

- Use beta-agonists to relieve symptoms

- If used >3 times per week introduce preventer (cromoglycate or if unsuccessful inhaled steroids)

- In intractable asthma use alternate-day oral steroids

- Treat acute attacks promptly with nebulizer, consider short course of prednisone

- If attack persists, admit for nebulizer treatment, intravenous steroids +/− aminophylline.

- In severe cases ventilation may be required

Checklist for review of a child with asthma

If the child is new to you or the clinic, check:
- ☐ The family's understanding of asthma and their ability to make adjustments in medications
- ☐ Inhaler technique
- ☐ Environmental control, especially smoking
- ☐ Accessibility of inhaler at school

At routine follow-up, review:
History
- ☐ Diary, or if unavailable ask about symptoms of cough and wheeze
- ☐ Frequency of reliever Rx
- ☐ Number of severe attacks
- ☐ Number of absences from school as a result of asthma
- ☐ Any activities restricted because of asthma

Physical examination
- ☐ Height and weight
- ☐ Examination of chest
- ☐ Consider checking inhaler technique

Investigations
- ☐ Peak flow measurement

Action:
- ☐ Advise on increasing or decreasing preventer treatment
- ☐ Consider changing device as child matures
- ☐ Counsel about particular issues such as life-style and independence

evidence of asthma on physical examination. In the child with chronic severe asthma the chest may take on a barrel shape and Harrison sulci (an anterolateral depression of the thorax at the insertion of the diaphragm) may be present (Fig. 2.25, p. 31). Clubbing of the fingers is rare even in severe asthma and suggests other causes of chronic obstructive lung disease.

Investigations

Pulmonary function tests other than peak flow measurements are rarely indicated. The long-term management of asthma is essentially clinically based.

Prognosis

Most children with asthma improve as they grow older. Preschool children who wheeze only with colds are likely to grow out of it in the early school years. The prognosis varies with the severity of the condition. Only 5% of those with mild asthma progress to develop severe disease. In contrast, 95% of those with severe disease continue to suffer as adults. After remission, asthma may recur in adulthood.

Issues for the family

Education

The family must learn to recognize the symptoms and signs of asthma, and the difference in action of the medications prescribed. They must know how to use the various inhalation devices and to identify when the child is too distressed to take the medication by the usual route. They must also learn the technicalities of peak flow monitoring and the importance of keeping an effective diary and utilizing it to make changes in treatment. Parents should be amenable to adapting the environment, but smoking may be the most important and difficult feature.

Although in the young child the parent must be responsible for the asthmatic management, it is important that the child learns how and when to use an inhaler independently by the time he or she starts school, and that more responsibility is gradually developed.

It does not seem that there is any particular advice to give the family regarding the prognosis for subsequent children being affected other than avoidance of smoking antenatally as well as postnatally. Although breast-feeding protects against the development of eczema in susceptible infants, no such clear connection has been established for asthma.

Psychosocial

Asthma too often is responsible for absences from school and interferes in full participation in both school and extra-curricular activities. Even when symptoms are controlled during the day, children perform poorly following disturbed nights. A particularly difficult period may be during adolescence when poor compliance or aerosol abuse may complicate the picture.

Asthma is a condition which can be frightening for the child and the family. This may lead to a tendency to overprotect the child. As emotional factors can trigger symptoms, this too can affect the functioning of the family. The role of the health professional is important in not only managing the physical symptoms of asthma but also to address these issues and maximize the chance of the child leading a full and normal life.

ASTHMA AT A GLANCE

Epidemiology

Commonest chronic respiratory condition. Some 10% of children are affected

Aetiology/Pathophysiology

Environmental factors cause bronchoconstriction, mucosal oedema and excessive mucus production in a genetically predisposed child

How the diagnosis is made

Diagnosis is clinical, based on recurrent or persistent cough/wheeze which is reversed by bronchodilators

Clinical features

History
- Recurrent episodes of cough/wheeze
- Nocturnal cough
- Dyspnoea
- History of atopy*
- Family history atopic disease*

Physical examination
- Normal chest exam between attacks
- Acute, often severe respiratory distress during attack
- Barrel shaped chest if long-standing asthma*
- Poor growth, delayed puberty if severe disease*

Investigations
- Reduced peak flow rate, improved by bronchodilators
- Hyperinflation on chest X-ray

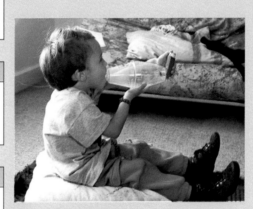

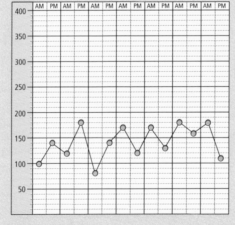

Peak flow chart

General management

Medication: involves 'preventers' and 'relievers' by delivery system appropriate for age (see Principles of Therapeutics Box p. 323)
Environmental control:
- no smoking in child's presence
- dust/mite free environment
Monitoring of asthma:
- home diary of symptoms and treatment
- peak flow meter
Education:
- understanding asthma
- competent use of inhalers
- environmental control
- self management
School:
- education of staff
- inhalers must be accessible
- monitoring of school performance, absences and compliance

Management of acute problems

Acute attacks need prompt treatment often by nebuliser and short course of steroids (see Principles of Therapeutics Box p. 323)

Points for routine follow up

Monitor
- symptoms of cough/wheeze
- activity levels
- school absence
- acute attacks
- growth
- chest exam
- peak flow rate

Prognosis

Asthma resolves over time for most children unless severe. Deaths still occur from asthma in the UK

NB *Signs and symptoms are variable

Issues at school

Given the prevalence of asthma, there are likely to be two or three children with asthma in any class. It is important that all teachers therefore have an understanding of the condition. In the young child the teacher must be able to recognize symptoms and help the child in administering his or her therapy.

It is critical that all asthmatic children have ready access to their inhalers. The older primary school child should be allowed to carry the inhaler around at all times, and certainly should have it with them for sports activities. The younger child should have it accessible in his or her tray—it will do no good locked in the teacher's drawer or the school office. Teaching staff need to understand that inadvertent use by the child or friends will cause no harm. A spare inhaler should be prescribed to be kept in school.

Staff at school can also be helpful in reporting symptoms to the parents or school nurse. This may be of particular value at secondary school, when poor compliance can be a particular issue

DIABETES MELLITUS

Prevalence

Diabetes occurs in one in 500 children. It is an important condition as it has such a major impact on the child and family in terms of daily life, the possibility of unpredictable emergencies and the severity of the medical problems that occur later in life.

Aetiology and pathophysiology

Aetiology

Diabetes mellitus is the medical condition that results from insulin deficiency. In childhood this almost always occurs as a consequence of failure of the beta cells in the islets of the pancreas. This aetiology contrasts with adult onset diabetes which usually results from a peripheral resistance to the action of insulin and high rather than low insulin levels occur.

The process by which the beta cells in the pancreatic islets of Langerhans are destroyed is yet to be elucidated. It is likely that the process is generated by environmental factors, possibly viral, which affect genetically susceptible individuals. An autoimmune process has also been implicated.

Pathophysiology

In order to appreciate the management of diabetes it is necessary to review normal glucose metabolism. Insulin in the normal individual is secreted in response to a rise in blood

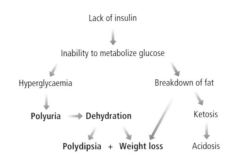

Fig. 10.8 Glucose metabolism and the clinical features (shown in bold) of diabetes.

glucose. Its release is finely modulated by the fluctuation in glucose levels which occur on eating and exercise, and are also under hormonal and neural influence. Insulin facilitates the utilization of glucose as energy for immediate use and its storage as fat for later use. In the fasting state, the fall in blood glucose cuts off insulin secretion, so allowing for mobilization of fat with resultant ketone production. The result is regular swings between the high insulin anabolic rate and the low insulin catabolic state.

In the diabetic individual the lack of insulin results in an inability to utilize glucose, causing hyperglycaemia and breakdown of fat. This is responsible for the clinical features of the untreated diabetic state (see Fig. 10.8).

High levels of blood sugar place the individual in a hyperosmolar state. The resultant osmotic diuresis causes polyuria and dehydration, precipitating thirst and polydipsia. Despite the high glucose levels the calories cannot be utilized and their loss in the urine causes weight loss. As insulin levels are low, fat is broken down to ketones and ketoacidosis ensues.

Management of the condition requires replacement of insulin. It is impossible to mimic the normal physiological state exactly; however, regular injections of insulin should maintain blood sugar levels near the normal range. This is important not only to avoid the immediate symptoms and dangers of hyperglycaemia, but also the long-term complications of diabetes.

Diabetic complications

There are four major long-term complications which occur in diabetes and which account for the major morbidity of the condition:
1 retinopathy (the commonest cause of blindness in developed countries);
2 nephropathy (affects 25–40% of diabetic individuals);
3 neuropathy;
4 heart disease.
Complications tend to occur some years after onset and therefore are uncommon in the childhood years. These complications have been shown to be directly related to the degree of long-term glycaemic control, and it is for this

reason that every effort must be made to maintain the child in as close to a euglycaemic state as possible.

In addition to these complications, hypothyroidism, other autoimmune diseases and coeliac disease occur more commonly in the child with diabetes.

Initial presentation of diabetes

In childhood diabetes symptoms are usually present for only a number of weeks before the diagnosis is made. This contrasts with adult onset diabetes where symptoms may occur for months or even years before diagnosis. Most children are diagnosed following recognition of the symptoms of polyuria, polydipsia, thirst and weight loss, although rarely they present in diabetic ketoacidotic coma. In young children polyuria may present as secondary nocturnal enuresis. Accompanying symptoms may include lethargy, anorexia and constipation, and if prolonged also vomiting, abdominal pain and the features of diabetic ketoacidosis (DKA) (see Fig. 10.13).

Physical examination is often not helpful but may confirm weight loss, and there may be signs of dehydration and the smell of acetone on the breath. The diagnosis is confirmed by the finding of hyperglycaemia, either on random blood sampling or by testing the urine for the presence of sugar. An elevated blood sugar is confirmation in itself, and no further tests such as fasting blood sugar or glucose tolerance tests are indicated.

Referral to a paediatric specialist team is always required. The child is usually admitted to hospital for a few days even if not in ketoacidosis, as intensive education is essential for both the child and the family.

Medical management at presentation

Correction of the metabolic state

Most children are admitted with hyperglycaemia and ketonuria, but not in frank ketoacidosis. Normoglycaemia is usually easily achieved by subcutaneous insulin injections and oral rehydration. If marked dehydration and ketoacidosis are present these demand treatment as described in Table 10.5.

Education of the child and parents

The diagnosis of diabetes involves a change in life-style, probably greater than any other chronic medical condition. The initial education period is crucial in establishing and maintaining these changes. By the end of this period the family should have acquired the following skills:
- insulin administration;
- blood glucose monitoring;
- testing urine for ketones;
- nutritional understanding and a dietary plan;
- an understanding of the relationship of food, insulin, exercise and infection;
- ability to identify and manage hypoglycaemic attacks;
- an understanding of the importance of good control;
- knowledge as to how to obtain advice at any time.

In addition, the school should have been visited to ensure that the staff likewise understand and are trained to cope.

The diabetic team

The team of professionals required to manage diabetes successfully in childhood usually consists of:
- a paediatrician with a special interest in diabetes;
- a diabetes nurse specialist;
- a dietitian;
- a social worker.

In some teams a psychologist or psychiatrist, chiropodist and dentist are also involved.

Management of diabetes

Goals of management

The goals of management in diabetes, as for any chronic condition of childhood, are to encourage the child to live as normal a life as possible, while accepting the limitations that good management of the condition allows (see also p. 316).

Practical management

Medication

Insulin preparations have varying durations of action (see Table 10.4). The goal of therapy is to approximate insulin

---

Goals of management
Diabetes

- Good metabolic control—maintaining blood glucose levels as normal as possible, without episodes of DKA and a minimum of hypoglycaemic events

- A good understanding of the condition by the family such that they can competently manage the child's diabetes and adjust insulin requirements to diet, exercise, stress and infection

- Minimize complications

- Normal growth and development with full participation in school and social activities

- Work towards the child taking maximal responsibility for his or her diabetes as appropriate for the child's age and intelligence

levels to physiological insulin secretion. This is achieved by mixing short and intermediate acting insulins. In the childhood years it is usually satisfactory if given twice daily although this may have to be increased during adolescence. The different types of insulin can be drawn up in the same syringe, or premixed preparations can be given.

Children usually require 0.5–1.0 units/kg, giving two thirds of the dose in the morning and one third at night. These proportions form a very rough guide and the dose needs to be adjusted on a regular basis according to blood glucose measurements which should be monitored regularly. Insulin is usually given before meals to match the rise in insulin with the rise in postprandial glucose. Figure 10.9 shows the relationship of blood glucose and insulin levels to meals and insulin injections.

Mode of delivery Insulin is given subcutaneously by syringe or by using preloaded insulin 'pens' (Fig. 10.10). The site of injection is unimportant, but children are encouraged to rotate the site between upper arms, thighs, abdomen and buttocks, in order to avoid lipoatrophy and lipohypertrophy which are unsightly and can affect absorption rates.

Other aspects of management

The other mainstay of treatment is diet. This is often seen to be a major restriction for the family, but in fact the requirements are simply a normal 'healthy' diet which is high in fibre in amounts sufficient to promote normal growth. However, as there is no physiological insulin response to eating, it is important that meals are taken at regular times through the day and of consistent amounts, in order to match postprandial glucose rises with the administration of insulin. Regular snacks are required in order to prevent blood glucose levels dropping between meals. High sugar foods must be kept to a minimum as they cause excessive swings in glucose levels.

In children as opposed to adults it is important not to adjust food intake to counteract rises in blood sugar, as this may jeopardize growth. Unless obesity is an issue, the child's requirements should be guided by appetite and hunger, and the dietary recommendations and insulin dose adjusted accordingly.

Families require the guidance of a dietitian, particularly in the early stages. In order to allow for flexibility and consistency, the family is taught to recognize foods as easily identifiable 10 g portions which allow for ready and sensible adjustments.

Monitoring the condition

Blood glucose monitoring and diary

Confirmation of symptoms and adjustments in insulin dose are guided by regular blood glucose monitoring (Fig. 10.11) using glucose testing strips and a monitor. The goal is to keep glucose levels as close to the normal range of 4–6 mmol/L as possible. Most children adjust to the demands of testing and it is usually recommended that it is carried out at least 3–4 times per day, 2 days per week, and whenever the child has symptoms of hypo- or hyperglycaemia. Results are recorded in a diary (Fig. 10.12) and allow for sensible adjustments in insulin dose to be made on a regular basis. If measurements are running high for a period, especially if the child is unwell, the family is taught to test for ketosis by measuring the level of ketones in the urine using Acetest strips.

Table 10.4 Types of insulin preparation and their action

Type of insulin	Onset	Peak	Duration
Short acting	30 minutes	2–4 hours	Up to 8 hours
Medium to long acting	1–2 hours	4–12 hours	16–35 hours

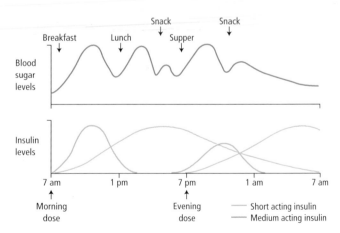

Fig. 10.9 Relationship of blood glucose and insulin levels to meals and insulin injections.

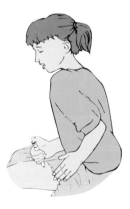

Fig. 10.10 Child injecting herself using a pen.

Unsafe sex can lead to pregnancy, sexually transmitted diseases including AIDS, and have a deleterious effect on future fertility.

The highest rate of sexually transmitted disease is found amongst adolescents. This in part is a result of the sexual behaviour characteristic of this age group, which includes multiple partners, failure to use barrier contraception, reluctance to consider that a partner may have venereal disease, and lack of communication skills to discuss the issue. There are also physiological differences that render the adolescent vaginal epithelium more susceptible to infection.

Gonorrhoea, chlamydia and human papilloma virus are the commonest sexually transmitted diseases in adolescence. HIV infection is on the increase, although because of the long latency period, it may not manifest itself in the teenage years. Risk factors for contraction of HIV include unprotected intercourse and intravenous drug use.

Dieting

A preoccupation with appearance and body shape is characteristic of adolescence. Dieting is an almost universal activity among teenage girls, and often takes the form of extreme starvation diets. Eating disorders are an increasing problem.

Table 11.3 Signs of drug taking

Sudden changes of mood
Loss of appetite
Loss of interest in appearance, school work, leisure interests
Drowsiness or sleeplessness
Furtive behaviour
Unusual stains/smells on clothing

A further concern is that girls as young as 8 or 9 years commonly have a distorted sense of body image, and are increasingly involved in dieting behaviour.

Physical changes in adolescence

Puberty can be defined as the process of gonadal maturation which results in the acquisition of secondary sexual characteristics, a growth spurt and fertility. These occur under the influence of the sex hormones (Fig. 11.1). Gonodatrophin releasing hormone (GnRH) is released from the hypothalamus and stimulates the synthesis of follicle stimulating hormone (FSH) and luteinizing hormone (LH) which in turn stimulate the gonads to produce testosterone or oestrogen.

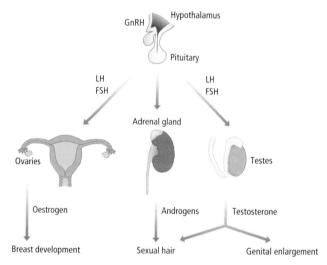

Fig. 11.1 Hormonal events leading to the development of secondary sexual characteristics.

Table 11.4 Common forms of substance abuse

Substance	Epidemiology	Effects	Physical signs
Solvent (sniffing)—toluene based glues, aerosols, fuel gases and solvents	Mainly boys 100 deaths per year from heart failure, suffocation and injuries	Intoxication, excitement, hallucination	Disorientation, slurred speech, blurred vision Skin irritation around the nose and mouth Solvent smells on breath or clothing
Cannabis (generally smoked as a hand-rolled cigarette)	Most widely used illicit drug	Pleasurable feelings of relaxation, altered sensory perception	Red eyes and tachycardia
Cocaine (sniffed through a tube or injected). 'Crack' refers to a less refined form of cocaine		Exhilaration, indifference to pain and hunger, residual depression and fatigue	Tachycardia, hypertension, hyperthermia Teratogenic effect on the fetus
Opiates (swallowing, injecting, sniffing and smoking)	Leading cause of drug related death Consequences of injecting include thrombophlebitis, AIDS and hepatitis B	Euphoria and contentment	Sedation, depression of respiration, heart rate and bowel activity Skin scars
LSD (oral)		Hallucinations	Disorientation, panic

These hormones are responsible for development of breasts and the uterus in girls and all the secondary sexual characteristics in boys. Androgens secreted by the adrenal glands are responsible for sexual hair in girls and contribute to sexual hair development in boys. The key ages at which pubertal events are usually seen are shown in Table 11.5.

For the purpose of clinical description puberty has been divided into five stages, known as Tanner stages. These range from Tanner stage 1 (prepuberty) to Tanner stage 5 (full maturity). They are useful for monitoring the progress of puberty in children where there are concerns about growth or puberty. The five stages for breast, gonadal and pubic hair development are illustrated in Fig. 11.2.

Pubertal development in boys

Puberty in boys usually starts between the ages of 11 and 14 years. The first sign is testicular enlargement, which is fol-lowed by pigmentation and thinning of the scrotum and growth of the penis. As puberty progresses pubic, axillary and facial hair develop, the voice deepens and the ability to ejaculate develops. The growth spurt, which is accompanied by an increase in body size and muscle bulk, occurs when puberty is well underway and is maximal from 14 to 16 years, reaching its peak 2 years after that of girls.

Pubertal development in girls

Puberty tends to start earlier in girls than boys. The first sign is usually breast budding which develops at around 10–11 years, and is followed by pubic and axillary hair development. The growth spurt occurs early, and is virtually completed by menarche (the onset of periods) which usually occurs at 11–13 years. The interval between onset of puberty and menarche is on average 2.0–2.5 years.

PROBLEMS OF PUBERTY

Delayed puberty

Puberty is defined as being delayed if there are no signs of puberty by the age of 14 in a boy, 13 in a girl or if menarche has not occurred by the age of 16 (Table 11.6). Adolescents may present either because of concerns about the absence of sexual development or because of short stature (see p. 56). The commonest cause of pubertal delay is maturational delay, which is commonly familial. Other causes to be considered are Turner's syndrome in girls, and anorexia nervosa or intense athletic training, both of which can

Table 11.5 Key ages in puberty

	Boys	Girls
Normal pubertal range from start to completion	11–16 years	10–14 years
First signs of puberty	Testicular enlargement	Breast budding
Precocious puberty	Onset <9.5 years*	Onset <8.5 years
Delayed puberty	Onset >14 years	Onset >13 years
Delayed menarche	—	Onset >16 years

* High likelihood of pathological rather than physiological cause for precocious puberty in boys.

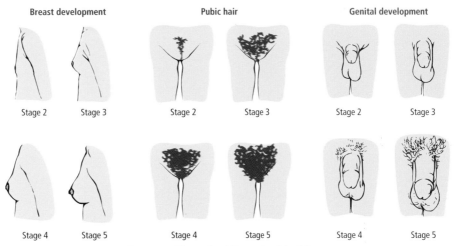

Breast development — Stage 2, Stage 3, Stage 4, Stage 5

Pubic hair — Stage 2, Stage 3, Stage 4, Stage 5

Genital development — Stage 2, Stage 3, Stage 4, Stage 5

Fig. 11.2 Tanner staging of secondary sexual characteristics.

Tanner stage 1 is prepubertal. Tanner stage 5 is adult.
Breast or genital development should be staged independently of pubic hair development

Table 11.6 Causes of delayed puberty

Boys and girls
Maturational delay (commonly familial)
Pituitary lesions
Gonadal failure
Chronic and severe disease

Girls
Turner's syndrome
Intense athletic training
Anorexia nervosa

Table 11.7 Causes of precocious puberty

Hypothalamic–pituitary
Maturational advance (true precocious puberty)
Central nervous system lesions

Ovarian
Premature thelarche

Adrenal
Congenital adrenal hyperplasia
Adrenal tumours

suppress the hypothalamus. Any chronic and severe disease can delay puberty, and rare causes include pituitary or gonadal failure.

Maturational delay (constitutional delay)

Maturational delay of puberty is commonly familial. Although a normal variant it can cause considerable distress, particularly in boys. The diagnosis is based on the pattern of growth (short but steady, see p. 58), a family history of delayed menarche in the women or delayed growth in the men of the family, a delayed bone age and the absence of any evidence of central nervous system pathology. Reassurance is usually all that is required, but if the adolescent (nearly always a boy) is suffering socially, puberty can be triggered by a low dose of testosterone given for a few months.

Turner's syndrome (see p. 59)

In Turner's syndrome, which is caused by an abnormality or absence of one of the X-chromosomes, puberty does not occur, as the gonads, which are just streaks of fibrous tissue, fail to secret oestrogen. Girls with Turner's syndrome should have been identified earlier in childhood because of short stature, but still occasionally present with delayed puberty. It is important to remember that many girls with Turner's syndrome are normal phenotypically and do not have the classic features of the syndrome, so a karyotype is indicated in any girl with either delayed puberty or short stature.

Precocious puberty

Puberty is defined as being precocious if secondary sexual characteristics occur before the age of 8.5 years in a girl or 9.5 years in a boy (Table 11.7). Pubertal signs may occur precociously as a result of premature activation of the hypo-

thalamic–pituitary axis ('true' precocious puberty) or inappropriate secretion of oestrogen or androgens. Precocious puberty in girls is usually idiopathic, but boys are far more likely to have an underlying pathological lesion, and so require especially thorough evaluation.

The child with precocious puberty suffers on two accounts. First he or she has to contend with physical, emotional and social changes at an inappropriately young age and, secondly, adult height is jeopardized as a result of premature fusion of the bones.

Approach to the child with precocious puberty

Activation of the hypothalamic–pituitary axis can be clinically distinguished from inappropriate secretion of the sex hormones alone. In the former the full picture of puberty occurs, whereas in the latter oestrogen secretion causes breast development but no pubic hair, and androgen secretion, pubic hair but no testicular or breast enlargement.

Accompanying features of precocious puberty (with the exception of premature thelarche) include acceleration of growth, advance of skeletal maturation and emotional changes.

Investigations should be directed by the findings on physical examination and should include hormone levels, a karyotype in girls, X-ray for bone age, pelvic ultrasound and computed tomography (CT) or magnetic resonance imaging (MRI) scan of the head.

Causes of precocious puberty

Premature thelarche

Premature thelarche (isolated premature breast development) is not uncommon and occurs in the first 2 years of life. It is a benign condition thought to be caused by a maturational aberration of the hypothalamic–pituitary axis. It does not cause acceleration of growth, and investigations are normal, although ovarian ultrasound may show a few small cysts. The breasts regress spontaneously over some months. Accidental ingestion of maternal contraceptive pills can also cause thelarche.

True precocious puberty

True precocious puberty refers to puberty that is triggered early by premature activation of the hypothalamic–pituitary axis. In girls, the underlying cause is usually idiopathic, but in boys there is commonly an underlying central nervous system lesion such as a tumour or trauma. Treatment includes therapy for the underlying lesion if there is one, and administration of a hormonal analogue which suppresses the secretion of the gonadotrophins.

Congenital adrenal hyperplasia

Congenital adrenal hyperplasia is an autosomal recessive disorder which results in a block in the adrenal production of corticosteroids. As a consequence, a build-up of androgenic precursors occurs, which can result in either ambiguous genitalia (detected at birth, see p. 239), or precocious development of pubic hair. Diagnosis is confirmed by the finding of elevated corticosteroid precursors, and treatment consists of life-long steroid replacement therapy.

Gynaecomastia

Gynaecomastia (breast development in boys) is very common, occurring in 65% of adolescent boys, and is thought to be caused by an oestrogen–androgen imbalance which occurs at puberty. It may be unilateral or bilateral and spontaneous regression occurs over time. Reassurance is usually all that is required, but if there is significant social embarrassment, hormonal or surgical treatment can be given.

Acne

Acne is virtually universal in adolescence. Its development is linked to the onset of sebaceous gland activity and the production of free fatty acids. Inflammation occurs as a result of colonization by micro-organisms.

Clinical features The skin lesions consist of a mixture of comedones (white heads and black heads), pustules and nodulocystic lesions, which may be interspersed with scarring. Lesions may be confined to the face or involve the chest and upper back. As adolescents become preoccupied with their appearance acne assumes great importance. It can cause much distress, may dominate life and even give rise to self imposed isolation.

Management Offering treatment for even mild acne can enhance self image and is therefore important. Diet plays no significant part in the development of acne, although a healthy diet should be encouraged for reasons of general health. Greasy cosmetic and hair preparations should be discontinued. Mild cleansing agents can help by drying the skin and suppressing skin flora. In more severe cases topical antibiotics and retinoic acid, which acts by eliminating the keratinous plug, may be required. The adolescent should be warned that all topical treatment requires several weeks to have an effect. In severe pustular or nodulocystic acne oral antibiotics (usually tetracycline) are indicated.

PSYCHOLOGICAL PROBLEMS OF ADOLESCENCE

Eating disorders

Eating disorders commonly begin as innocent dieting behaviour, which progresses to become a serious condition which may be life-threatening. Girls are far more commonly affected than boys, and the age of onset is decreasing so that as many as one fifth are under the age of 13 years. The eating disorders are characterized by an intense fear of becoming obese, and a distorted body image so that even emaciated affected individuals perceive themselves as being fat. In an attempt to achieve the desired weight there is a denial of hunger, preoccupation with food and bizarre eating behaviours.

Anorexia nervosa

Girls with anorexia nervosa restrict their intake of carbohydrate- and fat-containing foods by extreme dieting in order to control their weight. This is usually accompanied by excessive physical activity.

Clinical features An arbitrary definition of anorexia nervosa has been taken to be a loss of more than 20% body weight in relation to height. The clinical features found are those of malnutrition, with emaciation, amenorrhoea, constipation, dry skin, lanugo hair and hair loss. As body weight

EATING DISORDERS AT A GLANCE

Anorexia   Bulimia

Epidemiology

Girls principally affected
Prepubertal onset now more common

Aetiology/Pathophysiology

Bizarre eating behaviour associated
with a distorted body image and fear
of becoming obese

Clinical features

Anorexia nervosa
History
• extreme dieting (**a**)
• excessive physical activity (**b**)
• weight loss
• amenorrhoea
• constipation
Physical examination
• emaciation
• dry skin
• lanugo hair
• hair loss
• if severe — bradycardia, hypotension
and hypothermia

NB *Signs and symptoms are variable

Clinical features

Bulimia
History
• eating in binges (**c**)
• followed by induced vomiting (**d**) or
laxatives (**e**)
• symptoms of oesophagitis
Physical examination
• usually normal weight
• staining of inner surface of teeth*
• parotid swelling*

Confirmatory investigations

Not required

Differential diagnosis

Other causes of weight loss
Other causes of amenorrhoea

Management

Psychotherapy
Behaviour modification techniques
Nutritional rehabilitation

Prognosis

Can be life-threatening (mortality rates
up to 10%)

decreases bradycardia, hypotension and hypothermia are found.

Bulimia

The girl with bulimia has bouts of eating in binges and then purges herself by inducing vomiting or using laxatives.

Clinical features These girls, in contrast to anorexics, often are of normal weight or slightly obese. Oesophagitis, parotid swelling and staining of the internal surface of the teeth can occur as a result of frequent vomiting.

Management Eating disorders, particularly anorexia, can be life-threatening and mortality rates are as high as 10%, so the condition must be taken seriously. The approach involves a combination of psychotherapy, behaviour modification techniques and nutritional rehabilitation. Antidepressants are sometimes prescribed.

Depression and suicide

Adolescence is naturally a time of moods which swing from the depths of depression to the heights of elation. It is often difficult therefore to decide which adolescent is at risk for true depression. Factors associated with an increased risk include a disturbed or disrupted home life, poor functioning at school, low self esteem, antisocial and aggressive behaviour, substance misuse, stressful life events and a family history of affective disorder.

Suicide is increasing in incidence and is a leading cause of death in this age group. The method most commonly used in adolescence is ingestion of medication, either their own or a parent's. The seriousness of an attempt cannot be related to the lethality of the dose, but is related to the degree of premeditation and the likelihood of rescue.

Clinical features Depression has been defined as a persistently lowered mood, and misery that is severe enough to interfere with everyday life. It is accompanied by feelings of worthlessness, a sense of hopelessness, anxiety, pessimistic thoughts and often suicidal ideas or acts. The depressed adolescent may experience insomnia and difficulty falling asleep, sometimes to the extent of being awake all night and sleeping through the day, and appetite may be altered.

Falling school grades, increase in school absenteeism, and the use of alcohol and drugs are common.

Management Sources of stress should be identified and dealt with as far as possible. Counselling, psychotherapy and, where appropriate, family therapy may be helpful. The parents too need help, especially in dealing with uncooperative behaviour, and providing additional care and affection. At this age, treatment with antidepressants should only be prescribed by specialists.

Any attempt at suicide must be taken seriously as most successful suicides occur among those who have made earlier attempts. Short-term hospitalization is usually indicated to attend to pharmacological sequelae, to assess the psychosocial situation and to impress on the family the need to attend to underlying problems.

GYNAECOLOGICAL PROBLEMS

Menstrual complaints

Amenorrhoea

Amenorrhoea, or the absence of periods, may be primary or

DEPRESSION AND SUICIDE AT A GLANCE

Epidemiology

Suicide: leading cause of death in teenagers
Commonest method is drug ingestion
Risk factors
• disturbed home life
• poor functioning at school
• low selfesteem
• antisocial behaviour
• substance misuse
• family history of affective disorder

Clinical features

Insomnia and difficulty falling asleep*
Altered appetite*
School failure and absenteeism*
Alcohol and drug use*

NB *Signs and symptoms are variable

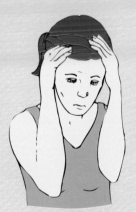

Management

Identify sources of stress
Counselling/psychotherapy for adolescent and family
Antidepressants with caution
Attempted suicide: hospitalize for medical treatment and psychosocial assessment

Prognosis

Seriousness of attempted suicide is related to the degree of premeditation and likelihood of rescue, rather than drug dose
Most successful suicides follow an earlier attempt

Table 11.8 Causes of secondary amenorrhoea

Physiological
Hormonal cycle immaturity
Stress
Intense athletic training
Pregnancy

Pathological
Anorexia nervosa
Chronic illness
Brain tumour
Hyperthyroidism

Table 11.9 Causes of vaginal discharge

Physiological
Poor perineal hygiene
Foreign body
Candida
Sexually transmitted diseases*

* Indicative of sexual abuse if found in a prepubertal child.

secondary. The term primary amenorrhoea indicates that menarche has never occurred, and is discussed on p. 349 (Delayed puberty). Secondary amenorrhoea refers to the cessation of periods for more than 3 months after regular cycles have been established. Its causes are listed in Table 11.8.

Most amenorrhoea in adolescence is physiological. After menarche it is usual for periods to be scanty or irregular for several months, and several months may elapse between periods. Stress, such as starting a new school, can disrupt periods, and girls undergoing intense athletic training can experience amenorrhoea as a result of hypothalamic–pituitary axis suppression. Pregnancy should always be considered as a cause of amenorrhoea in the teenage girl.

The commonest pathological cause of amenorrhoea is anorexia nervosa or dieting. Interestingly, the amenorrhoea can precede the weight loss. Any chronic illness can cause amenorrhoea, but particularly those associated with malnutrition or tissue hypoxia, such as diabetes mellitus, inflammatory bowel disease, cystic fibrosis or cyanotic congenital heart disease.

Approach to the girl with amenorrhoea

Evaluation of the girl with amenorrhoea should include a complete history, focussing on diet, potentially stressful events, exercise, sexual activity, medical history and neurological symptoms. Signs of anorexia nervosa, pregnancy and neurological abnormality should be sought on physical examination. Baseline investigations include a full blood count, plasma viscosity and pregnancy test, and if these are negative, gonadotrophin levels, thyroid function tests, pelvic ultrasound and imaging of the head should be considered.

Dysmenorrhoea

Adolescent girls commonly experience painful menstrual cramps, and dysmenorrhoea is the commonest cause of short-term school absenteeism. The mechanism is thought to

be caused by high levels of endometrial prostaglandins. Effective treatment can be given prophylactically using prostaglandin synthetase inhibitors. An alternative is the oral contraceptive pill, if contraception is desired.

Heavy periods

Excessive menstrual bleeding is most often secondary to the anovulatory cycles that normally occur in the first year postmenarche. Without ovulation, oestrogen unopposed by progesterone causes endometrial proliferation with eventual massive shedding. Hormonal treatment is required if there is anaemia or hypovolaemia. Other causes of heavy periods include bleeding disorders and aspirin ingestion.

Vaginal discharge (Table 11.9)

A normal physiological increase in vaginal discharge occurs in the year prior to menarche. In childhood, discharge secondary to poor perineal hygiene is common and may be accompanied by dysuria, frequency and pruritus. The treatment is as described for dysuria (p. 183). If the discharge is persistent and foul smelling a foreign body (usually toilet paper) should be suspected. In the prepubertal girl candida is not common, although may follow antibiotic therapy. Sexually transmitted diseases must be suspected in the sexually active girl, and a high index of suspicion maintained even in the prepubertal child as, if found, it is indicative of sexual abuse.

Pregnancy

It has been reported that almost 40% of sexually active teenagers become pregnant within 2 years of initiating intercourse, and over half result in live births. The increase in live births is particularly increasing among younger adolescents, many of whom become pregnant deliberately. Girls most at risk are those who lack self esteem, become sexually active early, come from unhappy or unstable backgrounds, and those in care.

Adolescent pregnancy carries increased risks for both the mother and the baby. Contributing factors obstetrically include late booking for antenatal care, poor attendance at clinic and antenatal classes, and poor nutrition. The babies tend to suffer from higher infant and perinatal mortality rates, an increased incidence of sudden infant death syndrome (SIDS), low birthweight (both pre- and post-term), gastrointestinal problems, accidental and non-accidental injury, behaviour problems and delayed psychomotor development.

The adolescent mother is more likely to suffer from post-natal depression, and is less likely to marry ultimately, finish her secondary school education or gain employment.

The problem of increasing numbers of teenage pregnancies is being addressed at a national level, and a reduction in levels is one of the targets of the governmental Health of the Nation initiative.

Abortion

Abortion remains a major form of contraception in this age group, and one third of teenage pregnancies end in legal abortion. Apart from the medical risks of abortion, there are considerable emotional effects for the teenage girl. Follow-up, careful counselling and support are particularly important as many become pregnant again within a year.

Contraception

More adolescents are engaging in sexual intercourse at younger ages, often without any form of contraception. Studies show that fewer than 50% of teenagers use any form of contraception at the time of first intercourse, and the lag between becoming sexually active and seeking effective contraception usually exceeds 1 year. Unfortunately the first visit to a family planning clinic is frequently because of a pregnancy scare.

Reasons why adolescents commonly fail to seek contraceptive advice include their conviction that sexual intercourse is an unpremeditated and infrequent act, fear that their parents will find out and doubt that any advice they seek will be confidential.

Information, access to contraception and motivation are all necessary for successful pregnancy prevention. Interestingly, in contrast to common expectations, sex education far from increasing sexual activity has been shown to delay the

Table 11.10 The advantages and disadvantages of various contraceptive devices during adolescence

Contraceptive device	Advantages	Disadvantages
Condom	Low price Available without prescription Little need for advanced planning Effective in preventing transmission of STD including HIV No side-effects	Less effective in preventing pregnancy Acceptance low in younger adolescents
Diaphragm and spermicide	No side-effects Effective in preventing pregnancy if adolescent is highly motivated Some protection against STD	Not adequately effective in preventing pregnancy if motivation is poor Must be fitted individually Interrupts spontaneity of sex Low acceptability in some girls Messy
Sponge	No prescription or fitting required Less messy than a diaphragm	Significant failure rate Need to be near source of water to insert Increased risk of toxic shock syndrome
Intrauterine contraceptive device (IUD)	Effective in preventing pregnancy Requires no motivation	Increased menstrual bleeding and dysmenorrhoea Increased risk of pelvic infection and future infertility
Oral contraceptive pill	Most reliable method if taken effectively Method unrelated to episode of intercourse Relief of dysmenorrhoea Decreased risks of benign breast disease, anaemia and ovarian cysts	Less suitable if intercourse is infrequent Post-pill amenorrhoea more common in adolescence Raises levels of high density lipoproteins (Major side-effects are exceedingly rare in adolescents)

STD, sexually transmitted disease.

onset of first intercourse, increase contraceptive use and reduce numbers of pregnancies. Advice to the teenager should be based on frequency and circumstances of sexual activity, past experience and compliance with both contraceptive and non-contraceptive chronic medications. The risk of any contraceptive method should be weighed against the risk of pregnancy, which for young adolescents is a significant one. If contraception is to be successful every effort must be made to individualize the method to the needs of the patient. The advantages and disadvantages of the various types of contraception for adolescents are shown in Table 11.10.

Parental consent is not required for the prescription of contraception, provided the doctor has grounds to believe that the adolescent is adequately mature enough to appreciate the risks (and benefits) of contraception.

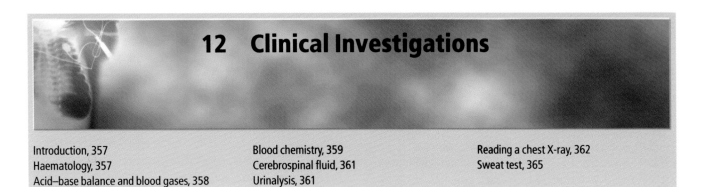

12 Clinical Investigations

Introduction, 357
Haematology, 357
Acid–base balance and blood gases, 358

Blood chemistry, 359
Cerebrospinal fluid, 361
Urinalysis, 361

Reading a chest X-ray, 362
Sweat test, 365

We should use investigations like a drunk man uses a lamp post; for support rather than illumination.

Anon.

Introduction

Investigations should only be requested to confirm a clinical diagnosis or, if indicated, after taking a careful history and performing a physical examination. Fishing for a diagnosis by ordering a battery of tests is poor medicine, an unacceptable use of resources and not in the best interests of the child. The student should understand the relevance of ordering commonly requested investigations.

It is important for the undergraduate to be able to interpret a number of investigations performed on children. In order to do this knowledge of the normal ranges for certain basic investigations is required and should be memorized. The importance of investigations is not simply to recognize if any value falls outside the normal range, but also to interpret the significance of the abnormality and how it influences diagnosis/management.

The normal ranges that are important for medical students to know are listed in the tables below, together with the significance of abnormalities.

Haematology

Normal values for the major haematological indices are shown in Table 12.1.

Haemoglobin

At birth the haemoglobin concentration is high with a mean of 18 g/dL, but falls rapidly to reach its lowest point at 2 months of age (range 9.5–14.5 g/dL) before increasing to a stable value at about 6 months. A low haemoglobin indicates anaemia (p. 89). Figure 12.1 shows how it should be investigated.

Mean cell volume

Mean cell volume (MCV) is a measurement of size of the red blood cell. In paediatrics, microcytic anaemia (MCV <76 fl) is the most common abnormality and is a result of either iron deficiency anaemia (p. 90) or thalassaemia trait (p. 92). An abnormally large red cell is rare and is most likely to be a result of folate deficiency. The MCV is normally high in the newborn for the first few weeks. A low MCV may precede a fall in haemoglobin level.

Mean cell haemoglobin

This refers to the amount of haemoglobin in the red cell and is usually low (hypochromic anaemia) in conjunction with microcytic anaemia.

Examples of pathology

The two most important types of anaemia occurring in paediatrics are discussed below. Table 12.2 shows the important differences in distinguishing the two conditions.

Microcytic hypochromic anaemia
The two likely diagnoses are iron deficiency anaemia and thalassaemia trait. To distinguish the two it is necessary to measure serum ferritin (low in iron deficiency anaemia) and perform haemoglobin electrophoresis (abnormal in thalassaemia trait). Lead poisoning is a rare cause of this type of anaemia and if considered a serum lead level is required.

Anaemia with reticulocytosis
This occurs as the result of haemorrhage or haemolysis. The reticulocyte count is increased indicating an effort by the bone marrow to replenish the destroyed red cells. In haemolysis there may also be evidence of jaundice (p. 128), either clinically or on measurement of an elevated unconjugated bilirubin (Fig. 12.1).

Increased white cell count (leukocytosis)
Systemic bacterial infection usually causes the white cell count to be raised ($15–30 \times 10^9$/L).

357

Table 12.1 Normal range for the major haematological indices for children of 6 months and older

	Normal range
Haemoglobin	11–14 g/dL
Haematocrit	30–45%
White cell count	$6.0–15.0 \times 10^9$/L
Reticulocytes	0–2%
Platelets	$150–450 \times 10^9$/L
Mean cell volume	76–88 (fl)
Mean cell haemoglobin	24–30 pg
Erythrocyte sedimentation rate (ESR)	10–20 mm in 1 hour

Table 12.2 Distinction between microcytic anaemia and anaemia resulting from haemolysis or blood loss (normal range)

	Microcytic hypochromic anaemia	Anaemia resulting from haemolysis or blood loss
Haemoglobin	Low	Low
Haematocrit	Low	Low
White cell count	Normal	Normal
Reticulocytes	Low	High
Platelets	Normal	Low
Mean cell volume	Low	Normal
Mean cell haemoglobin	Low	Normal

Table 12.3 Normal ranges for acid–base and blood gas measurements

Arterial pH	7.35–7.42
Arterial P_{CO_2}	4.0–5.5 kPa
Arterial P_{O_2}	11–14 kPa (lower values in neonates 8–10 kPa)
Arterial or venous bicarbonate	17–27 mmol/L

Table 12.4 Causes of acidosis and alkalosis

	Causes
Metabolic acidosis	Severe gastroenteritis
	Neonatal asphyxia
	Shock
	Diabetic ketoacidosis
Metabolic alkalosis	Pyloric stenosis
Respiratory acidosis	Respiratory failure of any cause
Respiratory alkalosis	Overventilation
	Overbreathing

The blood film shows that this is comprised mainly of excess polymorphonuclear granulocytes (neutrophils) with a preponderance of immature white cells (a left shift). These changes also occur as the result of severe stress or administration of corticosteroids.

Viral infection is usually associated with only a modest leukocytosis, but a preponderance of lymphocytes. In infectious mononucleosis characteristic atypical lymphocytes are seen in the peripheral blood film.

In leukaemia the white cell count is very high or very low and blast cells are usually seen in the peripheral blood film. Platelet numbers are often reduced.

Acid–base balance and blood gases

Normal acid–base and blood gas values are shown in Table 12.3.

Disturbances in acid–base chemistry occur as the result of either respiratory or metabolic disorders. Table 12.4 lists the causes of acidosis and alkalosis.

Blood pH

The acidity of blood is measured by pH. Normal pH range is 7.35–7.42 and measurements above this refer to alkalosis

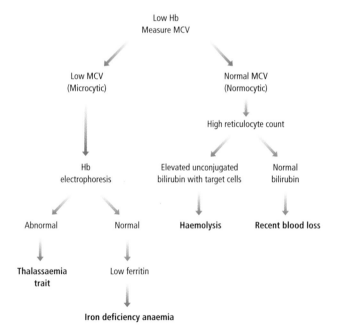

Fig. 12.1 Flow diagram to show investigation of anaemia.

Table 12.5 Changes in acid–base and blood gas values according to type of alkalosis or acidosis

	Metabolic acidosis	Metabolic alkalosis	Respiratory acidosis	Respiratory alkalosis
pH	Low	High	Low	High
P_{O_2}	Normal	Normal	Normal or low	Normal or high
P_{CO_2}	Normal or low*	Normal or high*	High	Low
Bicarbonate	Low	High	Normal or high*	Normal or low*

* Compensated state.

and values below it indicate acidosis. Whether the acidosis or alkalosis is metabolic or respiratory requires assessment of partial pressure of CO_2 and bicarbonate measurements (Table 12.5). A flow diagram for the interpretation of blood gas results is shown in Fig. 12.2.

P_{O_2}

The partial pressure of oxygen (P_{O_2}) in arterial blood indicates whether the child is hypoxic (low P_{O_2}) or hyper-oxic (high P_{O_2}). Generally the inspired oxygen can be adjusted to keep the child's P_{O_2} within the normal range (normoxic). Transcutaneous oxygen saturation monitoring is now widely used for continuous oxygen assessment.

P_{CO_2}

A high partial pressure of carbon dioxide (P_{CO_2}) indicates underventilation. This may occur in coma (p. 306) or caused by intrinsic respiratory disease such as respiratory distress syndrome (p. 247). A high P_{CO_2} will cause a respiratory acidosis (see Table 12.5).

A low P_{CO_2} in a mechanically ventilated child indicates that the machine's settings are too high for the state of the child's lungs. Rarely, overbreathing may occur in a sponta-neously breathing child as a result of hysteria. A low P_{CO_2} will cause a respiratory alkalosis (see Table 12.5).

Bicarbonate

This anion varies with acid–base status. In metabolic acidosis the serum bicarbonate is low. Examples of situa-tions where this occurs are neonatal asphyxia (p. 234) and diabetic ketoacidosis (p. 328).

In acute respiratory acidosis the bicarbonate may initially be normal, but then becomes elevated in an attempt to com-pensate and normalize the pH.

The only cause of metabolic alkalosis commonly seen in paediatrics is excessive vomiting as a result of pyloric stenosis (see below and p. 159). This causes an increase in bicarbonate (Fig. 12.2).

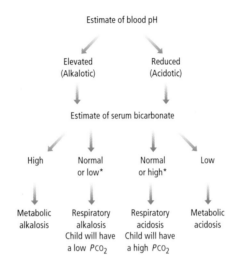

Fig. 12.2 Flow diagram to guide the interpretation of blood gas results.

Blood chemistry

Modern analytical blood chemistry investigations can be done rapidly on small volumes of blood by an automated process. One disadvantage of this is that the clinician receives results on all the variables that the machine is programmed to analyse. Consequently the result print-out may contain 12–20 different values. It is not necessary to memorize the normal ranges for all these variables, but it is important to know a limited number as shown in Table 12.6.

Blood urea and serum creatinine

Urea and creatinine are widely used as an index of renal function and/or vascular hydration.

Urea is a major metabolite of protein breakdown and is both filtered and reabsorbed by the kidneys. Its concentra-tion in the plasma is dependent on protein intake, state

Table 12.6 Normal ranges for basic clinical chemistry variables

	Normal range
Sodium	133–145 mmol/L
Potassium	3.5–4.7 mmol/L
Chloride	96–110 mmol/L
Bicarbonate	20–27 mmol/L
Creatinine	20–80 μmol/L
Urea	2.5–6.5 mmol/L
Glucose	3.0–6.0 mmol/L
Alkaline phophatase	Infant, 150–1000 unit/L
	Child, 250–800 unit/L

Table 12.7 Causes of hyper- and hyponatraemia

	Causes
Hypernatraemia	
Dehydration	Diarrhoea
	Fluid deprivation
Excess sodium intake	Inappropriate milk feed preparation
Hyponatraemia	
Sodium loss	Gastroenteritis with hypotonic fluid replacement
	Renal loss (renal failure)
	Cystic fibrosis (p. 176)
Water excess	Excessive IV fluid administration

of catabolism and renal function. Because its value is dependent on so many variables it is not a good measure of renal function. The commonest cause of an elevated urea is dehydration.

Creatinine is produced by muscles at a constant rate and is influenced far less by catabolism than urea. It is filtered by the glomerulus, but a proportion is also secreted by the proximal tubules. Nevertheless, creatinine clearance is a reliable measure of glomerular filtration rate and an isolated serum creatinine measurement is a much better index of renal function than urea.

Serum electrolytes

The normal range for serum electrolytes are shown in Table 12.6.

Sodium

In disease states sodium may be normal, increased (hypernatraemic) or low (hyponatraemic). These abnormalities are described under dehydration (p. 117). Causes for hypo- and hypernatraemia are shown in Table 12.7.

Potassium

Potassium is the major intracellular cation and is in relatively low concentration in the extracellular spaces. Artefactually high serum potassium levels may occur as the result of red cell haemolysis caused by keeping blood for too long in the container before analysis. If the blood is seen to be haemolysed when it is analysed then the serum potassium level will be unreliable.

Hypokalaemia most often occurs as the result of gastroenteritis or pyloric stenosis (see below).

Hyperkalaemia results from renal failure and increases as a result of metabolic acidosis. In diabetic ketoacidosis

(DKA) the serum potassium is high, but drops rapidly after the DKA is treated.

Alkaline phosphatase

In routine laboratory tests the alkaline phosphatase value represents a group of isoenzymes arising from bone and liver. In neonates the normal range may be up to four times that of the adult and gradually falls during childhood.

A high alkaline phosphatase may represent bone disease (particularly rickets) or, less commonly in children, cholestatic liver disease.

Examples of pathology

Dehydration

Three types of dehydration exist: hyper-, iso- and hyponatraemic. These are discussed in Chapter 4 (p. 117).

Diabetic ketoacidosis (p. 328)

The major metabolic and electrolyte abnormalities in DKA occur as the result of hyperglycaemia and ketoacidosis. The blood pH falls as a result of accumulation of ketoacids. As a consequence of the metabolic acidosis, the child attempts to compensate by hyperventilation (Kussmaul breathing, p. 306) which reduces the P_{CO_2}. The high blood sugar causes an osmotic diuresis which leads to progressive dehydration with increased creatinine/urea levels. The main biochemical abnormalities are therefore summarized as:

- pH   low
- P_{CO_2} low
- bicarbonate   low
- sodium   normal
- potassium   high
- creatinine/urea   high
- glucose   high.

Table 12.8 Normal cerebrospinal fluid values

Protein	0.15–0.4 g/L
Glucose	30–50% of blood glucose
Cells	<5 white cells
Pressure	<5 cmH$_2$O

Pyloric stenosis (p. 159)

In this condition vomiting causes excessive loss of hydrogen and chloride ions with increasing alkalosis. Because of the obstruction between stomach and duodenum, there is little sodium and potassium loss in the vomitus. Bicarbonate is increased and potassium is lost through the kidney in exchange for conserving hydrogen ions. The abnormalities seen in pyloric stenosis are:

- pH   high
- bicarbonate   low
- chloride   low
- potassium   low
- sodium   normal or low
- creatinine/urea normal or high.

Cerebrospinal fluid

Lumbar puncture should not be performed if there are signs of raised intracranial pressure as coning may occur (p. 110).

Meningitis can only be confirmed by obtaining cerebrospinal fluid (CSF) at lumbar puncture. The pressure of the CSF should be measured as the first drop of CSF emerges. This is most easily done by connecting a calibrated plastic tube to the needle and waiting for the fluid level to stabilize. The child must be quiet when the pressure is measured as crying will cause an artefactually high pressure to be recorded. Normal CSF pressure is <5 cmH$_2$O.

The normal range for protein and glucose in CSF is shown in Table 12.8. A blood sugar should be taken at the same time as the lumbar puncture to compare the plasma with CSF glucose (the normal ratio is 2–3 : 1).

The colour of the CSF should be described. It is normally absolutely clear and cloudiness suggests infection. Blood-stained CSF may occur as a result of intracranial bleeding or may occur as the result of a traumatic tap. This occurs if a blood vessel is penetrated by the needle on passage into the subarachnoid space. This can be determined by allowing the blood-stained fluid to drip into three successive containers. If the blood staining becomes less in successive containers then this is because of a traumatic tap, but if the blood staining remains uniform throughout the three containers this is likely to be because of intracranial haemorrhage. The results

**Distinguishing features
CSF investigation in bacterial and
viral meningitis**

	Bacterial meningitis	Viral meningitis
Cells	Polymorphs (in early stages cells may be absent)	Lymphocytes (in early stages polymorphs may be present)
Protein	High	Mildly elevated
Glucose*	Low	Normal
Gram stain	Organisms identified	No organisms seen
Culture	Positive growth (unless partially treated)	No growth

* Normal ratio of plasma : CSF glucose is 2–3 : 1.

obtained from the laboratory from CSF that is contaminated by blood as the result of a traumatic tap will reflect serum rather than CSF levels and will be unreliable.

Abnormalities found in the CSF as a result of viral and bacterial meningitis are shown in the Distinguishing features box, above.

Urinalysis

It is important that medical students are able to examine urine and perform urinalysis by using commercially available dipsticks.

Fresh urine should be collected into a sterile container from a midstream specimen if possible. A fresh bag is appropriate in young children and infants.

Observation

Look at the specimen in a clear test tube or equivalent container and comment on its colour and odour. In particular note the following:

Clarity Is the urine cloudy? (suggestive of infection).

Colour Red or brown urine is suggestive of haematuria. Red or pink colour suggests bleeding from the lower urinary tract. Coca-cola coloured urine is suggestive of blood loss from the kidneys.

Odour A smell of acetone indicates the presence of ketone bodies.

Dipstick testing

The dipstick contains a number of reagent blocks, each one about 5 mm². Depending on the stick there may be up to 10 reagent squares on the stick. The tests are all at best semiquantitative and so if quantitative information is required then the urine should be sent to the laboratory for analysis.

The only way to obtain definite data on the presence of a urinary tract infection is to count the cells under a microscope and to culture the urine and identify any bacterial colonies. The following procedure for dipsticking should be followed and is illustrated in Fig. 12.3.

1 Immerse the entire dipstick area (all the reagent squares) in the urine and remove the stick immediately.
2 Shake off excess urine from the stick.
3 Hold the strip in a horizontal position and compare the test areas with the colour chart label on the container. Many of the reagent squares require the result to be read at an exact time after the exposure to urine. This information is on the colour chart and is summarized below. Colour changes that occur after 2 minutes are of no reliability and should be discarded.

The times at which these blocks should be read are printed on the bottle and are summarized in Table 12.9.

Reading a chest X-ray

It is important to be able to describe the findings on inspection of a chest X-ray in a systematic manner. Undergraduates will not necessarily be expected to make the correct diagnosis, but for some conditions the signs are usually obvious.

In most cooperative children a posterior–anterior (PA) film is taken in inspiration. This means that the child stands with his or her chest against the X-ray plate and the X-ray beam is directed from the back through the chest to the plate. In sick children or neonates the film is usually anterior–posterior (AP) when the baby lies supine on the plate with the X-ray beam above. If the X-ray is AP it should be written on the film. Assume the film to be PA unless told otherwise.

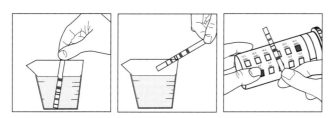

Fig. 12.3 Using the dipsticks for urinalysis.

For a complete radiological examination of the chest a lateral X-ray is necessary (see below). Normal appearances are shown in Fig. 12.4a.

Check technical factors

Identify the patient by the name on the X-ray, the date that the X-ray was taken and the orientation (right and left). Comment on whether the penetration is good, under- or overexposed. An underexposed film will appear more white with less contrast and an overexposed film will be blacker with the bones clear but little distinction between the heart and the lung fields. Penetration is ideal if the vertebrae can just be seen through the heart shadow.

Check that important anatomical landmarks have not been excluded including the costophrenic angles, the ribs and soft tissues into the root of the neck. Comment on attached lines, endotracheal tube, drains, etc.

Central positioning

Check whether the patient is standing square to the plane of the X-ray beam. This is apparent by looking to see whether the vertebral bodies and transverse processes are symmetrical. The clavicles and ribs should also be symmetrical. If there is rotation then the clavicles will appear asymmetrical. Estimating heart size or lung fields is unreliable in a rotated film.

Table 12.9 The timing and interpretation of dipstick urinalysis

Substance in urine	Time for block to be read	Comments
pH	Not critical	pH correlates with best colour match on card
Protein	Not critical	This is very sensitive and a trace or a '+' is usually not significant
Glucose	30 s	Specific for glucose not other reducing substances
Bilirubin	30 s	Any bilirubin in the urine must be further investigated
Ketones	40 s	Reagent block only reacts to acetoacetic acid which is always present in DKA
Blood	60 s	This is very sensitive and may be positive in clear urine. Quantification of haematuria by urine microscopy should be carried out if positive

DKA, diabetic ketoacidosis.

Inspection (see Fig. 12.4b&c)

Bony structures Comment on the ribs, clavicles and vertebral bodies. Is there any evidence of asymmetry or congenital abnormality? Count the ribs on both sides (12 pairs should be apparent). Missing ribs may occur as the result of cardiothoracic surgery or represent a congenital abnormality.

Diaphragms Both diaphragms should be clear and the right is normally higher than the left because of the liver position. Examine the costophrenic angles which should be clear and sharply defined. Look for air below the diaphragm, which is always abnormal.

Cardiac outline Measure the cardiac outline at its widest point and compare it to the widest diameter of the ribs. In infants the normal ratio of cardiac diameter to widest chest wall diameter is up to 0.6, and in older children a ratio of up to 0.5 is normal. Comment on the clarity of the cardiac outline. If the right border of the heart is obscured this suggests right middle lobe collapse/consolidation (Fig. 12.5 and 12.6b).

Lung fields The lung fields should be symmetrical and of uniform radiolucency. The only markings within the lung fields should be pulmonary blood vessels. Comment on the hilar shadows. It requires considerable experience to decide whether there is excessive hilar shadowing or whether this represents a normal chest X-ray appearance. Identify the horizontal fissure on the PA film (see Fig. 12.4b). Collapse/consolidation of a lung lobe can usually be seen by a focal opacity on the PA film (see Fig. 12.5a and Fig. 12.6). If there is deviation of the mediastinal shadow with lung

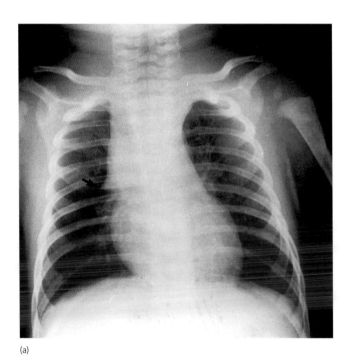

(a)

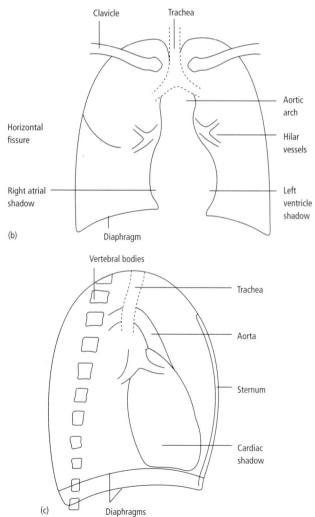

(b)

(c)

Fig. 12.4 (a) A normal PA chest X-ray. The thymus gland is seen as a 'sail shaped' shadow (indicated by the arrow). (b) Anatomical landmarks of a PA chest X-ray. (c) Anatomical landmarks of a lateral chest X-ray.

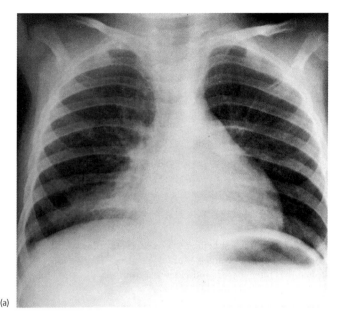

(a)

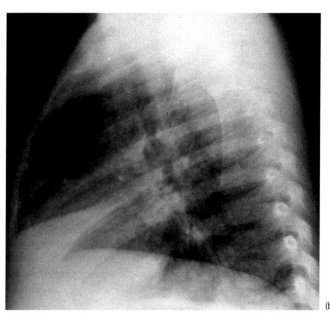

(b)

Fig. 12.5 Chest X-ray. (a) PA film showing collapse of right middle lobe with loss of definition of the right heart border. (b) The col- lapsed right middle lobe is seen as a wedge shaped shadow on the lateral film.

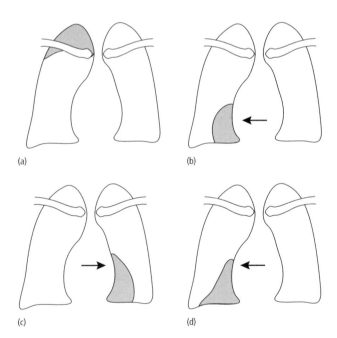

(a)   (b)

(c)   (d)

Fig. 12.6 Some commonly seen abnormal features of a chest X-ray film. The arrow represents possible deviation of the heart shadow which occurs with collapse rather than consolidation. (a) Right upper lobe collapse. (b) Right middle lobe collapse with loss of the right cardiac outline. (c) Left lower lobe collapse. (d) Right lower lobe collapse with loss of right diaphragm shadow.

field opacity this suggests collapse rather than consolidation. A lateral chest X-ray film is necessary to define precisely the area of lung collapse/consolidation (see below).

Small pleural effusions blunt the costophrenic angles and large effusions cause extensive radio-opacity in the affected lung field often with deviation of the mediastinal shadow to the opposite side.

Lateral chest X-ray

A lateral film should be included as part of a full radiological assessment of the chest. Interpretation of lateral chest X-rays

> **Focal points**
> **Evaluation of a chest X-ray**
>
> - Identify the film with name, date and laterality
>
> - Comment on quality of the film (exposure and rotation)
>
> - Examine bony landmarks and count ribs
>
> - Examine heart border. Comment on cardiomegaly and any lack of clarity of the heart outline
>
> - Examine lung fields. Comment on symmetry, clarity and any opacity. Comment on hilar regions
>
> - Examine lateral film

require some experience, but the various normal landmarks should be recognized (see Fig. 12.4c).

Sweat test

The sweat test is the definitive test for cystic fibrosis (p. 166). It is performed by stimulating a small part of the arm to sweat by pilocarpine iontophoresis (Fig. 12.7).

Collection of sweat

Two padded electrodes are applied either side of the child's forearm. The pad is soaked with pilocarpine which stimulates sweating locally. The pilocarpine is iontophoresed into the skin by passing a small electric current across the electrodes. Once this is carried out the electrodes are removed and sweat is collected by placing a clean preweighed filter paper square over the skin into which pilocarpine has penetrated. The filter paper should then be taped to the skin with a plastic covering to prevent evaporation of sweat and then the entire area bandaged with a crepe roll while sweat is collected over a period of at least 20 minutes. The filter paper is carefully removed. Clean plastic gloves must be worn during the entire procedure to avoid contaminating the filter paper with the examiner's own sweat. The filter paper is sent to the laboratory in an airtight plastic bag to prevent the sweat from evaporating. In the laboratory the filter paper is reweighed and both sodium and chloride measurements made.

The sweat analysis

On arrival in the laboratory the filter paper is weighed again

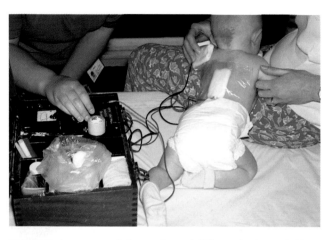

Fig. 12.7 A sweat test being performed. Pilocarpine is carried into the skin by low voltage electric current. The sweat is collected by filter paper and analysed for sodium and chloride concentration.

and the difference between the pretest weight and the final weight represents the amount of sweat collected. For the test to be valid, at least 100 mg of sweat must be collected. If the difference in weight is less than this then the test is invalid and should be repeated.

Measurement of both sweat sodium and chloride are necessary to exclude or confirm cystic fibrosis.

Diagnostic criteria for cystic fibrosis

- >100 mg of sweat.
- Sweat sodium >60 mmol/L.
- Sweat chloride >70 mmol/L.
- In cystic fibrosis the sweat chloride is usually higher than the sweat sodium value. In normal subjects the chloride is usually less than the sodium.

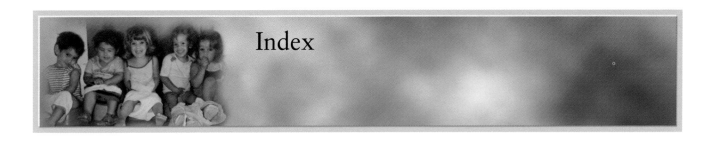

Index

Page numbers in **bold** refer to tables and those in *italic* refer to figures.

abdominal distension 237
abdominal examination 36–8
  acute abdominal pain 37, 134, **134**
  bowel obstruction 157
  evaluation
    focal points 38
  pyloric stenosis 157, *157, 159*
  rectal bleeding 172
  recurrent abdominal pain 145
  schema 38
abdominal migraine 149
abdominal pain, acute 132–7
  at a glance 135
  causes **133**, 135–7
    distinguishing features 138
  clinical features 133–4, **133**
  differential diagnosis 133, **133**
  evaluation
    focal points 134
  examination of abdomen 37, 134,
    134
  investigations 134, **134**
  management 135
  rectal examination 134
  see also recurrent abdominal pain
abdominal plain X-ray
  constipation 170, *170*
  intussusception 136
abortion 354
  consent issues 347
abscess 221
absent testis 88
accidents 310–12, 354
  adolescents 347
  prevention 50, **50**
N-acetyl-cysteine 310
acid–base balance 358–9, *359*
  normal ranges **358**
acidosis 358, **358**, *359*
acne 351
acrocyanosis 253
activated charcoal 310
active immunity 100
acute illness 100–41
  at a glance 101
  predisposing factors 100, **101**

presentation 100–1
  Baby Check illness rating score
    101, **101**
  older chidren **102**
  symptoms 100
acyclovir 110, 211, 342
ADD *see* attention deficit disorder
adenoidal hypertrophy 105
adenovirus 123
adolescents 345–56
  approach to communication 346–7
    guidelines 347
  asthma 323
  chronic illness impact 316
  consent to treatment 13, 347
  diabetes mellitus 330
  educational facilities 10
  epilepsy 336
  growth spurt 1, 2, 345, 348
  growth standards 20
  health care facilities 346
  health destructive behaviour 347–8
  health needs 346
  learning disability 283
  nutrition 10
  physical changes 345, 348–9
    see also puberty
  psychological problems 351–3
  psychosocial development 5, 345
  tasks 345–6, **346**
  vulnerable groups **346**
adrenal failure, acute 112, 113
adrenal hyperplasia, congenital 351
adrenaline 234, 304, 306
adventitious breath sounds 32
aggressive behaviour 293–4
air pollutents 120
alcohol intake 270
  adolescents 347
  brain growth effect 76
alkaline phosphatase concentration 360
  normal range **360**
alkalosis 358, **358**, *359*
allergies 15
  anaphylaxis 305
  asthma *see* asthma

rash 192
shock 303
vaccine contraindications 53
wheeze 120
allergy testing 319
allopurinol 342
ALTE (acute life-threatening episodes) *see*
  apnoea
ambiguous genitalia 239
amblyopia (lazy eye) 78
  at a glance 79
  neonatal screening 47
  treatment 78
amenorrhoea 353–4, **354**
aminophylline 124, 258, 259, 306, 322
ammoniacal (napkin) dermatitis 213
amoxycillin 109
ampicillin 105, 128, 227
anaemia 89–93
  cancer/cancer treatment 342
  causes 90–3, **90**
  clinical approach 90
  coeliac disease 166
  haematological investigations 357–8,
    358, **358**
  haemolytic jaundice 130
  hands examination 31, 33
  investigations 90, **90**
  microcytic hypochromic 357, *358*
  reticulocytosis 357
anal fissure 169, *170*, 172, 173, *173*
anal inspection 172
anal itching 183
analgesia 111, 311
anaphylactic reaction 201, 305–6
  at a glance 305
  management 306
anencephaly 237
angioneurotic oedema 201
ankle jerk reflex 24, *24*
anklylosing spondylitis 220
anorexia 133, 135, 145
anorexia nervosa 349, 351–2
  amenorrhoea 354
  at a glance 352
antacids 144, 148

anterior fontanelle 71
antibiotic prophylaxis
    cancer/cancer treatment 342
    infective endocarditis 83, 222, 338
    vesicoureteric reflux 111
antibiotic treatment
    acne 351
    acute epiglottitis 128
    acute post-streptococcal
       glomerulonephritis 189
    cough management 175
    cystic fibrosis chest infection 177
    diarrhoea 162
    impetigo 209
    infection in newborn 259
    infective endocarditis 222
    mastoiditis 229
    meningitis 110, 111
      neonate 257
    meningococcal septicaemia 113
    necrotizing enterocolitis 246
    osteomyelitis 222
    otitis media 105
    pneumonia 109
      neonate 250
    scarlet fever 196
    septic arthritis 115, 217
    septicaemia 305
    tonsillitis 104
    urinary tract infection 113
anticonvulsant medication 334–5, **334**
    side effects **335**
    teratogenic effects 337
antidepressants 353
antidiarrhoeal agents 162
antiemetic agents 162
antihistamines 201, 211, 306
antimetabolites 7
antipyretics 103, 104, 106, 222
aortic stenosis 83, 83, 222
    heart sounds 34, 82
apex beat 33, 34
Apgar score 232, **233**, 234
apnoea 121, 158, 179, 258–60
    at a glance 259
    causes 258–60, **258**
    central 258
    management 258
    obstructive 258
    primary 232
    resuscitation of newborn 232–3
    secondary 233
apnoea monitor 258, 314
apnoea of prematurity 259
appendicitis, acute 133, 135
    at a glance 136
    management 135
    peritonism 135
    rectal examination 134, 135
aqueductal stenosis 72
arthritis see joints swollen
ascites 37, 130, 132
aspiration of stomach contents 173
aspirin 103, 354
    poisoning 310
asthma 120, 121, 122–4, 318–24
    adolescents 323

aetiology 318
at a glance 123, 324
clinical features 32, 122
cough 174, 175, 176
definition 122
environmental control 320–1, 323
family issues 323, 324
    education 323
initial presentation 318–19
    allergy testing 319
    childhood 318–19
    infancy 318
management 122, 123–4, 319–24
    acute problems 321–2
    goals 319
medication 175, 319–21, 324
    administration routes 319–20,
      320, **320**
    principles of therapeutics 124,
      323
    step-by-step plan 319
pathophysiology 122, 318
peak flow monitoring 321, 321, 323
prevalence 318
prognosis 124, 323
psychosocial impact 323–4
respiratory failure 300
routine follow-up 322–3
    checklist 323
school issues 324
sputum 174
symptom diary 321, 322, 322, 323
triggers 318, 320–1
astigmatism 77
asymmetrical tonic neck reflex **26**, 26,
    278
ataxic gait 22
athlete's foot (tinea pedis) 210, 211
athletic training 349, 354
atopic dermatitis 201, 203–4
    advice for children 204
    at a glance 205
    clinical features 203–4, 203
    management 204
atrial septal defect 81–2
    heart sounds 34, 81
    prognosis 340
attention deficit disorders 295–6
    learning disability association 280,
      281
    management 295
autism 264, 265, 274
autoimmune thyroiditis (Hashimoto's
    syndrome) 58, 225
axillary lymph nodes enlargement 30

babies
    ear examination 29
    neurological assessment 25–7
      schema 24
    psychomotor development 3–4
Babinski reflex 24
Baby Check 101, **101**
Back to Sleep education campaign
    313, 314
bag and mask resuscitation 233, 233, 258
balloon valvuloplasty 83

barbiturates 307
    poisoning 310
barium enema 136
Barlow test 47, 239, 239
barrel chest 31, 31, 121
BCG vaccination 54
behavioural problems 149, 172,
    289–96, **290**
    chronic illness associations 315
    contributary factors **290**
    evaluation
      focal points **290**
      history-taking 289
    health education 50
    hearing loss association 284
    indicators of serious disturbance
      290
    learning disability association 282
    management 289–91
      guidelines 291
    protective factors **290**
    triggers 289
benign paroxysmal vertigo 180–1
benzyl penicillin 104, 114
beta-agonists 123, 319, 322
bicarbonate concentration 359
bile-stained vomitus 157, 240
    newborn 237
biliary atresia 251, 253
    hepatic cirrhosis association 132
    management 253
bilirubin metabolism 130, 130
birthmarks 206–7
birthweight 234
bite lesions 96, 96
blindisms 286
blindness see visual impairment
blood chemistry 359–61
    normal ranges **360**
blood gases 358–9, **359**
    neonatal respiratory distress 247
    normal ranges **358**
    respiratory failure 121
    wheeze 121
blood glucose measurement
    coma 307
    diabetes mellitus
      initial presentation 326
      monitoring 327, 328
    small baby 245
blood pH 358–9
    dehydration 117
blood pressure measurement 35, **36**
    cardiac pathology 80–1
blood in stool 172–3
    acute abdominal pain 133
    bacterial gastroenteritis 162
    causes **172**
    chronic diarrhoea 164
    clinical approach 172–3
    intussusception 136
blood transfusion reaction 305
blood urea 359–60
blood-stained vomitus 157
body fluids
    distribution 116
    intake/output balance 116

body temperature measurement 102
bonding 3
bone age assessment 2
bone marrow transplantation 342
bone scan 222
bow legs 89
bowel continence 172
bowel obstruction 7, 157, 158
    abdominal examination 157
    congenital 240
        aetiology 240, **241**
        clinical features 240, **241**
        newborn examination 237, 240
    constipation 170
Braille 287
brain abscess 151
brain stem evoked potentials 284
brain tumour 150, 151, **341**
brain stem death 308
BRAT diet 162
breast development 349
    isolated premature (premature
        thelarche) 350–1
breast milk 6
    anti-infective agents 7
    comparison with formula milk **8**
    excreted drug content 7
    iron content 91
breast-feeding 5–7, 71, 143, 161, 314,
    323
    advantages **7**
    contraindications 7, 225
    during oral rehydration therapy 118
    factors associated with success **6**
    stool pattern 168, 171
    technique 6–7
breast-milk jaundice 253
breath hydrogen test 164
breath sounds 32, 119
breath-holding spells 179–80
    at a glance 180
    cyanotic 179
    pallid (reflex anoxic seizures) 179–80
breathlessness
    cardiac pathology 80, 236
    haemolytic jaundice 130
    respiratory distress 121
    respiratory failure 300
British Diabetes Association 332
bronchial breath sounds 32
bronchial hyperreactivity 120
bronchiectasis 109, 125, 174, 176
bronchiolitis 124–5, 173, 176
    at a glance 124
    clinical features 125
    management 125
    respiratory failure 300
    wheeze 121
bronchitis 173–4, 176
bronchodilators 122, 125, 175, 318, 319
bronchoscopy 125, 175
bruises, non-accidental injury 96, 96
bulimia 352
    at a glance 352
bullying 16, 294
    management 294
burns 310–12

clinical assessment 311, *312*
    first aid 311
    non-accidental injury 96, 96
    principles of management 312
buttock wasting 36

café au lait spots 206, *207*, 270
caffeine 258, 259
calamine lotion 198
campylobacter gastroenteritis 162
cancer 340–4
    aetiology 340
    at a glance 344
    bone marrow suppression 342
    bone marrow transplantation 342
    chemotherapy 342
    diagnosis 340–1
        histology **341**
        staging **341**
    emotional support 342
    family issues 343
    immunosuppression 342
    initial presentation 340–1, **341**
        fever 220, 221, 222, 340
        joint swellings 219–20
        leg pain 155
    monitoring 343
    nutrition 342
    pathophysiology 340
    prevalence 340, **341**
    prognosis 343
    radiotherapy 342
    routine follow-up 343
    school issues 344
    surgical treatment 342
    therapy 341–4
        late consequences 343, *343*
        management goals 341
        metabolic consequences 342
        symptom management 342
candida infection 354
    AIDS opportunistic infection 224
    cancer/cancer treatment 342
    dysuria 183
    nappy rash 213, *215*
        management 214
    thrush (oral candidiasis) 213, 214,
        215, 221
cannabis **348**
captopril 338
carbaryl shampoo 212
carbohydrate requirements 5
cardiac arrhythmias
    syncope 181
    tricyclic antidepressant poisoning
        309
cardiac failure
    acute medical management 338
    clinical examination 80, 81
    congenital heart disease 83, 338,
        339–40
    shock 303
    wheeze 121
cardiac murmurs *see* heart murmurs
cardiac outline 363, *363*
cardiorespiratory arrest 298–9
    causes **299**

    principles of management 299
    treatment 298–9
cardiovascular system examination 33–5
    ausculation 34–5
    blood pressure 35
    evaluation
        focal points 35
    heart murmurs 80–1
    observation 33
    praecordium palpation 33–4
    pulse palpation 33
    schema 35
cataracts 27, 28, 270
    congenital 286, *286*
    neonatal screening 47, 235
catch-up growth 2, 61, 99
caustics ingestion 309, 310
CDH *see* hip dislocation, congenital
cefotaxime 110
cerebellar signs 150
cerebral oedema 307
cerebral palsy 245, 267, 277–80
    associated problems 278
        convulsions 140
        hearing loss 284
    at a glance 281
    ataxic 277
    causes 277, **277**
    clinical features 267, 277–8, *277*
    developmental assessment 39
    dystonic (athetoid) 277
    family impact 280–1
    gait disorders 22, 22, 89, 267
    genetic counselling 281
    global developmental delay 270
    intracranial haemorrhage 257, 258
    investigations 278
    kernicterus 251
    management 267, 278–9, *279*
        medication 279
        nutrition 279
        orthopaedic surgery 279
        principles 278, *279*
        routine review 279–80
    meningitis association 112
    muscle tone assessment 22
    muscle wasting 22
    presentation/diagnosis 278
    prevalence 277
    prognosis 267
    respiratory distress syndrome
        association 249
    schooling 281
    spastic 277
cerebrospinal fluid analysis 361
    meningitis 109–10
    normal values **361**
cervical adenitis 226–7
cervical lymphadenopathy 30, *30*, 104,
    225, *225*, 226, **226**
chemotherapy 94, 342
    immunization contraindication 51
    late consequences 343, *343*
chest deformity 31, *31*
    asthma 122, 323
    cystic fibrosis 176
chest examination 16, 31–32

cough 174–5
chest expansion assessment 32, 32
chest pain 155
    causes **155**, 156
    clinical approach 155–6
chest wall recession 31
    pneumonia 107, *107*
    respiratory distress 121
        neonatal 246, 248
        respiratory distress syndrome
        248
    respiratory failure 300
chest X-ray
    asthma 122, 322
    bronchiolitis 125, *126*
    congenital heart disease 83, 84, 254,
      338
    cystic fibrosis 177, *177*
    foreign body aspiration 124
    heart murmurs 81
    interpretation 362–4, *363*
        bony structures 363
        cardiac outline 363, *363*
        diaphragm 363
        evaluation
            focal points 364
        lateral film 364–5
        lung fields 364
        lung collapse/consolidation 364,
        364
    pneumonia 108, *108*
    respiratory distress, neonatal 246
    respiratory distress syndrome *248*
    transposition of great vessels 255
    wheeze 121
chicken pox (varicella) 192, 197–8
    at a glance 199
    clinical course **193**
    clinical features 197–8, *198*, 202
    complications 198
    management 198
    susceptibility with immune deficiency
      cancer/cancer treatment 342
      steroid therapy 231
child abuse 95–9
    characteristic features 96
    clinical evaluation 95–6
        focal points 96
        history taking 95–6
        physical examination 96
    developmental delay 271
    investigations 96–7, **97**
    management 56, 97, 98
    types **95**
    see also emotional abuse/neglect,
      non-accidental injury, non-
      organic failure to thrive, sexual
      abuse
child care 10
child development team 274, **275**
child health surveillance 44–99
    child protection 56
    detection of problems 45
    developmental examination 49
    growth 54–6
    physical examination **46**, 49, *49*
    problems detected 56–99

procedures 45–9, **46**
    screening 45–9
    professionals 44–5
    programme **46**
child health promotion 44–56
child health records 45
child with a disability 273–88
    at a glance 276
    breaking news 274
    education 274
        special/mainstream schools 275,
        276–7
        statement of educational needs
        275
    family impact 275–6
    financial benefits entitlement 275
    genetic counselling 274
    medical management 274
    presentation 273
    principles of management 274, 276
    referral to child development team
      274, **275**
    social services support 275
    voluntary organizations 275
child protection 56
Child Protection Register 56, 97
children at risk
    child protection 56
    growth monitoring 55
Chlamydia pneumoniae 176
chlamydial infection 176, 348
chloramphenicol 128
choanal atresia 260
cholestyramine 132
choreoathetosis 21
choroidoretinal degeneration 286
chromosome abnormalities 270
    learning disability 281
chromosome analysis 272
    delayed puberty 350
    global developmental delay 270
chronic illness 315–44
    adolescents 316
    amenorrhoea 354
    at a glance 318
    clinical approach 316–17
    coordination of care 317
    definition 315
    evaluation
      focal points 317
    family education 317
    family impact 316
    genetic implications 317
    growth effects 1, 130, 164, 166, 174,
      176
        failure to thrive 67
        short stature 57, 59
    growth monitoring 55
    management 316–17
        principles 317
    prevalence **316**
    psychosocial impact 315–16
        assessment 316, 317
        factors affecting adjustment **316**
    school life 315–16, 317–8
    sibling reactions 316
    social services support 317

voluntary/self-help organizations
    317
cisapride 158
cleft lip and palate 7, 105, 235, *236*
    clinical implications 235, **236**
    management 235
clinical examination 16
    abdominal system 36–8
    cardiovascular system 33–5
    developmental assessment 39–43
    ear 28–9, *29*
    evaluation
      focal points 21
    general observation 21
    growth assessment 17–21
    health surveillance **46**, 49, *49*
    musculoskeletal system 38–9
    neurological assessment 21–5
    respiratory system 31–2
    reticuloendothelial system 29–30
    throat 29, *30*
    visual system 25–8
clinical investigations 357–65
    acid–base balance 358–9
    blood chemistry 359–61
    blood gases 358–9
    cerebrospinal fluid 361
    chest X-ray 362–4
    haematology 357–8
    sweat test 364–5, *365*
    urinalysis 361–2
clubbing 21, 121, 130, 132, 145, 166,
  175, 176, 222, 323, 338
    causes **21**
    examination of hands 31, 33
coal tar preparations 206
coarctation of aorta 80, 83–4, 84, 222,
  236–7
    blood flow 236, *237*
    heart murmur 84
    pulse 33
    treatment in newborn period 236–7
cocaine **348**
codeine 175
coeliac disease 9, 166, *166*
    at a glance 167
    diabetes mellitus association 330
    failure to thrive 67
    jejunal biopsy 166, *166*
    malabsorption 164
    management 166
    short stature 59
        growth chart 64
cold sore 211, *211*
colic, infantile 143–4
    at a glance 144
    crying 142, 143–4
    management 144
collagen vascular disease 155, 220,
  221, 222
collapsing (waterhammer) pulse 33
colostrum 6
colour vision assessment 48–9
coma 306–8
    at a glance 307
    causes **306**
    depth assessment 306, **306**

coma *Cont'd*
    history taking 306
    investigations 307, **307**
    physical examination 306
    poisoning 310
    principles of management 308
    prognosis 308
    pupillary light reflex 306–7
    treatment 307–8
common cold 104, 105
communication 13
    adolescents 346–7
        guidelines 347
    cancer/cancer treatment 342
    clinical examination 16
    convulsions management 139–40
    history-taking 14–15
community paediatricians 45
    child protection 56
complex partial (temporal lobe)
    seizures 181, 332, 333
computed tomography (CT)
    cerebral palsy 278
    epilepsy 334
    headache 150
    hydrocephalus 72
    intracranial pressure elevation 72,
        150, 151
    pyrexia of unknown origin 221
    unconscious child 307
condylomata acuminata (venereal warts)
    209
congenital abnormalities 232, 240–1
congenital heart disease *see* heart disease,
    congenital
coning 110, 307, 361
consciousness level assessment
    306, *306*
    poisoning 309
consent to treatment
    adolescents 347
    contraception 13, 347, 356
    ethical issues 13
constipation 168–71, 172
    associated vomiting 157
    at a glance 171
    causes **169**, 170–1
        distinguishing features 169
    definition 168
    evaluation
        focal points 169
        history taking 169
        physical examination 169–70
    functional 170
    investigations 170, *170*
    management 170, **171**
    overflow diarrhoea/soiling 168, 172
    recurrent abdominal pain 145, 148
contact dermatitis 201, 203, 204
    clinical features 204, *204*
    management 204
continuous positive airway pressure
    (CPAP)
    apnoea in premature infant 258,
        260
    respiratory distress, neonatal 247
    respiratory distress syndrome 248

contraception 355–6, **355**
    consent issues 13, 347, 356
    see also safe sex
convulsions 306
    classification 332
    generalized 137–41, 332
        causes 140–1
        clinical approach 139–40, 335,
            337
        explanation for parents 139–40
        first aid 140
        medication 139, 140
        pathophysiology 138
        sequence of stages 138
        tonic-clonic (grand mal) 333
        trigger factors 138
    infantile spasms 21, 181, 333
    meningitis 109
    myoclonic 21, 181, 333
    neonatal 255–8
        at a glance 257
        causes 256–8, **256**
        hypoglycaemia 245
        investigations 256, **256**
        management 256
    partial seizures 332, 333
        complex (temporal lobe) 181,
            332, 333
    simple absence seizures 181, 333
    unconscious child 308
    see also epilepsy
coordination assessment 23, 23
corneal light reflex 27
coryza 104, 105
costochondritis 156
cough 173–7
    associated symtpoms 174
    asthma 318, 319
    causes **173**, 175–7
        distinguishing features 177
    characteristics 174, **174**
    chest examination 174–5
    evaluation
        focal points 174
        history taking 174
        physical examination 174–5
    investigations 175, **175**
    management 175
cough suppressants 175
counselling
    chronic illness 317
    depression 353
cover test 28, *28*
cow's milk protein intolerance 168, 173
    management 168
    wheeze 122
Coxsackie virus 198
crackles (creptitations) 32, 121, 127
cradle cap 203, 205, *206*
cranial nerve assessment 24
cranial nerve palsy 150
craniostenosis (craniosynostosis) 75, 76–7
crawling 39
creatinine phosphokinase 267, 268
creatinine serum level 359–60
creptitations (crackles) 32, 121, 127
cretinism 46

Crohn's disease 167, 168, 222
    clinical features 168
    joint swellings 220
    management 168
croup (acute laryngotracheobronchitis)
    127, 128, 301
    at a glance 129
    management 128
crying 4, 50, 142–4
    causes 143–4, **143**
    clinical approach 143
cryptorchidism 36, 87–8
    at a glance 88
    scrotal examination 37–8, 239
    testicular descent screening 47, *48*
Cushing's disease 58
Cushing's syndrome 58
cyanosis 33
    cardiac murmur 236
    cardiac pathology 80, 81, 338
    central 33, 253
    clinical examination 21
    hands examination 31
    neonatal 234, 253–5
    respiratory distress 121
        neonatal 246
    respiratory failure 300
    upper airway obstruction 127, 301
cyanotic breath-holding spells 179
cyclophosphamide 231
cystic fibrosis 106, 121, 166–7, *167*,
    176–7, 354
    at a glance 178
    clinical features 166–7, 176–7
    cough 174, 175
    dietary supplements 177
    failure to thrive 67
    genetic aspects 176
    investigations 167, 177
    liver disease 131
    malabsorption 176, 177
    management 167, 177
    meconium ileus 176
    neonatal hepatitis 253
    neonatal screening 176
    pancreatic insufficiency 164, 166,
        176
    pathophysiology 176
    prognosis 167, 177
    respiratory features 176, 177, *177*
    screening 49
    sputum 174, 177
    sweat test criteria 365
cystitis 148
cytomegalovirus 225
    intrauterine infection 244, 273,
        282
    neonatal hepatitis 253

day nurseries 10
deafness *see* hearing loss
death
    brain stem 308
    cancer-related 342
    ethical issues 12
decongestants 104
defaecatory pain 172, 173

dehydration 116–19, 157, 161, 184, 303, 306
    acute fluid loss estimation 118
    at a glance 119
    blood chemistry 360
    causes 119, 119
    evaluation
        focal points 118
        history taking 116
    hypernatraemic 116, 117
    hyponatraemic 116, 117
    investigations 117
    isonatraemic 116, 117
    maintenance fluid requirements
        estimation 118
    on-going fluid losses estimation 118
    oral rehydration therapy 118
    pathophysiology 116
    principles of management 119
    rehydration protocol 118
    severity assessment 116–17, *117*, **117**
    treatment 118, **118**
delayed puberty 349–50
    causes **350**
dental care 50
    health surveillance 78–80
dental caries 78–9, *79*, 150, 151
    prevention 79
dental development *3*
depression 353
    at a glance 353
desferrioxamine 92
development 1
    see also psychomotor development, developmental assessment
developmental abnormalities/delay 261–73
    at a glance 263
    causes 261, **262**
    cerebral palsy association 278
    child with a disability 273–88
    developmental assessment 261, 262
    evaluation
        focal points 262
        history taking 261–2
        physical examination 262
    global 268–70
    management 263
    presentation 261
    referral 263
    talking 263–6
    walking 266–8
    warning signs **42**, **43**, **262**
    see also global developmental delay
developmental assessment 39–43, 49, 261, 262
    essential milestones **42**, **43**
    fine motor development 40–1, *41*
    global developmental delay 270
    gross motor development 39, *40*
    health surveillance 49
    social development 42–3, *43*
    speech and language 42, *42*
        disorders 265
    warning signs **42**, **43**, **262**
dexamethasone 110

dextromethorphan 175
diabetes insipidus 184
diabetes mellitus 71, 184, 227, 325–31, 354
    adolescents 330
    aetiology 325
    at a glance 331
    brittle 328, *329*
    complications 325–6
        surveillance 330
    concurrent illness 330
    concurrent stress 330
    crisis management 330–2
    diet 327, 332
    education/advice 326, 329, 330
    family issues 326, 329, 330–2
    genetic aspects 332
    growth monitoring 55, 330
    honeymoon period 329
    hypoglycaemia 328–9, 330, 332
    initial presentation 326
    injection site inspection 330
    ketoacidosis 306, 326, 328, **329**, 330, 359
        blood chemistry 360
        treatment 328, **329**
    management 326–31
        acute problems 328–9
        goals 326
        principles of therapeutics 219
    medication 326–7, 327
        insulin preparations **327**
        mode of delivery 327, *327*
    monitoring 327–8
        blood glucose measurement 327, 328
        diary 327, 330
        glycosylated haemoglobin (HbA1c) 328, 330
    pathophysiology 325, *325*
    pregnancy 332
    prevalence 325
    prognosis 330
    routine follow-up 329–30
        checklist 332
    school issues 326, 332
    specialist referral 326
    support services 332
    voluntary/self-help organizations 317
diabetic clinic 329
diabetic nephropathy 325
diabetic neuropathy 325
diabetic nurse specialist 326, 332
diabetic retinopathy 325
    surveillance 330
diabetic team 326
diaphragm 363
diaphragmatic hernia 246, 250
    management 250
diarrhoea
    acute 160–2
        causes **161**, 162
        dehydration 116, 161
        evaluation
            focal points **161**
        investigations 161, **161**

        management 161–2
    acute abdominal pain 133
    AIDS opportunistic
        infection 224
    chronic 162–8
        associated symptoms 164
        causes **164**, 165–8
            distinguishing features 169
        evaluation
            focal points 164
            history taking 163–4
            physical examination 164
        investigations 164–5, **165**
        overflow/soiling 168, 172
        stool pattern assessment 164
    non-specific 165
    recurrent abdominal pain 145
diazepam 139, 140, 308, 309
    rectal administration 140, 141, 335, 337
dieting behaviour 348
    amenorrhoea 354
difficult behaviour 293–4
    management guidelines 290
digoxin 338
diphtheria 51, 104
    vaccine 51
disability
    assessment 274
    causes **274**
    see also child with a disability
discipline 290
diurnal enuresis 185
    causes 185–6, **185**
        distinguishing features 186
    evaluation
        focal points 185
DMSA radioisotope scan 113
dopamine 304
Down's syndrome 76, 105, 235, 270–1, 281, *281*
    at a glance 271
    clinical features 270, *271*, 274
    routine review 282
drowning 312
drug abuse 347, **348**
    signs **348**
drug allergy 306
dry powder delivery systems 320, *320*
DTP *see* diptheria, tetanus, pertussis
Duchenne muscular dystrophy 267–8
    at a glance 268
    genetic aspects 268
duodenal atresia 240, *241*
dysentery 172
dyslexia 265, 266, 295
    management 295
dysmenorrhoea 148, 354
dysmorphic syndromes/features 21, 60, 179, 183, 256
    failure to thrive 67
    global developmental delay 270
    learning disability 272
    newborn examination 235–6
    obesity 69
    small head (microcephaly) 76
dyspraxia 296

dysuria 182
    advice for girls 183
    causes 182, **183**

ear examination 28–9, *29*
    language/speech disorders 265
    see also hearing tests
eating difficulties 292
    management guidelines 292
eating disorders 10, 348, 351–2
    at a glance 352
    growth monitoring 55
    management 352
echocardiography 254, 255, 338
ectopic beats 33
ectopic testes *see* cryptorchidism
ectopic ureters 186
eczema 201
    see also atopic dermatitis
education 10
    see also school attendance/placement
ejection click 34
elbow dislocation 216–17, *217*
electrocardiogram (ECG)
    congenital heart disease 82, 83, 84,
        254, 338
    heart murmurs 81
electroencephalogram (EEG)
    epilepsy 334
    hysterical seizures 181
    indications with convulsions 139
    pallid breath-holding spells
        (reflex anoxic seizures) 180
electrolytes
    dehydration 117
    serum levels 360
        normal ranges **360**
emergency paediatrics 297–314
emergency presentations 297–8
    evaluation
        focal points 298
        physical examination 297–8, **298**
    initial assessment 297
    predisposing causes **298**
    presenting features **298**
    principles of management 298
    support for relatives 299
emotional abuse/neglect 99
    child protection 56
    global developmental delay 272
    language/speech disorders 265
    short stature 1, 57
emotional problems 289, **290**
    contributary factors **290**
        chronic illness 315
    evaluation
        focal points 290
        history taking 289
    headache 149
    management 289–91
        guidelines 291
    protective factors **290**
empyema 109
encopresis 172, 293
endocrine disorders
    failure to thrive 67
    growth monitoring 55

obesity 69
    short stature 58–9
energy requirements 5
enterobiasis *see* threadworms
enuresis 293
    diurnal 185–6
    nocturnal 186–8, 326
enuresis alarm 188
environmental factors
    asthma 120, 320–1, 323
    language/speech disorders 265
    walking delay 267
ephedrine nasal drops 104
epiglottitis, acute 127, 128
    airway obstruction 128, 128, 30i
    at a glance 129
    management 128
epilepsy 139, 181, 332, 333–7
    adolescents 337
    at a glance 336
    classification 332, **333**
    constraints on activities 335, 337
    definition 332
    driving licence 335, 337
    electroencephalography (EEG) 334
    family education 337
    initial presentation 333–4
    learning disability association 281,
        337
    management 334–7
        generalized convulsions 335,
        337
        goals 334
    medication 334–5, **334**
        side effects **335**
    monitoring 335
    physical examination 334, 335
    prevalence 332
    prognosis 335–7
    psychosocial issues 337
    radiological investigations 334
    routine follow-up 335
        checklist 337
    school issues 337
    seizures *see* convulsions
    types 333
        drug therapy **334**
    voluntary/self-help organizations
        317
Epstein–Barr virus 226, 227
erythromycin 52, 162, 196, 209
Escherichia coli 112, 162, 256, 258
ethical issues 11–13
    consent 13
    evaluation
        focal points 13
    ommission versus commission 12
    quality of life 12
    sanctity of life 12
    withdrawal of intensive care 12
ethnic minorities 11
eustacian tube dysfunction 105, 106
exchange transfusion 251
Ewing sarcoma **341**
exercise haematuria 190
expectorants 175
external cardiac massage 299, *299*

resuscitation of newborn 233
extracellular fluids 116
eye contact, mother-baby 4
eye strain 152

face, response to mother's 3
facial nerve (VII) assessment 24
factitious fever 221, 222
failure to thrive 61–7
    causes **61**
        genetic 67
        organic 62
    clinical approach 61–2
    congenital heart disease 338
    defining feature 61
    evaluation
        focal points 62
    food battles 10
    history 62
    HIV infection/AIDS 224
    investigations 62, **67**
    management 62
    neglect 96
    non-organic 62, 67–9, 99
        at a glance 68
        growth chart 66
        management 99
faints 178–82, **179**
    clinical approach 178–9
    causes
        distinguishing features,
          infants/preschool children 182
        distinguishing features, school-age
          children 182
    evaluation
        focal points 179
Fallot's tetralogy 253, 255, *255*
family centres 10
family history 16
    abuse/neglect 95–6
    asthma 122, 318
    atopic dermatitis 203
    congenital heart disease 80
    convulsions 140
    failure to thrive 62
    global developmental delay 270
    haematuria 189
    headache 149
    maturational delay 349, 350
    migraine 150, 151
    neonatal convulsions 256
    nocturnal enuresis 187
    psoriasis 203
    recurrent abdominal pain 145
    short stature 57, 58
    walking delay 266, 267
    wheeze 121
    see also genetic factors
family structure 11
family tree *16*
fat requirements 5
febrile convulsions 103, 138, 139, 140–1
    anticonvulsant medication
        indications 141
    at a glance 141
    first aid 141
    principles of management 141

recurrent 140, 141
    roseola 195
    shigella gastroenteritis 162
    status epilepticus 140
    treatment 139, 140–1
feed thickeners 144, 158, 160
feeding problems 237
    small baby 245–6
femoral pulse
    cardiac murmur 236
    newborn examination 236–7
femoral-radial pulse delay 80
fertility 345, 348
fetal alcohol syndrome 272, 274
fetal lung maturation
    growth retarded baby 244
    surfactant development 248
fever
    acute illness 102–3
    causes **102**
    convulsions *see* febrile convulsions
    evaluation
        focal points 103
        history taking 102–3
        physical examination 103
    following convulsions 139
    infections 103–15
        causes
            distinguishing features 116
        investigations 103, **103**
        malignant disease 340
        principles of management 103
        recurrent abdominal pain 145
        temperature measurement 102
    see also pyrexia of unknown origin
fifth disease 192, 196
    clinical course **193**
    clinical features 196, *197*, 202
fine motor development 40–1, *41*
fits 178–82, **179**
    causes
        distinguishing features,
            infants/preschool children 182
        distinguishing features school-age
            children 183
    clinical approach 178–9
    evaluation
        focal points 179
    see also convulsions
flat feet 89
flucloxacillin 217
fluoride supplements 8, 79
focal convulsive activity 139
folic acid supplements 237
fontanelle closure 71
fontanelle examination 25
food diary 62
food fads 289, 292
food sensitivity 306
    chronic diarrhoea 164
foreign body aspiration 106, *176*, 301
    at a glance 126
    clinical features 124, 176
    cough 174, 176
    investigations 175
    management 125, 176
    prognosis 125–6

    sputum 174
    stridor 127
    wheeze 120, 121, 125–6
formula feeds 7–9
    comparison with breast milk 8
    dehydration management 119
    preparation 8–9, 8
        hypernatraemic dehydration
            following errors 117
fractures, non-accidental injury 96–7, 97
fragile X 272, 274, 281
frog position 25, *25*
functional upper airway obstruction 260
fundoscopy 28
funnel chest (pectus excavatum) 31, *31*
funny turns 178–82, **179**
    causes
        distinguishing features,
            infants/preschool children 182
        distinguishing features, school-age
            children 182
    clinical approach 178–9
    evaluation
        focal points 179

gait assessment 21–2, 22
gait disorders 88–9
    causes 89, **89**
gastroenteritis 136, 156, 157
    abdominal examination 157
    at a glance 163
    bacterial 162
    causes 162
        distinguishing features 162
    dehydration 116, 118
    management 162
    non-specific diarrhoea following
        165
    reactive arthritis 217
    secondary lactose intolerance 165
    viral 162
gastrointestinal congenital
    anomalies 148
gastro-oesophageal reflux 148, 158
    associated vomiting 157
    at a glance 159
    barium swallow 158, *158*
    failure to thrive 62
    management 158
gaze positions 27, *27*
general practitioners 45
genetic counselling
    cerebral palsy 281
    child with a disability 274
    Duchenne muscular dystrophy 268
    hearing loss 286
    learning disability 283
genetic factors
    chronic illness 317
    diabetes mellitus 332
    growth 1, 59–60, 67
    visual impairment 286
    see also family history
genital disorders 85–8
    groin swellings 86–7
    impalpable testes 87–8

    scrotal swellings 85–6
genitalia examination 37–8
gestational age assessment 242
Giardia lamblia 148, 164, 168
glandular fever *see* infectious
    mononucleosis
global developmental delay 269–73
    associated conditions 270–3
    causes **269**
        distinguishing features 273
    clinical evaluation 269
        focal points 269
        history taking 269, 270
        physical examination 270
    investigations 270
    language/speech disorders 264
    management 270
glomerulonephritis, acute 196
    at a glance 190
    clinical features 189
    haematuria 188, 189
    Henoch–Schönlein purpura 199
    management 189–90
glue ear 29, *29*, 105–6
    conductive hearing deficit 265
gluten intolerance *see* coeliac disease
gluten-free diet 166
glycosylated haemoglobin (HbA1c)
    328, 330
goitre 225, 226, **226**
    thyroditis 228
gold therapy 218
gonorrhoea 348
Gower's sign 22, 268, *269*
grasp reflex 278
griseofulvin 210
groin lymph nodes enlargement 30
groin swellings 86–7
    causes **87**
grommets 106
gross motor development 39, *40*
growing pains 154
growth 1–2, 54–6
    adolescence 1, 2, 345
    at a glance 55
    catch-up 2, 61, 99
    determinant factors 1
    evaluation
        focal points 2
    infancy 1–2
    monitoring 55–6, **56**
        guidelines for concern 55–6
    organ 2
        at a glance 3
    patterns
        normal 54
        obese children 69, *70*
    preschool years 2
    school years 2
growth assessment 17–21, *17*
    centile chart interpretations 21
    head (occipitofrontal) circumference
        (OFC) 17
    height 17
    plotting measurements 21
    standards 17, *18*, *19*, *20*
    weight 17

growth disorders 56–68, 56
    abuse/neglect 96
    cardiac failure 80
    chronic diarrhoea 164
    chronic liver disease 130
    chronic lung disease 174
    coeliac disease 166
    cystic fibrosis 166, 176
    diabetes mellitus 330
    growth monitoring 56
    Hirschsprung's disease 169
    wheeze association 121
growth fall-off 61, 145
    causes 61
growth hormone 1
growth hormone deficiency 58–9
growth hormone treatment 57, 58
growth plate fracture 217
Guthrie test 47, 47
gynaecological disorders 353–6
    recurrent abdominal pain 145,
        148–9
gynaecomastia 351

H2 receptor antagonists 144, 148, 158
haematocolpos 148
haematological disorders 219–20
haematological investigations 357–8
    normal ranges 358
haematuria 188–90, 199, 222
    causes 188, 189–90
        distinguishing features 189
    evaluation
        focal points 188
        history taking 188
        physical examination 189
    investigations 189, 189
haemoglobin concentration 357
haemoglobin S 93
haemoglobinopathies
    anaemia 90
    screening 49
haemolytic anaemia 357, 358
haemolytic disease of newborn 253
haemophilia 155, 219–20
Haemophilus influenzae 105, 110, 115,
    127, 177, 222, 229
Haemophilus influenzae B 53, 128
    vaccine 53, 128
haemorrhagic disease of newborn 5
hand foot and mouth disease 198
hands examination 21, 21, 31, 33
Harrison's sulci 31, 31, 323
Hashimoto's syndrome (autoimmune
    thyroiditis) 58, 225
head injury 306
    non-accidental 96
head lice (pediculosis capitis) 212, 212
head (occipitofrontal) circumference
    (OFC) 17, 71, 72, 76
    centile charts 73–4
    newborn examination 234–5
head size abnormalities
    large head 71–5
    small head 75–7
headache 149–52
    associated symptoms 149

causes 149, 150–2
    distinguishing features 152
clinical approach 149–50
evaluation
    focal points 149
features of concern 150
management 150
psychosomatic 293
Heaf test 53
health destructive behaviour 347–8
health education 46, 50
health promotion 50
    adolescents 346
health surveillance see child health
    surveillance
health visitor 44, 291
    child protection 56
hearing aids 285–6
hearing loss 284–6
    associated problems 265, 284
    at a glance 285
    causes 284, 284
    cerebral palsy association 284
    clinical features 284
    communication skills 286
    conductive
        glue ear/otitis media 105, 106,
            265, 284
        treatment 285
    education 286
        school placement 286
    family impact 286
    genetic counselling 286
    hearing aids 285–6
    kernicterus 251
    language/speech disorders 264, 265
    learning disability association 281
    meningitis 111
    mumps 111, 227
    neurosensory 111, 285–6
    presentation/diagnosis 273, 284
    prevalence 284
    principles of management 284, 285
    risk factors 284
    visual impairment association 286
hearing tests
    audiological 265, 284
    distraction test 48, 48
    global developmental delay 270
    language/speech disorders
        investigations 265
    sweep audiometry 48
heart disease, congenital 106, 220,
    337, 338–9, 354
    aetiology 338
    at a glance 339
    diagnosis 338
    family issues 340
    infective endocarditis
        prophylactic antibiotics 222, 338,
            340
        pyrexia of unknown origin 221,
            222
    initial presentation 338
    management 338
    neonatal cyanosis 253, 254
        investigations 254

nutrition 338
    pathophysiology 338
    prevalence 337, 338
    prognosis 340
    routine follow-up 340
        checklist 340
    school issues 340
    wheeze 121, 125
heart examination see cardiovascular
    system examination
heart murmurs 34, 35, 80–4, 236, 338
    causes 80
    clinical examination 80–1
    diastolic 34, 35, 236
    evaluation
        focal points 80
        history taking 80
    grading 34, 35
    infective endocarditis 221, 222
    innocent (functional) 80, 81
        sites 81
    management 81
    pathological 80
        causes
            distinguishing features 84
            left to right shunts 81–2
            obstructive lesions 83–4
    systolic 34
heart rate 33, 33
heart sounds 34
heavy periods 354
heel-shin test 23, 23
height measurement 17, 17
Heimlich manoeuvre 125, 127, 302–3,
    302
Helicobacter pylori 148
hemiplegic gait 22, 22, 89, 267
Henoch–Schönlein purpura
    (anaphylactoid purpura) 172, 192, 199
    at a glance 201
    clinical features 199, 200, 202
    joint pain/swelling 217
    management 199
hepatic cirrhosis 130, 131, 132
    management 132
hepatitis A 131
hepatitis B 131
    chronic infection 132
    immunization 132
        neonate/infant 253
    neonatal hepatitis 253
hepatocellular carcinoma 132
hepatosplenomegaly 130–1, 179, 183,
    270
        HIV infection/AIDS 224
herpes simplex
    intrauterine infection 244
    meningoencephalitis 110
HIB see haemophilus influenzae B
hip dislocation, congenital 89
    at a glance 240
    examination 239–40
        Barlow test 47, 239, 239
        observation 239
        Ortolani test 47, 239, 239
    management 240
    risk factors 239

screening 47
Hirschsprung's disease 169, 170–1, 240, 241
  at a glance 242
  diagnosis 170
  management 241
  neonatal presentation 241
histamine 120
history taking 14–16
  interview 14–15
  problem list compilation 16–17
  structured format 15–16
HIV infection/AIDS 100, 223–4
  adolescent sexual activity 348
  at a glance 224
  breast-feeding 7, 224–5
  management 224
HLA B27 220
Hodgkin's disease 341
homelessness 11
housing conditions 11
human papilloma virus 348
hyaline membrane disease *see* respiratory distress syndrome
hydrocephalus 72, 75, 111
  at a glance 75
  head circumference centile charts **74**
  intracranial haemorrhage 258
  long-term follow-up 75
  prognosis 72, 75
hydrocoele 85
  anatomical development *86*
hydrocortisone 306
hydronephrosis 189, 241
  management 241
hydroxychloroquine 218
hyperactivity disorder 294
  learning disability association 281, 281
  management 294
hyperkalaemia **360**
hypermetropia 77, *77*
hypernatraemia 116, 117, 360
  causes **360**
hypertension 157
  coarctation of aorta 84
  haematuria 189
  headache 150, 151
  vomiting 157
hyperthyroidism 226, **226**
hyperventilation 181
hypocalcaemia 256
hypoglycaemia 183
  coma 307
  diabetes mellitus 328–9, 330, 332
  neonatal convulsions 245, 256
  small baby 244–5
hypokalaemia 360
hyponatraemia 116, 117, 360
  causes **360**
hypospadias 238–9, *238*
hyposplenism 225
hypothermia
  near-drowning 312
  small baby 244
hypothyroidism 226

acquired 58
  at a glance 59
clinical features 58
congenital 46, 272
  management 272
  neonatal screening 46–7, 272
failure to thrive 67
global developmental delay 270, 272
obesity 69
replacement thyroxine therapy `58, 228, 272
short stature 57, 58
signs **226**
thyroiditis 58, 228
hypotonia 237
  global developmental delay 270
  position at rest 25, *25*
  tone 25
hypoxic-ischaemic encephalopathy 76, 234
hysterical seizures 181

idiopathic recurrent abdominal pain 147
  at a glance 147
idiopathic thrombocytopenic purpura 192, 193, 199
  at a glance 202
  clinical features 199, *200*, 202
  management 200
imigrants 11
imipramine 188
immunity 100
immunization 51–4, 100
  contraindications 51, 53
  general guidelines 51
  schedules **51**
immunodeficiency 100, 106, 109
  cancer/cancer treatment 342
  chicken pox exposure management 197, 342
  HIV infection/AIDS 224
  immunization contraindication 51, 53
impalpable testes 87–8
  causes 87
  evaluation
    focal points 87
impetigo 209, *209*
inborn errors of metabolism 272, 274
indomethacin 250
infantile spasms 21, 181, 333
infants
  growth standards *18*
  nutritional requirements 5
infection 103–15
  anaemia 90
  coma 306
  convulsions 139
    see also febrile convulsions
  diarrhoea 161, 162, 164–5
  causes
    distinguishing features 116
  leukocytosis 357–8
  neonatal jaundice 253
  newborn 100, 258–9
    clinical features 259, **259**

nosocomial 258
  perinatally acquired 258
  small baby 246
predisposing factors 100, **101**
pyrexia of unknown origin 220
recurrent 222–4
  causes 223–4, **223**
respiratory failure 300
vomiting 156, 157
wheeze 120, 121, 124
see also septicaemia
infectious mononucleosis (glandular fever) 104, 225, 226, 227
  at a glance 228
  management 227
  pyrexia of unknown origin 221
infective endocarditis 222
  prophylaxis with congenital heart disease 83, 222, 338, **340**
  pyrexia of unknown origin 220, 221, 222
infertility 88
inflammatory bowel disease 167–8, 354
  chronic diarrhoea 164
  joint swellings 220
  pyrexia of unknown origin 220, 222
  recurrent abdominal pain 148
  short stature 59
influenza virus 106
infratentorial tumour 150
inguinal hernia 36, 85, 86, 87, 88
  anatomical development *86*
  at a glance 86
inguinal lymphadenopathy `87
injury *see* accidents
insect sting allergy 305
insulin `pen' 327, *327*
insulin preparations **327**
insulin therapy 326–7, *327*
intensive care withdrawal 12
intermittent positive pressure ventilation 233, 247, 248
intoeing 89, *89*
intracellular fluids 116
intracranial haemorrhage 72, 257–8
  idiopathic thrombocytpenic purpura 199, 200
  management 258
intracranial pressure elevation 71, 72
  coma 306
  fontanelle examination 25
  headache 149, 150, 151
    management 151
  investigations 72
  lumbar puncture contraindications 361
  papilloedema 306
  subdural effusions/haematoma 75
intrauterine growth retardation 241, 242–4
  asymmetrical 244, **244**
  at a glance 245
  catch-up growth 2, 61
  causes **244**
  failure to thrive 67
  hypocalcaemia 256

intrauterine growth retardation *Cont'd*
  hypoglycaemia 256
  management 244
  short stature following 60–1
    growth chart 63
  symmetrical 242–3, *244*, **244**
    prenatal infection 244–5
intrauterine infection
  brain growth following 76
  global developmental delay 273
  neonatal convulsions 256
  symmetrical growth retardation
    244–5
intravenous pyelography 185
intubation
  airway obstruction 127, 128
  anaphylactic reaction 305
  resuscitation of newborn 233
intussusception 135–7, *136*, 143, 162,
  172
  at a glance 136
  blood in stool 133, 136
  management 136
ipecacuanha syrup 310
ipratropium bromide 319
iron 5
iron deficiency anaemia 10, 49, 90–1, 357
  at a glance 91
  failure to thrive 62
  investigations 90, 357–8, *358*, **358**
  screening 49
iron salt therapy 91
irritability 25, 234, 237
irritable bowel syndrome 147–8
  management 148
Ishihara colour vision test 48–9
isonatraemic dehydration 116, 117
isoprenaline 304
itching (pruritus) 36, 211–13
  causes **211**
  jaundice 130, 132
  management 211
ITP *see* idiopathic thrombocytopenic
  purpura
IUGR *see* intrauterine growth
  retardation
IVP *see* intravenous pyelography

jaundice 36, 128, 130–2
  causes **130**, 131–2
  clinical features 130–1, **131**
  evaluation
    focal points 130
  haemolytic 130, 357
  hepatic 130
  infectious mononucleosis 227
  investigations 131, **131**
  obstructive 130
  prognosis 131
  see also neonatal jaundice
jejunal biopsy 166, *166*
jitteriness 234
joint examination 38–9
joint stiffness 216
joint swelling/pain 39, 214
  acute abdominal pain 133
  causes **215**, 216–20

clinical approach 214, 216
evaluation
  focal points 216
haematological/malignant disease
  219–20
Henoch–Schönlein purpura 199
inflammatory bowel disease 220
investigations 216, **216**
juvenile chronic arthritis 217–19
  at a glance 219
  clinical features 217–18, **218**
  management 218–19
  pauciarticular 218, *218*
  polyarticular 218
  systemic (Still's disease) 217

kernicterus (bilirubin toxicity) 251
Kernig's sign 100, 101, 103, 109
kidneys examination 37
knock-knees 69, 89
Koplick's spots 192, 193, *194*
Kussmaul respiration 306

labial adhesions 88
lactase deficiency 119
lactation 6, *6*
lactoferrin 91
lactose intolerance 164, 165–6
  management 166
language development 42, *42*
language disorder 265–6
  presentation 274
language/speech problems 263–6
  causes 264, 265–6
    distinguishing features 266
  classification **264**
  clinical evaluation 264–5
    focal points 264
  hearing loss 284
  speech delay 42
large baby, growth chart *65*, *67*
large head 71–5, 179, 183
  causes **72**
    pathological 72, 75
  evaluation
    focal points 72
laryngeal oedema 305
lead chelating agents 91
lead poisoning 90, 91
  anaemia 357
  recurrent abdominal pain 149
learning disability (mental retardation)
  60, 245, 272, 281–3
  associated problems 280
  at a glance 283
  behaviour management 282
  causes 281, **281**
  clinical features 267, 281
  early educational programmes 282
  epilepsy association 337
  family impact 283
  genetic counselling 283
  global developmental delay 268, 270
  hearing loss association 284
  idiopathic severe 274
  kernicterus 251
  language/speech disorders 264, 265

management 267, 282
  principles of management 282
meningitis association 111
presentation/diagnosis 274, 281
prevalence 281
routine review 282–3
school issues 282, 283–4
visual impairment association 286
walking delay 267
left to right intracardiac shunt 33,
  81–2, 109
leg pain 152–5
  causes 153–5, **153**
  clinical approach 152–3
  evaluation
    focal points 153
  investigations 153, **153**
  organic versus non-organic
    clinical features **154**
    laboratory tests **153**
  systemic disease associations 155
  traumatic 155
legal aspects 13
Legg–Calvé–Perthes disease 154, *155*
length, newborn measurement 234
let-down reflex 6
leukaemia 90, 94, 339, **341**
  acute lymphoblastic (ALL) 94
    at a glance 95
  cervical lymph gland enlargement
    225
  joint swellings 219
  leg pain 155
  management 94, 341
  pyrexia of unknown origin 222
  white cell count 358
leukocytosis 357–8
life-threatening events, acute 179,
  258, 312–14
  at a glance 313
  first aid 313
  investigations 313–14
  see also sudden infant death
    syndrome
limp 152–5
  causes 153–5, **153**
  clinical approach 152–3
  evaluation
    focal points 153
lip-reading 286
liver disease, chronic 130, 131, 132
liver examination 36, *37*
liver transplantation 131, 132
lobar collapse 106
loperamide 165
LSD 348
lumbar puncture
  coning 307, 361
  contraindications 361
  convulsions 139
  meningitis 109
    neonate 257
  unconscious child 307
lung abscess 109
lung consolidation/collapse 106,
  364, *364*
  chest percussion 32

lung disease, chronic 174, 175
    investigations 175
        respiratory distress syndrome
            association 249
        wheeze 121, 125
lymph node enlargement
    axillae 30
    clinical examination 29–30
        evaluation
            focal points 30
    groin 30
    infectious mononucleosis 227
    neck 30, 224
    rubella 195
lymphoma 225, **341**

macrocephaly *see* large head
maculopapular rash 192, 193
magnetic resonance imaging (MRI)
    cerebral palsy 278
    epilepsy 334
    headache 150
    hydrocephalus 72
    intracranial pressure elevation 72,
        150, 151
    pyrexia of unknown origin 221
    unconscious child 307
malabsorption
    chronic diarrhoea 164
    cystic fibrosis 176
    failure to thrive 67
    hepatic cirrhosis 132
    recurrent abdominal pain 148
malathion 212
malnutrition 1, 354
    brain growth effect 76
    catch-up growth 2
    failure to thrive 62
    immunodeficiency 100
    vomiting 157
malrotation 148
mannitol 307
mastitis 7
mastoid process swelling 225, *225*, **226**
mastoiditis 105, 229
masturbation 292–3
maturational delay
    delayed puberty 349, 350
    language/speech disorders 265
    short stature 57, 58
MCU *see* micturating cystourethrogram
mean cell haemoglobin 357
mean cell volume 357
measles 53, 109, 192, 193–4
    at a glance 195
    clinical course **193**
    clinical features 193, *194*, 202
    complications 193
    immunization 53, 193
    treatment 194
measles encephalitis 193–4
measles mumps rubella (MMR)
    vaccination 53, 192
mebendazole 183, 213
meconium ileus 176
melaena 172
menarche 349

meningismus 162
meningitis 53, 109–11
    antibiotic treatment **111**
    at a glance 110
    bacterial 109, 110
    brain growth effect 76
    causes **109**
    cerebrospinal fluid analysis 361
    clinical features 109
    coma 306
    complications 111
    coning 110
    convulsions 139
    diagnosis 109–10
    differential diagnosis 109
    intracranial pressure
        elevation 25
    management 110, 257
    nasopharyngeal carriage eradication
        110
    neonatal 109, 110, 256–7
    partially treated 110
    presentation 101
    principles of therapeutics 111
    splenectomy association 225
    viral 109, 110
    vomiting 156, 157
meningocele 237
meningococcal septicaemia 113–15, 192,
    193, 198
    antibiotic prophylaxis in contacts
        114
    at a glance 115
    clinical features 114, 202, 303
    management 114, 198
    principles of therapeutics 114
    prognosis 115
    rash 198, *198*
    shock 303
menstrual complaints 353–4
mental retardation *see* learning disability
mesenteric adenitis 134, 137–8
    management 138
    recurrent abdominal pain 148
    tonsillitis association 104
metabolic acidosis 358, 359, **359**
    hypernatraemic dehydration 117
    resuscitation of newborn 234
metabolic alkalosis 358, 359, **359**
metabolic disorders 179, 183, 272
    global developmental delay 270
metered inhalation devices 123, 320,
    321
methionine 310
methotrexate 218
methylphenidate 295
metronidazole 168
microcephaly *see* small head
micrognathia 260
micturating cystourethrogram
    urinary tract infection 112
    vesicoureteric reflux 112–13, *113*
migraine 149, 150–1
    at a glance 152
    clinical features 150–1
    management 151
    recurrent abdominal pain 149

milestones 3, 4, 39, **42**, 43
    see also developmental
        assessment
mineral requirements 5
MMR *see* measles, mumps, rubella
mobility development 4
molluscum contagiosum 209, 210, *210*
Mongolian spot 207, *208*
Moro reflex 25, *26*, 237, 278
morphine 311
mother and toddler groups 10
mother-baby interaction 3–4
motor maturation delay 267
movement
    neurological assessment 21, 25
    newborn examination 234
mumps 53, 225, 226, 227
    at a glance 229
    clinical course **193**
    complications 111, 227
    vaccine 53
mumps meningoencephalitis 110, 227
Munchausen by proxy 98
murmurs *see* heart murmurs
muscle bulk assessment 22
muscle power assessment 23
muscular dystrophy 267
musculoskeletal chest pain 156
musculoskeletal examination 38–9
    joint swelling 216
Mycoplasma pneumoniae 109, 176
myelomeningocele 237
myoclonic seizures 21, 181, 333
myopia 48, 77, *77*

naevus flammeus (salmon patch) 207,
    208
nail-biting 292
naloxone 233, 310
nappy rash 213–14
    ammoniacal dermatitis 213
    at a glance 214
    candida 213, 215
    causes **213**
        distinguishing features 214
    psoriatic 214, *215*
    seborrhoeic 214, 215
nasal obstruction 104
National Poisons Unit 309, 310
near-drowning first aid 312
nebulizers 123, 319, *320*
neck stiffness 100, 101, 103, 109
neck swellings 225–9, *225*
    causes **225**, 226–9
    cervical lymph glands 225, *225*, 226,
        226
    clinical approach 225-226
    evaluation
        focal points 226
        history taking 225–6
        physical examination 225–6, *226*
    investigations 226, **227**
    mastoid 225, *225*, **226**
    parotid glands 225, *225*, **226**
    thyroid gland 225, 226, **226**
necrotizing enterocolitis 246
neglect 95

neglect *Cont'd*
   child protection 56
   failure to thrive 62, 96
   global developmental delay 270,
     272
     management 272
   language/speech disorders 265
   physical examination 95–6
   social history 96
Neisseria meningitidis 110, 113, 304
neonatal asphyxia 234
   feeding problems following 246
   metabolic acidosis 359
   principles of management 234
neonatal cyanosis 234, 254
   at a glance 255
   causes 253, 254–5, **254**
   management 254
neonatal hepatitis 253
neonatal infection *see* infection
neonatal jaundice 250–3
   at a glance 252
   causes **250**, 252–3
   clinical significance 251
   hepatic 251
   history taking 251
   infection 253
   investigations 251, **251**
   pathophysiology 250
   physical examination 234, 251
   posthepatic 251
   prehepatic 250
   premature infant 252
   principles of management 251
   treatment 251
neonatal meningitis 109, 110, 256–7
neonatal mortality rate 232
neonatal pneumonia 250
neonate 232–60
   resuscitation 232–4
   terminology in statistics 232, **233**
   see also newborn examination
nephrotic syndrome 229
   at a glance 230
   clinical features 229, 230
   investigations 230, **230**
   management 230–1
   relapse 231
nerve palsies 22
neural tube defects
   associated hydrocephalus 72
   at a glance 238
   newborn examination 237–8, 237
   preventive folic acid supplements
     237
neuroblastoma **341**
neurocutaneous syndromes 273
neurodegenerative disorders 272, 274
neurofibromatosis 273
   café au lait spots 206, *207*
neurogenic bladder
   diurnal enuresis 185, 186
   spina bifida occulta 185, 186
neurological assessment 21–5
   babies 25–7
     schema 26
   coma 306

convulsions 139
coordination 23, *23*
cranial nerves 24
developmental abnormalities/delay
   262
   gait abnormalities 21–2, *22*
   global developmental delay 270
   muscle bulk assessment 22
   muscle power 23
   observation 21–2
   older child 24
   reflexes 23–4
   schema 26
   sensation 23
   tone 22, *23*, 25
   walking delay 267
neurological disorders
   hearing loss association 284
   newborn examination 237
neuromuscular disorders 22
newborn examination 232, 234–40
   technique 234–5
     history 234
     measurements 234–5
     observations 234
     physical examination 235, *235*
night terrors 180, 292
nightmares 291–2
nightwalking 289
nipple trauma 6
Nissen fundoplication 158
nitrofurantoin 113
nitrogen wash-out test 254, *254*
nits 212, *212*
nocturnal enuresis 186–8, 326
   at a glance 187
   causes **188**
   management 188
non-accidental injury 97–8, 306, 354
   at a glance 98
   child protection 56
   clinical features 97, 98
     bone injuries 96–7, 97
     hidden head injuries 96
     shaking injury 75
     skin lesions 96, 96
     subdural haematoma 75
   developmental delay 272
   prognosis 98
   skeletal survey 96–7
non-organic failure to thrive 67, 68, 99
non-organic pain 147, 156
non-specific viral exanthem 192
non-specific viral infection 106
non-steroidal anti-inflammatory
   drugs 218
nose–finger test 23
nosocomial infection 100
   newborn 250, 258
nursery school 10
nutrition 5–10
   adolescents 10
   cancer/cancer treatment 342
   cerebral palsy 279
   congenital heart disease 338
   diabetes mellitus management 327,
     332

   growth effects 1
   health education/promotion 50
   infancy 5
     breast-feeding 5–7
     evaluation
       focal points 9
     formula feeds 7–9
   preschool years 9–10
   principles of healthy eating 10
   promotion of good bowel habits
     171
   school years 10
   weaning 9
nystatin 214

obesity 1, 9, 10, 56, 61, 68–71
   at a glance 71
   causes **69**
   clinical approach 69
   evaluation
     focal points 69
   growth patterns 69, *70*
   medical complications 71
   prevention 71
objects, contact with 4
obstructive apnoea 259–60
   management 260
occupational therapy 296
   cerebral palsy 279
ocular movement assessment 27
oedema 36, 166, 229
   haematuria 189
   nephrotic syndrome 229–31
ophthalmoscope 28
opiates 7, **348**
opisthotonus 24, *25*
optic atrophy 286
oral rehydration therapy 118, 161
orchitis 227
organomegaly 237, 241
Ortolani test 47, 239, *239*
osteogenesis imperfecta 96
osteomyelitis 155
   at a glance 223
   clinical features 222
   management 222
   pyrexia of unknown origin 221,
     222
   septicaemia 303
osteosarcoma **341**
otitis media 29, *29*, 104, 105–6, 143, 151,
   156
   associated diarrhoea 161, 162
   associated eustacian tube
     dysfunction 105
   at a glance 106
   clinical features 29, 105
   complications 105
   conductive hearing loss 48, 265, 283,
     284
   glue ear 29, 105–6
   management 105
   mastoiditis 229
   secretory 48, 105–6, 284
   septicaemia 303, 306
ovarian cyst 149
oxytocin 6

pain, non-organic 147, 156
pain relief 12
pallid breath-holding spells (reflex anoxic seizures) 179–80
pallor 89
    causes 90
    shock 303
palmar erythema 132
palmar grasp reflex 26, 26
pancreatic enzyme supplements 167, 177
pancreatic insufficiency
    chronic diarrhoea 164
    cystic fibrosis 166, 176
papilloedema 306
paracetamol 103, 104, 140, 150
    poisoning 310
parachute reflex 26, 26, 26
parainfluenza virus 124, 128
parasitic infestation
    chronic diarrhoea 164–5, 168
        management 168
    recurrent abdominal pain 148
parent-held child health records 45
parental rights 13
parents' role in health surveillance 45
parotid glands swellings 225, 225, 226
partially sighted child see visual impairment
parvovirus B19 196
passive immunity 100
passive smoking 50, 173, 174, 175
    wheeze 122
patent ductus arteriosus 222, 250, 250
    clinical features 33, 250
    management 249
    prognosis 340
pauciarticular juvenile chronic arthritis 218, 218
    clinical features 218
Pco₂ 359
peak flow assessment
    asthma 122, 321, 321, 323
    wheeze 121, 122
pectus carinatum (pigeon chest) 31, 31, 33
pectus excavatum (funnel chest) 31, 31
pediculosis capitis (head lice) 212, 212
pelvic inflammatory disease 148
pelvic mass 185, 186
pelviureteric junction obstruction 241
penicillamine 218
penicillin 109, 189, 193, 196, 198, 225, 227, 231, 250
peptic ulcer 148
perinatal history 15–16
perinatal infection 100
perinatal mortality rate 232, 354
peritonism 133, 134, 135
peritonsillar abscess (quinsy) 104
periventricular leukomalacia 257, 258
permethrin 212
persistent pulmonary infiltrates 224
personal health record 14
pertussis (whooping cough) 51–2, 109, 157, 174, 176
    acute wheeze 120, 124
    at a glance 52

clinical course 193
    vaccine 52
petechial rash 109, 114, 191, 192, 193
pharyngitis 29, 104
phenobarbitone 256
phenylketonuria
    global developmental delay 272
    neonatal screening 47, 47, 272
phimosis 88
phosphate balance 5
phototherapy 251, 252
physical exercise 69
physiotherapy 279
pigeon chest (pectus carinatum) 31, 31, 33
pigmented naevi 206, 207
pituitary tumour 150
pizotifen 151
PKU see phenylketonuria
plantar reflex 24
plantar warts 208, 209
play development 4
play patterns 4
playgroups 10
pleural effusion 109
    chest percussion 32
pneumocystic carinii pneumonia 224, 342
pneumonia 106–7, 134, 176, 306
    AIDS opportunistic infection 224
    at a glance 109
    causative organisms 107
    chest X-ray 107, 108
    clinical features 108–9
    complications 109
    management 109, 250
    newborn 250
    predisposing factors 106
    pyrexia of unknown origin 220
    sites of chest recession 107, 108
pneumothorax 109
Po₂ 359
poisoning 306, 309–10
    agents 310, 310
    at a glance 311
    clinical approach 309–10
    suicide attempts 309, 310, 353
polio 52
    vaccine 52–3
polyarticular juvenile chronic arthritis 218
    clinical features 218
polycystic kidneys 189
polydipsia
    dehydration 116
    diabetes mellitus 326
    psychogenic 184
    thirst 184
polyuria 183–5
    causes 184–5, 184
    clinical approach 183–4
    diabetes mellitus 326
    thirst 184
popliteal angle 25, 25
port-wine stains 207, 209, 270
Portage system 282
posseting 156, 159–60

post-nasal drip 176
posterior fontanelle 71
posterior urethral valves 148, 186, 241
post-streptococcal disease 105, 196
    glomerulonephritis 188, 189
    reactive arthritis 217
postural drainage 177
potassium serum levels 360
Potter's syndrome 241
poverty 11
    associated morbidity 11
praecordium thrill 33–4
precocious puberty 350–1
    causes 350–1, 350
    clinical approach 350
prednisolone 322
pregnancy 354–5
    anticonvulsant medication 337
    diabetes mellitus 331
premature infants 232, 241, 242
    age correction for growth 21
    apnoea 258
    associated disorders 242, 243
    at a glance 244
    feeding problems 245
    functional upper airway obstruction 260
    immune function impairment 100, 246, 258
    intracranial haemorrhage 257
    neonatal jaundice 252
    patent ductus arteriosus 249–50
    respiratory distress 246–50
        causes 246
    respiratory distress syndrome 248
    retinopathy of prematurity 246
premature thelarche 350–1
prepuce retractability 88
preschool child
    growth 2
        standards 19
    nutrition 9–10
    psychomotor development 4
primary apnoea 232
primary school 10
primitive reflexes 26, 26, 26
    persistence 278
processus vaginalis persistent patency 85
prolactin 6
promethazine 198
propranolol 151
prostaglandin therapy 236, 254, 255
protein intolerance 164
protein requirements 5
pruritus see itching
pseudomonas infection 177, 258
    neonatal pneumonia 250
pseudosquint (false strabismus) 78, 78
psoriasis 203, 205–6
    clinical features 205–6, 206
    family history 203
    management 206
    nappy rash 214, 215
psychiatrist referral 291
psychogenic abdominal pain 147
psychogenic enuresis 186

psychogenic headache 149
psychogenic polyuria/polydipsia 184
psychogenic urinary frequency 184
psychological problems
    adolescents 351–3
    obesity 69, 71
psychologist referral 291
psychomotor development 2–5
    adolescents 5
    baby 3–4
    preschool child 4
    school-age child 5
    warning signs 262
    see also developmental
        assessment
psychosocial factors
    failure to thrive 62, 67–8
        at a glance 68
        growth chart 66
    growth effects 1
    short stature 57, 61
psychosomatic symptoms 293
puberty 348–9
    boys 349
    delayed 349–50, **350**
    girls 349
    hormonal events *348*
    key ages **349**
    precocious 350–1, **350**
    Tanner stages 349, *349*
pulmonary flow murmur 81
pulmonary stenosis 84, *84*
    heart sounds 34
    prognosis 340
pulse palpation 33
    cardiac pathology 80
PUO *see* pyrexia of unknown origin
pupillary light reflex 27
    coma 306–7
purpuric rash 192, 198–200
    septicaemia 304, 305
        meningococcal 114
pyelonephritis 113
    pyrexia of unknown origin 221
    recurrent abdominal pain 148
    vomiting 156, 157
pyloric stenosis 159, *160*, 359
    abdominal examination 157, *157*,
        158
    at a glance 160
    blood chemistry 361
    clinical features 159
    dehydration 116
    management 159
    vomiting 156, 157
pyrexia of unknown origin 102, 220–2
    causes **220**, 222
    evaluation
        focal points 220
    investigations 221, **221**
    temperature chart 221, *221*
pyrogens 102

quality of life 12
quinsy (peritonsillar abscess) 104

radiofemoral delay 33

radiotherapy 342
    late consequences 343, *343*
Ramstedt procedure 159
range of movement 39
rashes 190–201
    acute onset 191–3, **192**
        causes
            distinguishing features 202
        clinical course **193**
        evaluation
            focal points 192
        generalized 193–7
        management 193
        purpuric 198–200
        vesicular 197–8
        wheals 200–1
    chronic *see* skin lesions, chronic
    clinical approach 190–1
    descriptive terms 191
reaching for objects 4
reactive arthritis 217
reciprocating games 4
records 45
recovery position *140*, 308, *308*
rectal biopsy 170
rectal bleeding *see* blood in stool
rectal examination 37
    acute abdominal pain 134, 135
    blood in stool 172
    chronic diarrhoea 164
    constipation 170
    diurnal enuresis 185
    recurrent abdominal pain 145
recurrent abdominal pain 144–9
    causes **145**
        organic versus nonorganic **146**
    chronic diarrhoea association 164
    evaluation
        focal points 145
        history taking 144–5
        physical examination 145
    gastrointestinal causes 148
    gynaecological causes 148–9
    idiopathic 147
    investigations 145, **146**
    management 145
    non-organic **146**, 147–8, 293
    organic **146**, 148–9
    urinary tract causes 148
recurrent infection 222–4
    causes **223**
red eye 27
red reflex 27
    neonatal screening 47, *47*
reflex anoxic seizures 179–80
reflex epilepsy 138
reflexes
    neurological assessment 23–4
        babies 25–6
    primitive 26, **26**, *26*
reflux nephropathy (renal scarring) 111,
    113
reflux oesophagitis 142, 143, 144
refractive errors 77, *77*
regurgitation 159–60
renal failure, chronic
    anaemia 90

polyuria 185
    short stature 59
renal scan 185
renal tumour 188, 189
respiratory acidosis **358**, 359, **359**
respiratory alkalosis **358**, 359, **359**
respiratory distress 31, 121, 174
    asthma 122
    chest recession *31*
    coma 306
    newborn 246–50
        at a glance 247
        causes 246, **246**, 247–50
        clinical features 246
        cyanosis 254
        management 246–7
        pneumonia 250
        respiratory support 247
respiratory distress syndrome 244, 246,
    247–9, *248*
    aetiology 248
    at a glance 245
    chest X-ray 248
    clinical evaluation 248
    complications **249**
    management 249
respiratory failure 300
    airway obstruction 127
    at a glance 301
    causes **300**
    investigations **300**
    principles of management 301
    smoke inhalation 311
    treatment 300
    wheeze 121
respiratory rate 31, **31**
    newborn examination 234
respiratory support
    acute wheeze 121, 124
    apnoea of prematurity 258
    emergency paediatrics 298–9
    respiratory distress, neonatal 247
    respiratory distress syndrome 248
    respiratory failure 300
    resuscitation of newborn 233
respiratory syncytial virus 120, 124, 318
respiratory system examination 31–2
    auscultation 32, 119
    evaluation
        focal points 32
    observation 31
    palpation 31–2
    percussion 32
    schema 33
respiratory tract anomalies 173
rest position 25
resuscitation
    acute life-threatening events 313
    cardiorespiratory arrest 299, *299*
    drowning 312
    emergency presentations 297, 298–9
        support for relatives 299
    external cardiac massage 299, *299*
    newborn 232–4
        moderate depression 233
        primary apnoea 232
        principles of management 234

risk factors 232, **233**
resuscitation
    secondary apnoea 233
        severe depression 233–4
    septicaemia 305
    shock 304
    thermal injury 311
reticuloendothelial system examination 29–30
retinal haemorrhages 75, 76
retinoblastoma **341**
retinoic acid 351
retinopathy of prematurity 246, 286
    management 246
retractile testes 87
Reye's syndrome 103
rhabdomyosarcoma **341**
rhesus incompatibility 253
rheumatic fever 196
rhonchi 32, 121, 127
    see also wheeze
ribavirin 125
rifampicin 110, 114
right ventricular hypertrophy 33, *34*
ringworm (tinea) 210, *210*, *211*
rooting reflex 6
roseola 192, 195
    clinical course **193**
    clinical features 195, 202
rotavirus gastroenteritis 162
rubella (German measles) 30, 53, 192, 193, 194–5
    at a glance 196
    clinical course **193**
    clinical features 195, *195*, 202, 225
    complications 195
    immunization 53, 195
    intrauterine infection 53, 195, 244, 273
    joint pain/swelling 217
rumination 156

safe sex 224, 347–8
salbutamol 123, 319
salicylate poisoning 310
salicylic acid ointment 206
salmonella gastroenteritis 162
sanctity of life 12
scabies 203, 211–12, *212*
    management 212
scabies mite 211, 212, *212*
scalds 311–12
    first aid 311
scalp infection 30
scarlet fever 192, 195
    at a glance 197
    clinical course **193**
    clinical features 195, *196*, 202
    complications 196
    management 196
school attendance/placement
    asthma 325
    cancer 344
    child with a disability 274, 275, 276–7
    chronic illness 315–16, 317–8
    congenital heart disease 340

diabetes mellitus 326, 332
epilepsy 337
hearing loss 286
learning disability 282, 283–4
visual impairment 287, 288
school failure 295
    causes 295–6, **295**
school health education/promotion 50
school non-attendance 294–5
    causes **294**
school nurse 44–5
    child protection 56
school refusal 294–5
school-age child
    growth 2
        standards *20*
    nutrition 10
    psychomotor development 5
    social development 5
school-based problems 289, 294–5
scoliosis 31, 89
    clinical examination 38, *38*
screening 45–9, **46**, 272
    antenatal for congenital heart disease 338
    colour vision 48–9
    congenital hip dislocation 47
    congenital hypothyroidism 46–7
    cystic fibrosis 49, 176
    haemoglobinopathies 49
    hearing tests 48, *48*
    phenylketonuria 47, *47*
    red reflex 47, *47*
    sickle cell anaemia 93
    test criteria 45
    testicular descent 47, *48*
    visual acuity 48, *49*
scrotal examination 37–8
scrotal swelling 85–6
    causes **85**
        distinguishing features 87
    clinical approach 85
    evaluation
        focal points 85
scrotal transillumination 85
seborrhoeic dermatitis 201, 203, 205
    clinical features 205, *206*
    cradle cap 203, 205, *206*
    management 205
seborrhoeic nappy rash 214, *215*
secondary apnoea 233
secondary school 10
secondary sexual characteristics 345, 348
seizures *see* convulsions
self-help organisations 317
self-injurious behaviour 281
sensation assessment 23
septic arthritis 115–16, 216, 217
    clinical features 115, 217
    hip joint 154
    investigations 217
    management 115, 217
    shock 303
septicaemia 305
    AIDS opportunistic infection 224
    pneumonia 109
    pyrexia of unknown origin 221

shock 304–5
splenectomy association 225
'setting sun' sign 72
sex education 355
sex hormones 348, 348
sexual abuse 96, 99, 170, 209, 354
    child protection 56
    clinical features 99, 172
    investigations 97
    management 99
sexual activity 345, 347–8, 354, 355, 356
sexual hair development 349
sexually transmitted disease 348, 354
    consent issues 347
shapes recognition 4
shigella gastroenteritis 162
shock 303–5
    at a glance 304
    causes **303**, 304–5
    dehydration 116, 303
    history taking 303
    investigations 303, 303
    meningococcal septicaemia 113–14
    physical examination 303
    principles of management 304
    prognosis 304
    signs 303
    treatment 304
short stature 55, 56–61
    causes **57**
        chronic illness 59
        endocrine 58–9
        genetic 59–60
        intrauterine growth retardation 60–1, *63*
        physiological 58
        psychosocial 61
    delayed puberty 349
    evaluation
        focal points 57
        physical examination 57, 58
    history 57
    investigations 57, **58**
    management 57
    maturational delay 57, 58
    normal variant 58
sickle cell anaemia 92–3
    at a glance 93
    clinical features 93
    joint pain/swellings 220
    leg pain 155
    management 94
    screening 49, 94
sickle cell trait 93
SIDS *see* sudden infant death syndrome
sign language 286
simple absence seizures (petit mal) 181, 333
single parenting 11, 289, 347
sinus arrhythmia 33
sinusitis
    headache 150, 151
    pyrexia of unknown origin 221
sitting 39, *40*
skeletal dysplasias 60
skeletal survey 96–7

skin grafting 311
skin lesions 36, 190–1
  chronic 203
    causes
      distinguishing features 207
  clinical approach 190–1
  descriptive terms 191
  discrete 207–11, **208**
    causes
      distinguishing features 211
  types **191**
  see also rashes
skin problems, chronic 201, 203–11, **203**
sleep-wake cycles 3
sleeping pattern establishment 291
sleeping problems 50, 291–2
slipped capital femoral epiphysis 71,
  154–5
  clinical features 155
slow rising pulse 33
small baby 241–6
  associated problems 244–6
    feeding 245–6
    hypoglycaemia 244–5
    hypothermia 244
    infection 246
    intracranial haemorrhage 257
    necrotizing enterocolitis 246
    retinopathy of prematurity 246
  blood sugar assessment 245
small for gestational age (SGA) 242
  feeding problems 246
  hypoglycaemia 244
  immune function impairment 246
  management 244
  short stature following 57
small head (microcephaly) 75–7, 179, 183
  causes **76**
  clinical approach 76
  evaluation
    focal points 76
  global developmental delay 270
smile 4
smoke inhalation 311
smoking 174, 175, 321, 323, 347
Snellen chart 48, *49*
social development 42–3, *43*
  adolescent 5
  early vocalisation responses 4
  effects of abuse/neglect 96
  playing with other children 4, 5
  school-age child 5
social disadvantage 10–11
social history 16
  abuse/neglect 95–6
social interaction 2–5
social services support 275, 317
sodium balance
  dehydration 116, 117
  infancy 5
sodium bicarbonate 234
sodium cromoglycate 319
sodium requirements **118**
sodium serum levels 360
soiling 172
solvent abuse **348**
soy milk formula 166, 168

spacer devices 123, 319, *320*
spastic diplegia *277, 278*
  gait 22, *22*, 89, 267
spastic hemiplegia 277–8, *277*
  gait 22, *22*, 89, 267
  neurological assessment 26
spastic quadriplegia *277, 278*
spasticity 22
special registers 45
speech development 4, 42, *42*
  abnormalities *see* language/speech
    problems
  early vocalisation responses 4
  preschool child 4
speech therapy 265, 266
  cerebral palsy 279
spider naevi 36, 130, 132
spina bifida 22, 237
  associated hydrocephalus 72
  at a glance 238
spina bifida occulta 237, 238
  clinical features 238
  neurogenic bladder 185, 186
  spinal cord tethering 238
spleen examination 36–7, *37*
splenectomy 225
sputum 174
  cystic fibrosis 177
squint (strabismus) 77–8
  assessment 28
  causes 77
  clinical approach 77–8
  corneal light reflex 27, *27*
  cover test 28, *28*
  'false' 78, *78*
  latent 28, 77, *78*
  management 78
  non-paralytic 78
  paralytic 78
stammering (stuttering) 265
Staphylcoccus 115, 209
  toxin 304
Staphylcoccus aureus 177, 217
Staphylcoccus epidermidis 258
Staphylcoccus pyogenes 222
star charts 290
statement of educational needs 275,
  282
status asthmaticus 123
status epilepticus 138, 308–9, **309**, 333
  at a glance 309
  clinical features 309
  febrile convulsions 140
  management 139, 309
steam inhalation treatment 127
steatorrhoea 130, 166
stereotypic behaviour 281
steroid excess
  obesity 69
  short stature 58
steroid therapy 218
  acute asthma attack 322
  anaphylactic reaction 305
  fetal lung maturation stimulation
    248
  immunization contraindication 51
  immunodeficiency 100

inhaled 319
  airway obstruction 127, 128
  asthma 123
  croup 128
  meningitis 110
  nephrotic syndrome 230
  topical 203, 204, 205, 206, 213, 214
stiff gait 22
stitch 156
stool pattern **163**, 168
strawberry naevus (superficial
  haemangioma) 206, *208*
streptococcal infection
  cervical adenitis 225, 226
  impetigo 209
  newborn 258
    meningitis 256
    pneumonia 250
    septicaemia 304
  scarlet fever 196
  tonsillitis 104
  see also post-streptococcal disease
Streptococcus pneumoniae 105, 106
Streptococcus pyogenes 222
Streptococcus viridans 222
stress
  amenorrhoea 354
  crying in babies 143
  diabetes mellitus management 330
  eating problems 292
  enuresis 186, 293
    nocturnal 187
  recurrent abdominal pain 145, 147
  tension headache 150
stress incontinence 186
stridor 31, 119, 120, 126–8, 301, 305
  airway obstruction 127
  causes **126**, 128
    distinguishing features 128
  clinical approach 127
  investigations 127, **127**
  pathophysiology 126–7
  principles of management 128
  treatment 127–8
Sturge–Weber syndrome 207, 273
Stycar rolling ball test 27
subacute bacterial endocarditis *see*
  infective endocarditis
subacute sclerosing encephalitis (SSPE)
  194
subdural effusions 75, 111
subdural haematoma 75
  chronic
    developmental delay 272
    headache/intracranial pressure
      elevation 151
suboccipital lyphadenopathy 30, 195
suck reflex 245
suction 233
sudden infant death syndrome 258,
  312–14, 354
  at a glance 313
  definition 312
  overheating 312, 314
  pathophysiology 312–13
  prevention 314
  sleeping position 312

Back to Sleep education campaign 313, 314
sugar malabsorption 164
suicide/attempted suicide 353
   at a glance 353
   poisoning 309, 310, 353
sumatriptan 151
surfactant administration therapy 249
surfactant development 248
sweat test 167, 175, 177, 365
   sweat analysis 365
   sweat collection 365
sweep audiometry 48
symptom diary
   asthma 321, 322, 322, 323
   chronic diarrhoea 164
   cough 174
   diabetes mellitus 327, 330
   epilepsy 335
   headache 149
syncope 181
syphilis 244
systemic juvenile chronic arthritis (Still's disease) 217, **218**
systolic ejection murmur 81

tall stature 55–6, 61
teasing at school 294
teenage health clinics **346**
teething 79–80, 142
temper tantrums 50, 293
   management guidelines 293
temporal lobe (complex partial) seizures 181, 332, 333
temporal lobe epilepsy 140, 141
tendon jerks
   assessment 23–4
   babies 25
tension headache 149, 150
   at a glance 151
   management 150
terbutaline 123, 319
testicular descent screening 47, 48
testicular maldescent see cryptorchidism
testicular torsion 85–6
testicular tumour 88
tetanus 51
tetracycline 7, 351
thalassaemia 92
   at a glance 92
   screening 49
   treatment 92
thalassaemia trait 90, 92, 357
theophylline 124, 258, 259
thin child 56
thirst
   diabetes mellitus 326
   polyuria/polydipsia 184
threadworms (enterobiasis) 148, 183, 212–13
   diagnosis 212–13, 213
   treatment 213
throat examination 29, 30
thrush (oral candidiasis) 213, 215
   management 214
   pyrexia of unknown origin 221

thumb-sucking 292
thyroiditis 227–8, 228
thyroid cancer 225, 228
thyroid gland palpation 226
thyroid gland swelling 225, 225, 226, **226**
thyroid hormone 1
thyroxine therapy 228, 272
tics 181–2
time out 291, 293
tinea capitis 210, 210
tinea corporis 210, 210
tinea pedis (athlete's foot) 210, 211
toddler diarrhoea 165
toewalking 89
toilet training 186
tone
   cerebral palsy 278
   neurological assessment 22, 23
     babies 25
     popliteal angle measurement 25, 25
tonsillar exudate 104, 104
tonsillitis 104–5, 134, 161
   acute follicular 104, 104
   at a glance 105
   chronic 104
tonsils examination 29
topical cortiosteroid therapy 203, 204, 205, 206, 213, 214
TORCH infection
   intrauterine infection 244–5
   neonatal convulsions 256
toxoplasmosis 225, 244, 273
trace element requirements 5
tracheal position 31–2, 32
tracheostomy 302, 311
transient synovitis 153–4
transposition of great vessels 254–5
   clinical features 255
   management 255
   neonatal cyanosis 253, 254
traumatic haematuria 188
traumatic joint pain/swelling 216–17
traumatic leg pain 155
tricyclic antidepressants poisoning 309, 310
trigeminal nerve (V) assessment 24
trimethoprim 111
truancy 294, 295, 347
   management 295
tuberculosis 53–4, 176, 220
   AIDS opportunistic infection 224
   at a glance 54
   BCG vaccination 54
   breast-feeding 7
   Heaf test 53
tuberous sclerosis 140, 273
Turner's syndrome 59–60, 60, 67, 350
   at a glance 60
   delayed puberty 349, 350
   short stature 57
tympanic membrane appearances 29, 29

ulcerative colitis 168, 222
   joint swellings 220
   management 168

ultrasonography
   coarctation of aorta 237
   congenital hip dislocation 240
   diurnal enuresis 185
   hydrocephalus 72
   hydronephrosis 241
   intracranial pressure elevation 72
   intussusception 136
   pyrexia of unknown origin 221
   pyrloric stenosis 159, 160
   spina bifida occulta 238
   urinary tract infection 111
umbilical hernia 36, 237
undescended testes see cryptorchidism
unwanted habits 292–3
upper airway obstruction
   acute epiglottitis 127, 128
   anaphylactic reaction 305
   complete 125, 127
   croup (acute laryngotracheobronchitis) 128
   emergency presentation 125, 127, 300–2
     at a glance 302
     clinical approach 301–2
     principles of management 302, 303
   neonatal apnoea 260
   stridor 119, 127
   wheeze 119
upper respiratory tract infection 103–4, 173, 175–6
   cervical lymph gland enlargement 225
   diarrhoea association 161, 162
   nasal obstruction 104
ureteric reimplantation 113
urgency incontinence 186
urinalysis 361–2
   dehydration 117
   dipstick testing 362, 362, **362**
   diurnal enuresis 185
   haematuria 189
   jaundice 130
   observation 361
   polyuria/frequency 184
urinary calculi 148, 188
urinary frequency 182–5
   causes 184, **184**
   clinical approach 183–4
urinary symptoms 183–90
urinary tract congenital anomalies 111
   diurnal enuresis 186
   haematuria 188
   investigations 185
urinary tract infection 103, 111–13
   at a glance 112
   clinical features 111–13
   diagnosis 111
   diarrhoea association 162, 165
   diurnal enuresis 185–6
   dysuria 183
   follow-up 111, 112
   frequency 184
   haematuria 188
   investigations 112, 113
   principles of management 113

urinary tract infection *Cont'd*
    pyrexia of unknown origin 220
    recurrence 113
    recurrent abdominal pain 145, 148
    renal function following 113
    treatment 111–13
    vesicoureteric reflux 110, 111–13
urinary tract obstruction 148
urine specimen collection 111
uroscopy 185
urticaria (hives) 200–1, *201*, 202

vaginal discharge 354, **354**
valve areas palpation 34, *34*
varicella *see* chicken pox
varicella encephalitis 198
varicella pneumonia 198
vasopressin 188
venereal warts (condylomata acuminata) 209
venous hum 81
ventriculoperitoneal shunt 72
ventriculoseptal defect 82–3, *83*, 222
    at a glance 82
    heart murmurs 34, 83
verrucas 208, *209*
vesicoureteric reflux 113–14
    antibiotic prophylaxis 111, 113
    at a glance 114
    clinical features 113
    diagnosis 111
    grading *113*
    management 113
vesicular breath sounds 32
vesicular rashes 197–8
viral arthritis 217
viral gastroenteritis 162
viral hepatitis 131–2
    at a glance 132
    causal agents **131**
viral infection, non-specific 106
    wheeze 120, 121, 124
visual acuity assessment 27
    global developmental delay 270
    Snellen chart screening 48, *49*
visual development 4
visual evoked potentials 287
visual fields assessment 27–8, *28*
visual impairment 286–8

associated problems 286
    hearing loss 284
    learning disability 281
at a glance 287
causes 285–6
clinical features 286
definitions 285
diabetic retinopathy 325
    surveillance 330
education 287
    mobility training 288
    school placement 288
family impact 288
practical management 287–8
presentation/diagnosis 286–7
prevalence 285
principles of management 287, 288
visual system examination 27–8
    fundoscopy 28
    health surveillance tests 77–8
    observation 27
    ocular movements 27
    squint assessment 28
    visual acuity assessment 27
    visual field 27–8, *28*
vitamin K 5
vitamin requirements 5, 9
vitamin supplements
    cystic fibrosis 167
    hepatic cirrhosis 132
vocalisation 4
voice, response to 3
vomiting 156–60
    acute abdominal pain 133
    associated symptoms 157
    causes **157**, 158–60
    clinical approach 156–7
    dehydration 116, 157
    evaluation
        focal points 157
    recurrent abdominal pain 145
    worrying features 158

waddling gait 22, *22*
waking at night 291
walking 39, *40*
walking delay/disorders 266–8
    associated conditions 267–8

causes **266**
    distinguishing features 268
clinical evaluation 266–7
    focal points 266
warts, common 208, *209*
water requirements 5, **118**
waterhammer pulse 33
Waterhouse–Friderichsen
    syndrome 114
weaning 9
    evaluation
        focal points 9
weight loss/poor weight gain
    buttock wasting 36
    chronic diarrhoea 164
    coeliac disease 166
    dehydration with acute
        diarrhoea 161
    diabetes mellitus 326
    malignant disease 340
    polyuria/frequency 184
    recurrent abdominal pain 145
    vomiting 157
weight measurement 17, *17*
    dehydration assessment 117
wheals, acute 200–1
wheeze 31, 32, 119–25
    asthma 318, 319
    at a glance 122
    causes 120, 122–6
        distinguishing features 128
    history taking 120–1, **121**
    investigations 121
    management 122
    pathophysiology 120, *120*
    physical examination 121, **121**
    triggering events 120
Wilm's tumour 188, **341**
withdrawal of treatment
    ethical issues 12, 13
    Royal College of Paediatrics and
        Child Health Guidelines 12–13
Wood light examination 210

xanthine derivatives 124, 258, 259, 319

zidovudine 224–5
zoster immunoglobulin
    prophylaxis 197